Communication Research on Expressive Arts and Narrative as Forms of Healing

Communication Research on Expressive Arts and Narrative as Forms of Healing

More Than Words

Edited by
Kamran Afary
Alice Marianne Fritz

LEXINGTON BOOKS
Lanham • Boulder • New York • London

Published by Lexington Books
An imprint of The Rowman & Littlefield Publishing Group, Inc.
4501 Forbes Boulevard, Suite 200, Lanham, Maryland 20706
www.rowman.com

6 Tinworth Street, London SE11 5AL, United Kingdom

British Library Cataloguing in Publication Information Available

Library of Congress Cataloging-in-Publication Data

Names: Afary, Kamran, 1957– editor. | Fritz, Alice Marianne, 1972– editor.
Title: Communication research on expressive arts and narrative as forms of healing : more than words / edited by Kamran Afary, Alice Marianne Fritz.
Description: Lanham : Lexington Books, [2020] | Includes bibliographical references and index. | Summary: "This collection, edited by Kamran Afary and Alice Marianne Fritz and authored by contributors with experience as educators, artists, and licensed therapists, integrates communication, therapy, and pedagogy to explore the role and efficacy of expressive arts therapies."— Provided by publisher.
Identifiers: LCCN 2020011215 (print) | LCCN 2020011216 (ebook) | ISBN 9781793602688 (cloth) | ISBN 9781793602695 (epub)
Subjects: LCSH: Art therapy. | Narrative therapy.
Classification: LCC RC489.A7 E973 2020 (print) | LCC RC489.A7 (ebook) | DDC 616.89/1656—dc23
LC record available at https://lccn.loc.gov/2020011215
LC ebook record available at https://lccn.loc.gov/2020011216

Contents

Acknowledgments

The editors would like to thank the chapter contributors for their thoughtful and creative work; your pioneering analyses and collaborative spirit made this volume possible. Thanks also to Lexington Books editor Nicolette Amstutz for the invitation to submit a proposal, her patience in working with us, and her vision to see the importance of expressive therapies in the current historical moment, when different community-building modes of communication are sorely needed.

Kamran Afary also thanks coeditor Marianne Fritz for initiating this collaboration with her research on rap music as a healing modality and for her thoroughness and care in editing the chapters and providing constructive feedback to all chapter contributors. Thanks also to Cal State LA for an Office of Research, Scholarship, and Creative Activities (RSCA) Award that gave me more time to work on writing a chapter and editing the collection. Thanks also to Sam Brawand for copyediting the manuscript before its submission, providing many helpful suggestions to contributors, and working on the index.

Finally, we would like to thank our subjects, respondents, informants, and participants for allowing us to tell their amazing stories, without which there would be no book.

Introduction

Kamran Afary and Alice Marianne Fritz

As the director of Parks and Recreation in East Los Angeles, a friend of ours oversees a summer acting workshop for children ages seven to seventeen years. Last summer, an eleven-year-old boy named "Arturo" enrolled in the workshop, along with eighteen other young boys and girls. Although initially quiet and withdrawn, Arturo gradually became more comfortable interacting with the other budding young actors in the group. Toward the end of summer, the children all participated in a theatrical production that showed parents and relatives what they had been working on during the five weeks leading up to that culminating event. The day after the showcase, our friend received an email from Arturo's parents. They wanted to tell him something of their gratitude, their amazement, at the change they saw in their son. "He has friends now!" they wrote in the email. For Arturo, speaking to other kids is, as his parents know only too well, highly atypical behavior: Arturo is autistic.

A young woman we know gives informal talks at various youth shelters, counseling centers, and anywhere else she senses her words may resonate with audiences who are haunted by traumatic episodes she herself has endured. Since the age of two, "Nia" has been alternately raised by a capricious aunt and various foster homes, that take her in each time the tides of her aunt's familial largesse ebb. Nia speaks openly about the molestation she has experienced both in her aunt's household and in foster care. Listening to her stories, one apprehends a disturbing motif of abuse: an uncle who habitually walks in on her showers "by mistake," an older male at one of the foster homes who forces Nia to undress in front of him, or sometimes worse. The tone of Nia's voice, as she relates such repulsive scenes, is initially jarring: there is not the slightest hint of despondence or self-pity; rather, her voice is matter-of-fact, her manner quietly assertive. She looks forward enthusiastically to each speaking engagement. To her, they pose not the threat of relived traumas, as one might expect, but rather the opportunity to confront, transform, and overcome those negative events by speaking about them to an empathetic audience. One senses that Nia is a woman who has found her inner strength from sharing with others her most painful memories.

The ability to communicate feelings and ideas to others in our social worlds is the sine qua non of mental health wellness. Mental health disturbances such as depression or anxiety are often the result when individuals are deprived of the ability to convey their thoughts to sentient listeners, such as happens with prisoners placed in solitary confinement. Frank J. Elgar, Wendy Craig, and Stephen J. Trites (2013) found that among adolescents, open communication with parents or stepparents significantly reduces internalizing problems (for example, depression, suicidal ideation) and externalizing problems (for example, physical aggression, vandalism), while promoting emotional well-being, prosocial behavior, and life satisfaction. For many people, the need to converse with others is strongest during times of emotional distress (Janoff-Bulman, 1992). Emotionally charged events appear to trigger individuals' need to discuss the situation, and the intensity of the emotion appears to be correlated with how often the episode is shared with others (Rimé, Herbette, & Corsini, 2004). The death of a loved one is an extremely distressing event for the survivors, and among individuals who had lost a family member or close friend to suicide, it was found that those who tended to talk about distressing issues had lower levels of grief compared to those not prone to self-disclose their problems (Levi-Belz & Lev-Ari, 2019). While contradictory evidence exists with regard to the effects on emotional well-being of disclosing distressing information, Eileen Kennedy-Moore and Jeanne C. Watson's (2001) review of relevant research led the authors to propose that the benefits of expressing negative feelings are not experienced immediately after the disclosure but emerge over time, and are enhanced when the expression is to an empathetic listener and when it is accompanied by the expression of positive feelings. Individual differences also influence the degree to which people feel better after expressing negative feelings. For some people, expressing their feelings to others can ease any anxieties over having those feelings, provide insight into those subjective emotions, and strengthen the bond between expresser and listener (Kennedy-Moore & Watson, 2001).

Even writing about traumatic life events (without knowing who will read the narrative) has been shown to improve individuals' self-perception, manifesting as greater acceptance of one's positive and negative qualities, stronger feelings of control over one's environment, and motivation to achieve deeper personal growth (Hemenover, 2003). Indeed, the fundamental premise of traditional talk therapy is that "when people put their emotional upheavals into words their physical and mental health seems to improve markedly"

(Smyth & Pennebaker, 1999, p. 70). Accordingly, the underlying telos of all therapies is to facilitate a client's self-expression (Malchiodi, 2005). However, individuals exhibit differences in their ability, willingness, or skill in talking or writing about the troubling or traumatic life events they encounter, and the limitation of traditional talk therapy is directly related to constraints on individuals' capacity to verbalize their emotions, experiences, memories, and perceptions, constraints that are not only individual but also social and cultural. Some problem-focused individuals, due to age, or to physical or mental illness, may lack the capacity to put their troubling thoughts into words (Malchiodi, 2005). Others may have endured traumatic events and are reluctant to relive painful memories by narrating them verbally (Malchiodi, 2005). For individuals with compromised verbal capability, an arts-based intervention offers alternative modes to communicate feelings and ideas. For example, Paula Rylatt (2012) reported positive outcomes from using creative therapy sessions with patients with diminished verbal ability due to dementia, most markedly in terms of the patients' observed levels of pleasure and enjoyment.

In terms of culturally constructed barriers to self-disclosure, there are sectors of society for whom an open acknowledgment of their emerging identities may carry prohibitive connotations or stigma; talking about one's anxieties and fears may, for instance, be considered effeminate and inappropriate for "real men" among certain populations. Whether the willingness or ability to communicate is due to physical, social, cultural, or individual factors, expressive arts activities may be a viable, alternative mode of communication for some people.

Cathy A. Malchiodi (2005) defines expressive therapies as "the use of art, music, dance/movement, drama, poetry/creative writing, play, and sandtray within the context of psychotherapy, counseling, rehabilitation, or health care" (p. 2). While the term is sometimes used to refer to integrative interventions that combine multiple artistic modalities (for example, Rogers, 2001), our use of the term encompasses both multimodal and unimodal contexts. Our choice of this term reflects an emphasis on the self-expressive opportunities that arts-based therapies encourage and facilitate. Beyond clinical interventions, the use of expressive modalities and embodied performance practices have also emerged in educational settings. All of those activities, whether in clinical, classroom, or informal, everyday settings, allow individuals to express their thoughts and emotions via what expressive arts therapy pioneer Margaret Naumburg (1955) called a "form of symbolic speech" (p. 437).

Self-expression through performance or creative arts as a therapeutic activity is by no means a novel idea. Early texts offer clues to how ancient peoples used art, music, and drama for mental health maintenance and restoration, and the use of art by psychotherapists in the 1930s and 1940s to promote mental wellness further legitimized creative activities as a treatment modality (Malchiodi, 2005). Likewise, during the late twentieth century, the field of communication studies witnessed the rise of dramatistic, narrative, and performance approaches to the study of social interactions in the works of Kenneth Burke, Walter Fisher, and Erving Goffman. Indeed the rise of performance studies as an interdisciplinary field reintroduced performance not only as a product but also as a process and a mode of inquiry. Expressive narrative practices have brought psychoanalytic theories out from strictly clinical encounters into educational research in order to provide space for faculty and students alike to explore social identities through the lens of critical cultural studies, ethnography, and community theatre practices.

Cases like Arturo's and Nia's, discussed above, far from being rare anomalies, have been frequently documented, whether anecdotally or within the research literature. Today, the numbers of mental health professionals, counselors, and educators who believe in the value of and wish to incorporate expressive arts modalities into their work continue to multiply. The current interest among Communication scholars and educators to introduce more creative, even playful, activities and practices into their pedagogical repertoire is demonstrated by the theme of "Communication at Play" that was chosen for the annual conference of the National Communication Association in 2018. Also symptomatic of the increasing popularity of expressive arts therapy and performance pedagogies among researchers and practitioners is the current proliferation of related professional associations, university programs, and, of course, books examining this form of embodied scholarly research.

A NEW FOCUS FOR EXPRESSIVE THERAPY

Since numerous volumes have already been written about expressive therapies, at this point, is there room for further discussion? Much of the scholarly work on the subject is generated within the discipline of psychology. From that vantage point, the value of expressive arts therapy lies chiefly in its power to stimulate a client's imagination and to unlock the portal to the unconscious (though the field of psychology is, of course, by no means monolithic, the generalization here refers to the focus of adherents of the psychodynamic and humanistic approaches). Importantly, from a psychoanalytic standpoint, the creativity involved in artistic activities allows access to the unconscious, which is usually barred from conscious scrutiny (Halprin, 2003). Other researchers and practitioners have taken a more aesthetic approach and directed their focus on the artwork itself, or the creative process (Levine, 2004a). Not that this perspective puts pressure on clients to produce work that is beautiful in the conventional sense; rather, its objective is to help clients let go of control through the whimsical nature of art-making (Levine, 2004b). To these two foci of previous scholars, in this collection, we train our attention on a third key factor underpinning the argument for using expressive arts therapeutically. An attempt to more fully describe what happens when arts practices are integrated into both therapeutic and educational settings, and to explain why the activity is often experienced by its participants as liberating and healing, yields a tripartite model whose central components are *imagination/creativity*, *artistic production*, and *communication*. It is our position that the importance of the communication aspect of expressive arts therapies warrants a discussion of such interventions by scholars working within the domain of Communication Studies.

When individuals, who are stuck on some problem or haunted by some trauma, engage in art-making, they mine for imaginative material from the lode of the unconscious, craft those inner impulses into an external form perceptible by others, then present the result to an observer. In the last step, as the audience/reader/therapist examines the artistic production, the meanings expressed through the artwork find an audience, and a communication is received. Natalie Rogers (2001), daughter of the famous humanistic psychologist and herself a practitioner of person-centered expressive arts therapy, encapsulates the process thus: "We express inner feelings by creating outer forms. When we express these feelings in visible forms, we are using art as a language to communicate our inner truths" (p. 163). The revelatory process may then continue with a dialogue about the product between the art creator and the observer (that is, through verbal discussion) until the problem-bound person achieves insight into the self or finds personal and social meaning (Malchiodi, 2005). Hence, the communication aspect of expressive therapies is not restricted to the symbolic expression inherent in producing an artistic artifact or experience, but is also constituted by the client/therapist or student/teacher discussions afterward. Given the centrality of communication as a feature of expressive therapies, a stronger emphasis on this aspect is warranted.

Communication is central to identity formation; people craft an identity for themselves by explaining their lives to others in narrative form. Dan P. McAdams (1996), proposing a more holistic framework for studying personality, describes three levels that constitute the individual person: a level consisting of context-invariant trait attributes, a second level consisting of a wide assortment of motivational constructs that are influenced by contextual and developmental factors, and finally, a third level consisting of the stories that individuals tell about themselves—it is "the level of identity as a life story" (p. 306). These stories string together temporally and episodically fragmented elements to establish a telic trajectory, such that a person's past is shown to have laid the foundations for their present, which in turn will make possible the person's future (McAdams, 1996). The self histories people share may vary depending on the audience, inflected by a need to manage the impressions of and attain status among consequential others (McAdams, 1996). These narratives are also informed by macrocontextual factors, reproducing "prevailing patterns of hegemony in the economic, political, and cultural contexts wherein human lives are embedded" (McAdams, 1996, p. 307). Expressive arts modalities may offer opportunities for participants to share their life story. Provided the therapist or educator can offer participants a space that is perceived as safe and judgment-free where they can engage in expressive arts activities, any self narratives that emerge may be less constrained by the need to impress. Moreover, the liberating potential of expressive arts may even help individuals recognize details in their life story that betray an internalization of hegemonic assumptions. Contemporary discourse in psychology on the construction of social identities encourages mental health professionals and educators to use an intersectional and ecological approach in creating space for the cocreation of identities in therapeutic and educational encounters (APA, 2017).

Another facet of communication-via-art-making that is usually absent from talk therapy is that of *play*. As Stephen K. Levine (2004b) pointed out in *Principles and Practice of Expressive Arts Therapy: Toward a Therapeutic Aesthetics*, in order for either therapy or art-making to be productive, "they must be carried out in an attitude of playfulness, open to possibilities and discovery" (p. 71). For a verbal dialogue between individuals to transpire successfully, there must be a rational presentation of ideas, appropriate turn-taking, and the selection and ordering of words in accordance with rules of syntax. Conversely, to immerse oneself in an artistic activity is to temporarily distance oneself from the world of reason and rules. Only when such playful letting go is allowed to take place can a person speak the lines, play the musical notes, assume the postures, or draw the shapes as they organically surface in the imagination, without judgment or fear of appearing silly to others. Even for individuals who are willing and able to verbally discuss their issues of concern, an artistic activity such as play acting, making music, creative movement, or drawing provides another outlet for symbolic communication to complement educational or therapeutic dialogue. All of the expressive modalities discussed in this collection are activities that most people experience as inherently enjoyable; besides being outlets for symbolic speech, then, they constitute opportunities for participants to, quite simply, have fun.

To summarize the discussion thus far, the gratification participants derive from engaging in expressive arts activities in educational and therapeutic settings is not only due to the unshackling of their imagination and repressed memories, or the inherent pleasure of producing a work of art, but also is largely explained by the expression, unconstrained by the rules governing verbal or written language, of hitherto uncommunicated, or even uncommunicable, ideas and emotions. While a psychological perspective privileges the imagination/creativity, and an aesthetic approach focuses on the artwork, an understanding of expressive arts therapy that highlights the communication aspect is needed. Specifically, what is missing from the extant literature is a book that assembles together in one collection the examinations of different expressive modalities and their praxis in performance research, classroom settings, and therapeutic encounters, written for readers studying or working in diverse disciplines, including communication studies and psychology. The present collection takes an interdisciplinary approach, with chapters written by mental health professionals and scholars in communication studies and other areas in the humanities. This allows for a more thorough exploration of the *expressive* aspect of expressive arts therapies.

A NEW PERSPECTIVE ON IDENTITIES

The expansive range of research topics and approaches in this collection of essays has benefitted from more contemporary discourses on intersectionality, critical cultural studies, and performance studies. The emergence of these three interdisciplinary modes of research and practice has transgressed the academic and professional boundaries that previously separated research and teaching in psychology, theatre studies, and communication studies (Madison & Hamera, 2006; Sajnani, 2013; Tilsen & Nylund, 2016). Modernist psychological models of personality development in the early part of the twentieth century were built on universal cultural forms and essentialized identities that did not provide much self-reflexivity on the way hegemonic cultural narratives shape normative identities, assign social roles, and thereby marginalize, deny, or erase recognition to those who do not fit those roles and identities. Consequently, a great deal of the focus was on diagnosing pathologies and identifying abnormalities, dysfunctions, and disorders. Narrative and performance paradigms prompted a greater search for diversity, difference, and agency. This process has had a long and complex history involving numerous theorists and schools of thought. Burke's (1945) dramatism in *A Grammar of Motives* created a shift in the way rhetoric and (Aristotle's) poetics were reframed as inseparable models of human social interaction, as performances. Goffman's (1959) *Presentation of Self in Everyday Life*, a dramaturgical model of social analysis, greatly expanded Burke's work and added a new understanding of social stigmas and normative practices. Fisher's "The Narrative Paradigm" provided a more rigorous taxonomy of concepts and categories to account for how humans process complex information through narrative. Augusto Boal's (1979) *Theatre of the Oppressed* developed the category of the *spectactor* who has agency in writing the script of their lives, which in turn inspired a new generation of artist-activists with skills to promote social and political change.

Among critical cultural studies practitioners there is widespread agreement that popular culture is a potent force in promoting dominant and subjugating narratives that shape identities and relationships in contemporary society. These narratives include capitalism's fragmentation and alienation of forms of labor, patriarchal forms of family that devalue women and children's agency and autonomy, Eurocentrism(s) that erase indigenous cultures and their contributions, heteronormativity that stigmatizes alternative forms of sexual and gender expression, along with uncritical sciences that promote these norms in medicine and psychology (Hadley, 2013; Tilsen & Nylund, 2016). The chapters in this collection address how research and teaching with creative arts modalities can also shape the narratives of what it means to be healthy individuals, or how people develop their identities in terms of ability, gender, race, and sexuality. Several chapters explore how the art forms deployed in educational and research practices can themselves be complicit with dominant and subjugating narratives, and point out alternative ways in which researchers and educators can be more vigilant in practicing new forms of social justice communication.

This book includes essays by scholars who are well-respected within the fields of psychology, theatre studies, and communication studies. The contributors constitute a spectrum of practicing artists, mental health professionals, and academic researchers. The diversity among the book's contributors is not limited to their discipline, training, and profession, but is reflected as well in the authors' social and cultural identities and backgrounds. The contributors write from and about a multiplicity of cultural perspectives, consonant with the cultural diversity of students in today's classrooms. The populations that these authors work with and/or write about cover a similarly diverse range, from students who are fighting for social justice and change, to prisoners who are taking a communication studies class while serving life sentences.

THE ORGANIZATION OF THIS BOOK

The eleven chapters that follow are grouped in two parts offering examples of emerging models of research and practice that turn to performance and expressive art modalities. The essays in Part I, "Performance and Drama," cover the intentional use of drama, performance, and theatre arts (including puppeteering and ventriloquism) in several settings with different populations to achieve psychological growth and change. Both in therapeutic settings and in the classroom, embodied dramatic activities provide a space for participants to create representations of abstract concepts or to weave their stories with textbook readings. Through dramatic enactments, the depth and breadth of inner experience can be actively explored and interpersonal relationship skills can be enhanced. Through embodied interaction, participants can expand their repertoire of dramatic roles, strengthen their own life roles, and learn to privilege improvisation. In the classroom, the use of creative drama enactments provides the context for participants to weave their stories with textbook readings. Participants can expand their repertoire of dramatic roles to find that their own life roles have been strengthened.

The insights he has gained in teaching at a state prison are at the heart of chapter 1, Kamran Afary's, "A Narradrama Approach to Teaching Communication." Prisons are paramilitary institutions that reinforce an atmosphere of toxic masculinity and silence expressions of vulnerability and of emotions. Building upon student-prisoners' prior work in making amends and practicing restorative justice, Afary describes a series of narradrama exercises in his interpersonal communication course that culminated in the production of several performances attended by family members, journalists, university trustees, prison staff, and other prisoners. The chapter argues for the incorporation of structured performance exercises as a way to deepen self-awareness, build healthier interpersonal relationships, and to help abolish dehumanizing prison conditions.

Mady Schutzman's chapter 2, titled "More Than Human," advocates for a reexamination of the histories and theories of puppeteering and ventriloquism as a way to open up an aesthetic space that is at one and the same time playful and creative, whether in educational or clinical contexts, in which communal and/or individual afflictions may be rescripted. Schutzman is interested in further developing the theatrical modes that Boal employed to bring about replacement or intervention in his agenda for social healing and political change. Moving beyond the usual iterations of drama, she assesses the use of puppetry and ventriloquism as modalities that are at once liberating and fun. Schutzman discusses how puppets create an ambivalence for performers and audiences that is at once both human and more than human. An exciting and unique feature of this chapter is that it provides several classroom or workshop exercises for students and participants.

Reflecting on fifteen years of Forum Theatre facilitation with Lesbian, Gay, Bisexual, Trans, Two-Spirited, Intersex, Queer, and additional sexual orientations (LGBT2SIQ+), gender non-conforming (GNC), and other targeted communities, Jessica Bleuer's "Theatre for Revolution or Theatre for Healing? Forum Theatre with LGBT2SIQ+ and Other Targeted Communities" (chapter 3) shines a spotlight on Forum Theatre's ability to make visible and minimize oppression, while developing tools for relational healing and revolution. Using information gathered from participants at three separate locations, Bleuer shows how advocacy projects aimed at reducing microaggressions on campus can use dramatization and the enactment of narratives to identify the oppressive forces in our environments, and to foster a healthier queer self-concept.

Often used as warm up exercises by other adherents of Boal, Image Theatre takes center stage in Bonny McDonald's "Two Snapshots: Staging Image Theatre as a Healing Art" (chapter 4). An educator who works with a racially mixed student population, McDonald makes a case for using Image Theatre as a form of activist intervention in its own right, to facilitate conversations about sensitive topics and to help students draw connections between their own immediate concerns and broader social problems. Through Image Theatre's facilitator-guided exercises, participants create images to symbolically convey thoughts or experiences, which then generate, in an organic manner, discussions between participants as they speculate on the images' meanings. McDonald describes her own variations of Image Theatre exercises and how she uses them to help students engage with a given topic more freely and on a deeper level.

The last essay in this section (chapter 5), "*Eyas* on the Prize: Mapping the Relaunch of Performance at the University of Houston-Clear Lake," reflects on the value of Performance Studies itself, using a case example of an academic community's efforts to reinstate the discipline at an institution that had previously cut the program to triage institutional resources. Andrea Baldwin's autoethnography attests to the importance of a performance program for both students and faculty at the University of Houston-Clear Lake (whose school mascot is a hawk, hence the "eyas" in the title, which refers to a baby hawk—an important motif not only because it represents the institution described in the chapter, but also because it functions as a metaphor for the author's own journey, from a new hire to a valued member of the community). Baldwin traces her efforts to rebuild such a program at an institution that favors STEM disciplines, and the resulting psychological rewards for students as they participated in performance-based classes and festivals, and even for the community at large, as they witnessed the fruits of the students' labors.

Individuals in a liminal state, homogenized by a common lack of formal titles and properties, "tend to develop an intense comradeship and egalitarianism" (Turner, 1970, p. 95), resulting in a system of relationships wherein social rank is unimportant, an alternative social arrangement Victor Turner calls *communitas*. Within the liminal space of the play rehearsal or performance, participants must work collaboratively so that one line feeds the next, an action by one actor motivates that by another, and a believable dramatic universe is created for the audience. As Baldwin shows in her chapter, exposure to theatre and performance helped the author's students form bonds with each other and with students of performance studies from other institutions. Falling squarely in the path of the devastating 2017 hurricane, Harvey, much of Houston was flooded, and homes, vehicles, and businesses were severely damaged. In one way or another, every Houston resident was affected by the tragedy. Ultimately, in the wake of Harvey, a performance piece by the author's students, in which they documented how they had been impacted by that natural disaster, proved to have cathartic effects that extended beyond the performers themselves, to touch the audience members who had also endured that shared tragedy.

Part II, "Narrative, Art, Dance, and Music," shifts to an exploration of the healing aspects of music, dance, mask-making, and storytelling. The liberating possibilities associated with music is the focus of the first trio of chapters in Part II. Unified by their belief that music is a preferred form of expression as well as therapeutic modality for many individuals, the authors of chapters 6, 7, and 8 offer evidence in their essays to support this claim. The remaining chapters in this part (9, 10, and 11) discuss the expressive modalities of dance/movement, art (mask-making), and storytelling/writing narratives.

While there is substantial variation in the way they use music in their work, and in the theoretical approach in which they ground their practice, music therapists in the United States and worldwide share a common recognition of the pleasure stimulated by music engagement as its fundamental attribute that can ultimately produce therapeutic outcomes. Whether the session involves improvising music in a group setting, performing precomposed music, creating original music or lyrics, or simply listening to prerecorded music (Malchiodi, 2005), it is crucial that the client does, in fact, experience the music as pleasurable, relaxing, or stimulating.

Chapter 6, "'Hip-Hop Just Saved Me': Rap Music Engagement as a Music-Based Intervention for Substance-Addicted Youth," coauthored by Alice Marianne Fritz and Kamran Afary, reinforces the argument that hip-hop music is a preferred medium of some youth. Looking beyond the inherent artifice of clinical settings, this chapter presents a case example in which a group of hip-hop identified youth organically create their own version of a "self-help group" through regular gatherings for the purpose of composing rap lyrics. "Performance" often occurs spontaneously and without the formal trappings people tend to associate with the word. Fritz and Afary's chapter provides an illustration of this, highlighting for readers the quotidian performances of rap songs by a group of friends for no other audience than each other, a performance prompted solely by their own love of the art form rather than the mandate of a professional therapist or substance abuse counselor. That some in the group, specifically the youth whose story is foregrounded in this chapter, derive psychotherapeutic benefits from those "spittin' sessions" that help them resist relapsing into substance addiction is a fortuitous secondary effect, unanticipated by those in the group.

As a team comprised of a psychologist and a hip-hop artist specializing in a postmodern form of narrative practice, Travis Heath and Jacobo Mesa Ramirez use a narrative and lyrical collaborative form to creatively reconstruct, enact, and lyricize the performance of a client-preferred treatment modality. In this narrative/lyrical-form, chapter 7, "Preferred Cultural Mediums of Healing: Rapping into Identity," Heath and Mesa Ramirez narrate a dialogical chronicle of interactions with Jay (a pseudonym), a justice-impacted youth struggling to extricate himself from his predicament by using hip-hop lyrics as a preferred form of creative dialogue. Many in today's youth populations view hip-hop as not merely a musical genre that is relevant to their lives, but as a lifestyle that is part of their construction of a preferred identity. However, as is the case with many trends and phenomena embraced by youth, hip-hop music is often seen as frivolous or even nocuous by more conservative groups, including some mental health professionals. The chapter by Heath and Mesa Ramirez holds particular salience for therapists and educators who wish to create an environment in which the client's/student's preferences are respected, and in which they have an equal voice in deciding on the form an intervention will take. The chapter ends with a brief section on the history of Narrative Therapy, a postmodern non-pathologizing approach developed by Michael White and David Epston that informs the work by Heath and Mesa Ramirez.

In chapter 8, "Music Therapy: An Ethnographic Approach to Understanding How Music Therapists and Adolescent Patients Communicate and Perform Community," Melanie Frontz Kramer and Kurt Lindemann investigate how music therapists address both micro- and macro-level patterns of communication during group sessions to encourage the performance and construction of a sense of community for adolescents. Kramer and Lindemann address the pressures on neurodivergent adolescents to fit into society's mold of normal, and demonstrate how through music therapy they can overcome feelings of stigma and of alienation, and thereby develop their sense of connection, togetherness, autonomy, and identity/expression. Building on Goffman's (1959) notion of performance of identity, Kramer and Lindemann explore how developmental disabilities, neurological limitations, and emotional and behavioral challenges are particularly stigmatized in contemporary society. Feeling pressured to fit into society's mold of *normal* causes such adolescents to further alienate themselves when what they really need is to experience a sense of community, which can occur through expressive arts forms of communication.

Dance/movement therapy (DMT) is grounded in the view that the body holds "memories" of feelings or experiences that may be difficult or impossible to verbalize, but may be conveyed metaphorically through movement (Meekums, 2010). Gregory J. Langner's "Comfort and Catharsis: Critical Reflections on Therapeutic Dance Practice" (chapter 9) focuses on this therapeutic modality, explored within the context of staged dance productions. A tenet commonly subscribed to by DMT practitioners is that when dancers work on a stage production, they are simultaneously working on issues in their personal lives, since dancers' inner lifeworld is inevitably made concrete through movement (Halprin, 2003). Interviews with professional dancers, filtered through his own experiences as a dancer and choreographer, provide Langner with evidence to build a case for dance performance as an activity that can help facilitate emotional and psychological well-being through catharsis when the body's expressive impulses and conscious desires connect with others in synchronous meditative movement.

As Anna K. Griggs, Meara H. Faw, and Laura H. Malinin point out in "The Art of Love: Using Participatory Community Arts Engagement to Facilitate Relational Maintenance among Couples with Dementia" (chapter 10), one of the most poignant consequences of Alzheimer's disease is its gradual disabling of a sufferer's ability to communicate with others. This diminished or altered capacity to communicate negatively impacts the sufferer and their interpersonal relationships, especially with family members, for whom the deteriorating communication with their loved one is likely extremely distressing. While there is currently no known cure for this debilitating disease, the authors propose that arts engagement constitutes a potentially satisfying and adaptive activity for individuals with the diminished memory and mobility caused by Alzheimer's and similar conditions. The main focus of this chapter, however, is on how arts engagement may have adaptive effects on relational maintenance between sufferers and their caregivers. Through their research, based on eight weeks of observational data, Griggs, Faw, and Malinin demonstrate how dyads collaborating on a mask-making activity use communicative strategies to maintain their relational intimacy. The authors highlight how the setting, a therapist-led mask-making workshop, encouraged the use of certain strategies. As such, this chapter constitutes an important contribution to the as yet inadequate examination of the effects of arts engagement on relational variables.

The final chapter in this collection looks at the clinical space of the hospital to discover the everyday narratives within. Elizabeth Spradley's "Storying Clinical Interactions: Narrative Medicine as an Artistic Intervention in Medical Training and Education" (chapter 11) presents findings from a thematic analysis of stories published by medical students and practitioners in the medical humanities journal *The Intima*, focusing on what functions the storytelling process serve for the authors. Spradley argues that medical students and practitioners, who are often taught to believe they can best perform their jobs by prioritizing empiricism and scorning humanism, can, in fact, gain valuable insights by documenting their professional experiences in the wholly humanistic form of narratives. By storying their work lives, the contributors to *Intima* acknowledge their own, very human, insecurities as budding medical professionals, open up a site of resistance to hegemonic entrenched medical practices, learn more self-reflexivity regarding the impact of their own behavior on their patients' stories, and facilitate emotional healing and community-building with their colleagues. The chapter concludes with a clear blueprint for how the medical field can embrace and implement storytelling in its curriculum and training for medical students.

In sum, the essays in this collection hone in on the communication aspect of expressive arts modalities to help scholars and students gain deeper insights from each of those modalities in conducting research and scholarly activity in a more integrated way. This book is deliberately wide in scope, exploring a variety of therapeutic expressive media through different qualitative methodologies, and reflecting the diverse voices of scholars and practitioners writing from a multiplicity of backgrounds and about a range of populations and settings. Many of the most widely-recognized and practiced creative modalities are represented within this work: drama, music, dance movement, art, and narrative approaches.

* * *

WHO THIS BOOK IS FOR: EDUCATORS, STUDENTS, AND PRACTITIONERS

Educators

Contemporary pedagogy is shifting away from a strictly lecture-based format to include more embodied methods of learning. Performance in some form is increasingly being used to engage students' interest and to supplement and enhance the learning of course content. Educators who wish to incorporate performance-based activities, such as writing song lyrics, writing and performing skits, drawing, etc., into their teaching may also find this book a useful source of inspiration. Several of the authors have included instructions for how to introduce performance-based exercises into the classroom, which may be adapted by the imaginative educator to accommodate a variety of academic subjects.

Among the contributors are instructors who currently teach various courses in the communication studies discipline, including Communication Theory, Qualitative Research Methods, and Performance Studies, among others. Other contributors teach ecological and multicultural approaches to the practice of narrative and drama therapies. These scholars are sensitive to the kind of resources that would best serve their students' needs when used as a supplementary text, and have written their chapter with those needs in mind. While some chapters in the present collection may be less conventionally structured than others, we present these experimental pieces alongside more conventional ones to show the range of possibilities for qualitative inquiry.

Students

This book is intended to be a useful resource for both upper division undergraduate- and graduate-level students taking courses in Communication Studies, Psychology, Sociology, Theatre Arts, and other related disciplines. The chapters are written in language that, while scholarly, is nonetheless accessible for students at the aforementioned grade levels. Knowledge of theoretical foundations supporting the use of the various expressive arts modalities in therapeutic and educational settings is not assumed, but rather, brief and straightforward descriptions of theories are provided when they are brought up. Additionally, the essays in this collection highlight multiple forms of creative classroom and therapeutic practices. Many students have a conception of "performance" or "art," etc. as productions that are showcased in theatres or work that hangs in galleries. The contributors write about artistic activities and products that occur in quotidian settings and are created by individuals who may not necessarily be institutionally-credentialed artists and performers. This enables students to understand the potential healing capacity of making or experiencing art in their own everyday lives. Finally, the essays collected here depict contemporary research with different populations to provide students a guide for doing their own fieldwork and examples with which to model their own projects. Students looking for inspiration or guidance to help them write their term papers will find this a useful book that provides examples of research that could be done in various fields. Informed by theories of performance studies and expressive arts modalities in therapeutic and educational settings, this collection particularly addresses a much-needed gap in available readings assigned to students in health communication.

Practitioners

Although written by scholars, the audience for this collection is by no means limited to an academic audience. Counselors, social workers, therapists, and others in the helping professions who are considering incorporating creative activities into their work with clients will find these essays a source of inspiration and practical guidance.

REFERENCES

American Psychological Association (APA). (2017). Multicultural guidelines: An ecological approach to context, identity, and intersectionality. Prepared by the Task Force on Re-envisioning the Multicultural Guidelines for the 21st Century. APA Council of Representatives. Retrieved from http://www.apa.org/about/policy/multicultural-guidelines.pdf

Boal, A. (1979). *Theatre of the Oppressed* (C. A. McBride & M.-O. L. McBride, Trans.). New York, NY: Urizen Books.

Burke, K. (1945). *A grammar of motives*. Englewood Cliffs, NJ: Prentice Hall.

Elgar, F. J., Craig, W., & Trites, S. J. (2013). Family dinners, communication, and mental health in Canadian adolescents. *Journal of Adolescent Health*, *52*(4), 433–438. http://dx.doi.org/ 10.1016/j.jadohealth.2012.07.012

Fisher, W. R. (1985). The narrative paradigm: An elaboration. *Communication Monographs 52*(4), 347–367. https://doi.org/10.1080/03637758509376117

Goffman, E. (1959). *The presentation of self in everyday life*. New York, NY: Doubleday.

Hadley, S. (2013). Dominant narratives: Complicity and the need for vigilance in the creative arts therapies. *Arts in Psychotherapy*, *40*(4), 373–381. https://doi.org/10.1016/j.aip.2013.05.007

Halprin, D. (2003). *The expressive body in life, art, and therapy: Working with movement, metaphor, and meaning*. New York, NY: Jessica Kingsley Publishers.

Hemenover, S. H. (2003). The good, the bad, and the healthy: Impacts of emotional disclosure of trauma on resilient self-concept and psychological distress. *Personality and Social Psychology Bulletin*, *29*(10), 1236–1244. https://doi.org/10.1177/0146167203255228

Janoff-Bulman, R. (1992). *Shattered assumptions: Towards a new psychology of trauma*. New York, NY: Free Press.

Kennedy-Moore, E., & Watson, J. C. (2001). How and when does emotional expression help? *Review of General Psychology*, *5*(3), 187–212. https://doi.org/10.1037/1089-2680.5.3.187

Levi-Belz, Y., & Lev-Ari, L. (2019). "Let's talk about it": The moderating role of self-disclosure on complicated grief over time among suicide survivors. *International Journal of Environmental Research and Public Health, 16*(19), 3740–3753. https://doi.org/10.3390/ijerph16193740

Levine, S. K. (2004a). Introduction. In P. J. Knill, E. G. Levine, & S. K. Levine (Eds.), *Principles and practice of expressive arts therapy: Toward a therapeutic aesthetics* (pp. 9–13). Philadelphia, PA: Jessica Kingsley Publishers.

Levine, S. K. (2004b). The philosophy of expressive arts therapy: *Poiesis* as a response to the world. In P. J. Knill, E. G. Levine, & S. K. Levine (Eds.), *Principles and practice of expressive arts therapy: Toward a therapeutic aesthetics* (pp. 15–74). Philadelphia, PA: Jessica Kingsley Publishers.

Madison, D. S., & Hamera, J. (Eds.). (2006). *The SAGE Handbook of Performance Studies*. Thousand Oaks, CA: Sage Publications.

Malchiodi, C. A. (2005). Expressive therapies: History, theory, and practice. In C. A. Malchiodi (Ed.), *Expressive therapies* (pp. 1–15). New York, NY: Guilford Press.

McAdams, D. P. (1996). Personality, modernity, and the storied self: A contemporary framework for studying persons. *Psychological Inquiry*, *7*(4), 295–321. https://doi.org/10.1207/s15327965pli0704_1

Meekums, B. (2010). *Dance movement therapy: A creative psychotherapeutic approach*. Thousand Oaks, CA: Sage Publications.

Naumburg, M. (1955). Art as symbolic speech. *The Journal of Aesthetics and Art Criticism*, *13*(4), 435–450. https://www.jstor.org/stable/426931

Rimé, B., Herbette, G., & Corsini, S. (2004). The social sharing of emotion: Illusory and real benefits of talking about emotional experiences. In I. Nyklíček, L. Temoshok, & A. Vingerhoets (Eds.), *Emotional expression and health: Advances in theory, assessments and clinical applications* (pp. 27–41). New York, NY: Brunner-Routledge.

Rogers, N. (2001). Person-centered expressive arts therapy: A path to wholeness. In J. A. Rubin (Ed.), *Approaches to art therapy: Theory and technique* (2nd ed., pp. 163–177). New York, NY: Brunner-Routledge.

Rylatt, P. (2012). The benefits of creative therapy for people with dementia. *Nursing Standard*, *26*(33), 42–47. https://doi.org/10.7748/ns2012.04.26.33.42.c9050

Sajnani, N. (2013). The Body Politic: The relevance of an intersectional framework for therapeutic performance research in drama therapy. *Arts in Psychotherapy*, *40*(4), 382–385. https://doi.org/10.1016/j.aip.2013.05.001

Smyth, J. M., & Pennebaker, J. W. (1999). Sharing one's story: Translating emotional experiences into words as a coping tool. In C. R. Snyder (Ed.), *Coping: The psychology of what works* (pp. 70–89). New York, NY: Oxford University Press.

Tilsen, J., & Nylund, D. (2016). Cultural studies methodologies and narrative family therapy: Therapeutic conversations about pop culture. *Family Process*, *55*(2), 225–237. https://doi.org/10.1111/famp.12204

Turner, V. (1970). *The ritual process: Structure and anti-structure.* Piscataway: NJ: Aldine Publishing.

Part I

Performance and Drama

Chapter One

A Narradrama Approach to Teaching Communication

Kamran Afary

Since fall 2016, California State University, Los Angeles, where I teach in the Department of Communication Studies, has been offering nearly fifty student-prisoners at nearby Lancaster Prison the opportunity to earn a bachelor's degree by taking Communication Studies courses.[1] In this chapter I argue for the use of Narradrama exercises as part of an instructional program for prison populations to promote psychosocial healing among the students. I use already published and publicly available writings by the Lancaster cohort and interviews with respected drama therapists also working with prisoners posted on YouTube as a case study to support this argument. Along with presenting the argument and evidence, I also provide detailed instructions on how educators could incorporate Narradrama into the classroom.

In spring 2020, sixteen of them, all members of the first cohort, are planning to graduate. At least four or more have left the prison and are now studying on campus and plan to walk at the graduation ceremony. Each year since 2017, we have had a convocation ceremony at the prison with honored invited guests and family members to mark the beginning of the academic year by celebrating the students' achievements. Each year the students choose to honor their transformative educational experience by creating performances based on their Narradrama class exercises: reflections on the material that we study which includes a discussion of the course concepts along with a personal experience. These writing exercises and reflections were further developed into short images, sculptures, or scenes for longer pieces that we developed into scripts and longer performances based on the themes. Narradrama is a relatively recent model of an expressive therapeutic approach that combines insights from postmodern narrative and drama therapy techniques. Although primarily used by mental health practitioners, it is increasingly used by educators in educational settings. This is the first time, to my knowledge, that a Narradrama approach has been used in working with prisoners.

In 2017 Cal State LA was one of sixty-seven postsecondary institutions to participate in the Second Chance Pell Program (Dowdell, 2015), and the only one that offered a bachelor's degree in Communication Studies. This one-of-a-kind degree program was the result of several years of creative collaboration by many participants across the university who were dedicated to abolishing the dehumanizing environments created by mass incarceration and the prison-industrial complex.[2]

This work is also made possible by the prisoners' own two-decades-long initiative in the creation of a progressive education *A-Yard,* initially called *Men for Honor Yard* (MacDonald & Williams, 2019). Prison reform policies initiated by the state of California that moved away from "tough on crime" policies which gutted earlier rehabilitative programs also freed up some of the state's budget for more educational programming (Widdoes, 2016). As the Vera Institute of Justice has suggested: "education is key to improving many long-term outcomes for incarcerated people, their families, and their communities—including reducing recidivism and increasing employability and earnings after release" (diZerega, 2017).

I started teaching Interpersonal Communication in spring of 2017 to a cohort of twenty-two students. We faced challenges and received much support from the prison staff to ensure proper arrangements for access to classrooms in a maximum-security prison and to bring teaching resources to a place where internet access was not readily available. But once inside the classrooms, we found a new reality behind bars: We met face-to-face with students who had lived "inside" for ten, twenty, thirty, or more years. Most of our students were sent to prison for life because of a crime they committed at a very early age, most during their teens. Here we found a welcoming, engaged, and deeply enthusiastic group of students who were eager to inquire, and to pose questions about communication theories and practices. Many of them had already taken college courses and were building on the knowledge and skills they had mastered. Several of our students were social justice activists working on some form of restorative justice project. Many had made their amends to victims long ago and were focused on contributing and being of service to other prisoners and to the outside world.

The writings quoted in this chapter are mostly from a peer-reviewed student academic journal, *Colloquy, 13* which we edited (Afary, Chee, & Dechaine, eds., 2017). Throughout the semester, students wrote reflections, reviews, and poems that were initially read aloud in class. These writings then became the basis for scenes, enactments, sculptures, and scripts. Excerpts from two performance scripts, *Imagine That* and *A Fresh Start*, were published by my colleague and collaborator, Elizabeth Malone (2019), who worked in several prisons and had produced a play on a day in the life of three women prisoners. The student-prisoner writings were a testament to their readiness to engage with what the discipline of communication studies has to offer and contribute to a dialogue on social justice.

As we advocate for more college education opportunities for incarcerated people, we also discover the unique ways in which those who are in prisons are ready to create more dialogic forms of social engagement.

LITERATURE REVIEW

Much has been written about the benefits of offering educational programs in prisons to reduce the rates of recidivism. Alternative forms of prison pedagogy have been studied by numerous scholars (Behan, 2014; Bumiller, 2013; Davidson, 1995; Davis, 2013; Gaskew, 2015; Germain, 2014; Goldberg, 2015; Hartnett, Wood, & McCann, 2011; Higgins, 2007; Zoukis, 2014). The question of whether it is even possible to offer radical education that advocates for the abolition of the system of mass incarceration (Alexander, 2010) inside a prison has also been discussed in more detail (Rafay, 2013). Similarly, the PCARE Collective (2017) has explored the complex issues that arise when one questions the prison-industrial complex and yet participates in educational programs that may legitimize its practices. Both Tony Platt (2018) in *Beyond The Walls* and John Sloop (1996) in *The Cultural Prison* have questioned the presumptions about our society's notions of punishment by tracing the history of concepts of punishment, how prisons serve to legitimize inequities, and why efforts to reform prisons with educational programs have led to expanding rather than contracting the net of social control. Others such as Jodie Lawston and Gabriel Jones (2011) chronicled their attempts to offer prison courses that raise critical consciousness and pose questions about the structural analysis of prisons. James Kilgore (2011) offers an account of introducing Paulo Freire's (1970) model of pedagogy in prison settings. Rebecca Sanford and Johanna Foster (2006) focus not only on classroom practices but the components and potential pitfalls in developing and implementing college-in-prison *programs*. Jim Thomas (1995) catalogued many of the problems involved in teaching in maximum-security prisons, while pointing out the irony that unconventional settings can both subvert, and yet stimulate, creative teaching strategies. Maria Torre and Michelle Fine (2005) and Erica Meiners (2009) advocate for stretching the limits of affirmative action programs to include prison higher education. The latter's empirical research shows the benefits of access not only to inmates, but to transforming prison environments and helping children of prisoners.

Performance as research methodology and as practice has been useful in both analysis of the social construction of identities in prison and in documenting collaborative projects between student-prisoners and outside communities (Baim, 2007; Deal, 2014; Clements, 2004). Randall Wright (2014), for example, uses Goffman's concept of performative spaces to examine the various forces (discourses and institutional processes) that shape student-prisoner identities. McCann (2019) also deploys a performance lens to analyze prison visits by students. Jean Trounstine (2008), who worked for a decade with women prisoners producing plays, argues for the need to go beyond prison education when funding can "lead to coercive expectations" (p. 674) of *correcting* the character of prisoners. The work of many theatre activists teaching conflict management through performance has been informed by Patricia Sternberg's *Theatre for Conflict Resolution* (1998), and Michael Rohd's, *Theatre for Community, Conflict & Dialogue* (1998). The transformative power of performance has also been studied by other scholars (Fischer-Lichte, 2008; Fennessey, 2000).

A work by communication studies scholars that has influenced my research and writing of this chapter on prison activism is the edited volume *Working for Justice: A Handbook of Prison Education and Activism* (Hartnett, Novek, & Wood, 2013). Of particular significance to my work is a chapter by Jonathan Shailor (2013) that describes in detail an innovative teaching method and process in carceral settings. In addition, scholarship on performance ethnography provides strong arguments for incorporating performance not only as activity, but also as research methodology for academic work by students and teachers alike (Denzin, 2017; Conrad, 2008; Hamera, 2011; Madison, 2018). Together these works provide a matrix to support this chapter's exploration of the efficacy of using drama therapy techniques to teach interpersonal communication in a prison classroom.[3]

Communication studies owes a debt of gratitude to the work of a group of scholars and activists who call themselves the Prison Communication, Activism, Research, and Education Collective (PCARE). The PCARE Collective initially came together in the United States in 2005, which ran programs in twelve different states from Arizona to Wisconsin. PCARE's numerous publications and newsletters contain many testimonials from prisoners on the transformative nature of its programs. Included are descriptions of best practices and an inventory of how citizenship can be enhanced with the arts, education, and activism. In "Working for Justice in the Age of Mass Incarceration," the editor's essay in *Working for Justice*, introduces the collection of writings on prison education and activism, and Stephen Hartnett, Eleanor Novek, and Jennifer Wood (2013) encourage readers to "use our words to solve problems, to seek restoration rather than retribution" (p. 2). Their handbook contains ten essays that demonstrate how activist teachers and scholars work in prisons and with communities to build new relationships that do not rely on incarceration.

Shailor's (2013) chapter, "Kings, Warriors, Magicians, and Lovers," provides an example of teaching in prison using psychoanalytic approaches, cultural performances, and meditation. Shailor (2013) uses Jungian archetypes (Jung, 1991) to help students reflect on different forms of "hegemonic masculinity" (p. 13). He argues that by exploring these archetypes one can gain insight into the shadow sides of the students' personality structure and help the student become a more productive person (Shailor, 2013, p. 14). His work is complex and multidimensional involving several layers of pedagogy, from reading Jung to watching popular films, developing character analysis, and creating alternative performances. Shailor (2013) argues that far from providing rehabilitation, prisons reinforce toxic forms of domination and violence (p. 14). Aggression, shaming, and humiliation permeate the shocking failure of prison cultures, he points out. As an alternative, Shailor (2013) has developed a model called the "Theater of Empowerment" to validate and nurture the humanity of those who are incarcerated. Working with Shailor's (2013) approach, prisoners learn to let themselves be more vulnerable and present. By making performance available to audiences such as family members and limited members of the public, student-prisoners gain new social and communication skills.

A second essay in this volume by David Coogan (2013), "Writing Your Way to Freedom: Autobiography as Inquiry in Prison Writing Workshops," provides both a model of how to create new empowering narratives by prisoners and a warning and critical review of where prison autobiographies from the 1960s and 1970s went wrong.

Norman Denzin (2017) writes that researchers can no longer rely on traditional concepts of performance in their work and need to create "spaces for a merger of praxis, ethnography, rhetoric, and activism in public (and private) life" (p. 45). He argues for the urgency of this task because new political economic realities have created conditions in which "any person is at risk of arrest, of becoming a victim, a prisoner, at best collateral damage in a global space where performance principles and technological rationality regulate daily life" (Denzin, 2017, p. 45). This is particularly true of prison education programs where traditional research resources are made unavailable due to the many layers of institutional sanctions. Utilizing performance as activity in the classroom and as methodology in research is not a luxury, but a necessity. In an essay on performance ethnography, Diane Conrad (2008) also argues for incorporating performance as a process of knowledge production and as a method of representing research that enables students to "engage in reenacting moments from real life that express, interpret, and re-present their ideas" (p. 610). This work can also lead to stronger analysis or interpretation of research. Conrad (2008) argues that *acting out* is a process that is both critical and analytic. By playing a role, students can explore the experiences of an *as if* character both from the inside and outside.

INTERPERSONAL COMMUNICATION, IDENTITIES, AND EDUCATION

In teaching interpersonal and health communication at Lancaster Prison, the topics that most resonate with me and the relationships I have developed with my students are greatly shaped by my own past life experiences. Before training as a drama therapist, my graduate research was in performance studies both at Cal State LA and at Northwestern University. Working with mentors such as Judith Hamera (2011) and Dwight Conquergood (2013), I learned to pay close attention to cultural performances, rites of passage, and rituals that each individual participates in to form a personal and social identity. Our identities are constituted by the ways in which we perform, both individually and collectively, notions of race, gender, sexuality, and class. In addition, my training in performance studies included from the very beginning techniques adapted from experimental theatre, performance art, and creative drama, while also drawing on a host of other disciplines from cultural anthropology to postmodern theory.

My personal experiences were also decisive. I was born into a highly patriarchal Iranian family where my role as *the only son* was hyper-defined at the moment of my birth. Very little negotiation of gender identity was allowed in my culture with its relentless micropolicing of gender roles in everyday life. The gender identity script was written before I was born and I was expected to follow it to the letter. I rebelled in every way possible, often without having a language to describe what I was opposing. As I became an activist in the United States in my early twenties in civil rights issues, I started to question many of these assumptions about binary gender norms, racial and social class hierarchies, and heteronormative sexualities. I was introduced to feminist thought and activism through my sisters' struggles against patriarchal norms and for gender equality. In the process, I came to a greater understanding of how various forms of toxic masculinity are constructed in our cultures. I also found ways in which I could both break out of the straightjacket of these norms, and yet, in some crucial areas, remain deeply committed to some of the ethical principles of my culture of origin. In that sense, I had my own experience of reconstructing a new sense of gender identity and breaking from various forms of toxic masculinity. This was all before the fields of gender studies and queer studies had a name. I carry this sense with me in my interactions with incarcerated students.

The interdisciplinary fields of genders and sexualities studies are a relatively new area in the academic world. The original inspiration for these fields came from the discipline of Women's Studies, which was developed primarily in the 1970s, and taught women that their gender was not just a fixed biological condition, but also one that was socially, politically, and culturally constructed. Feminist historians then delved into centuries of history to show how notions of femininity had evolved through time and in different societies. They also showed that feminine characteristics were not innate qualities but ascribed to women, and internalized by them. In this way a little girl was taught how to be a *proper woman*, and therefore, patriarchal society's desired expectations from women (dependent, submissive, sexually subservient to men in power) were achieved.

In recent years, genders and sexualities studies have attempted to delve into how different forms of masculinity are also socially, politically, and culturally constructed. Just because patriarchy has ruled for centuries does not mean men have been exempt from the straightjackets that have defined how they ought to act as men and what constitutes proper behavior for a *real man*. The study of genders and sexualities was not pioneered by heterosexual men but by gay, lesbian, queer, and transgender scholars and activists. In over a century of struggle, gay men, in particular, gradually established the fact that men who aspired to a different "regimes of sexuality," to use Michel Foucault's (1990, p. 129) famous term, or desired to interact with others in ways that were traditionally defined as more feminine, had a right to do so and were men, if they chose to identify as such. Yet the field can still be considered in its infancy, as evidenced by the recent controversy over a statement by the American Psychological Association that "understanding how boys and men experience masculinity is an important cultural competency" (APA, 2018, p. 8).

When I started teaching incarcerated students at the California State Prison, I sought to draw upon all these different strands of my background, the field of performance studies, feminist studies, genders and sexualities studies, interpersonal communication studies, my own personal journeys, and finally, drama therapy. As I hope this chapter shows, the result can be inspiring, both for my students and for me.

As an instructor, my first goal was to help students build their interpersonal communication skills and, in the process, find their own language. We worked together as they found new analogies and metaphors for the academic concepts we read in the assigned textbooks. We also worked on when, where, and how one might use these different discourses. Students then applied these insights to the performances they created, using their own informal and personal language as much as possible, and in the process created a language that was saturated with their experiences.

Drama therapy in general, and Narradrama in particular, are known for their cathartic potential. Through the process of Narradrama, participants reflect on their life experiences in an indirect way, and the results are often the release of strong and repressed emotions, which then can bring about significant psychological relief from internalized pains. By engaging in a type of *reflective learning*, the participants come to identify turning points in their lives, which may then lead them to construct new identities for themselves, and move away from the one that was imposed on them by their parents, their community, or their society as a whole. Below, I will discuss four of my students, who were paroled in 2018–2019 after going through Cal State LA's bachelor's program in communication studies, and whose writings reflect the creation of this synthesized and alternative identity. Some of their observations were submitted for publication to *Colloquy*, a journal of the Department of Communication Studies at Cal State LA. In fall 2017 *Colloquy* published their selected writings in a special feature issue (Afary, Chee, & Dechaine, 2017). Some of these writings were subsequently developed into performance scripts. This process of reflecting on their experiences, writing them down, and finally seeing their work published proved to be of dramatic help to the students in shaping new identities as writers. Looking at their printed work, in conjunction with others, they came to a better understanding of themselves and also gained a new respect for themselves and their fellow inmates who were now all published authors. The selections below focus on the interpersonal communication skills the students were able to demonstrate in their writings, skills that they had painstakingly developed over time, and were now able to demonstrate in a way that contributed to their release from prison.

An inmate who is eligible for parole is asked to write a formal application. Parole boards are concerned with several issues in reading these applications. They want to know if the inmate has experienced and can demonstrate remorse for the action that led to their incarceration. They also want to know about the inmate's plans and the availability of support upon release. They like to hear about new and productive activities by the inmate, and most of all they want to know if the inmate can fully integrate into society once they are released.

Clifton Lee Gibson was released from prison in the summer of 2019 after serving a twenty-three-year sentence. He worked toward his bachelor's degree in prison and included much of the work he produced in his courses in his parole application. Cal State LA has created a comprehensive program for parolees, which includes a chapter of the Rebound Project on campus, and arrangements with nearby half-way houses for some former inmates. Since his release Gibson has been working full-time as a counselor, taking classes full-time on campus, and working part-time as a student editor for *Communication Studies Prison BA Journal*, an academic journal that publishes writings by prisoners. In one assignment he summed up a course in interpersonal communication with this autoethnographic poem that develops a preferred narrative of his life:

From interpersonal communication, my mind began expanding
Family life and choices took on a whole new understanding
Poor country folk, was my *subculture's* foundation
Happy faces littered with internal tears of *maladaptive marginalization*
Behind one of our *Johari's windows* were pain and suffering
Hidden and under a closed system we were buffering.
What was disclosed and what was not
In a difficult situation, I was caught
Coercive power was my predominate socialization
Arguments and fights linked emotions with communication
I became witty, sarcastic, violent with no empathy in place
Conflict became dominating and integrating with a negative face . . . I drug regrets behind me with secrecy rules
I was stuck in muck till I developed coping tools
Through inner and higher education
I began regulating my self-talking conversation
Emotional intelligence started to grow
My kindness and core-self began to show
No longer was the solution violence or moping
I have been armed with problem and emotion-focused coping.
Seeking healthy solutions displayed by men
Now both parties may walk away with a win-win. (Gibson, 2017, p. 108)

In prison, Gibson facilitated a series of prison workshops, which were called Masks of Masculinity. He helped his fellow inmates discuss various forms of *toxic masculinity*. This concept refers to common masculine norms that can be harmful to men, as well as to the women and children around them, and to society as a whole. He learned that certain idealized forms of masculinity can have a highly destructive and harmful effect on the individual and on those around them, and often lead to violence. Many inmates find out through performance rehearsals that they were first caged by the notion of how they had to portray a tough male persona, a characteristic that was ultimately unattainable and destructive, before they were incarcerated by the state.

Toxic masculinity operates by suppressing one's emotions. Men learn to mask their emotions and maintain an appearance of *hardness*. Most importantly, toxic masculinity encourages the use of violence as an indicator of power, a violence often directed at more vulnerable members of one's own community including women and children, boys and girls. Toxic masculinity thereby feeds the continuing epidemic of domestic violence, young adult gang violence, and contributes to systemic incarceration. The prison regime often reinforces these violent stereotypes and thus contributes to the continuation of the vicious circle.

Brad Arrowood, another former inmate, addressed a second aspect of toxic masculinity. Arrowood served twenty-seven years in the California State Prison system before he was released on parole in 2018. Like Gibson, he included some of the materials he created for our classes in his parole application. In Lancaster Prison, Arrowood was a master post-traumatic stress disorder (PTSD) service dog trainer. Since his release, in addition to taking courses on campus, he has also started a new business training PTSD service dogs in Los Angeles. Individuals who have experienced violence and trauma in their lives and suffer from PTSD benefit greatly from working with a trained dog that can help them better cope with fear and anxiety.

Arrowood writes about "communicating comfort and support" in a prison context. He describes the difficulty of expressing emotional support in the prison setting and in the process illuminates an often-hidden dimension of how prisoners become lay caregivers to one another. (See Hook & Geist-Martin, 2018 for research on development of support among incarcerated women.) And yet the same inmates who nurture others must outwardly project the stereotypically tough image of masculinity, so they can survive in prison:

> In prison, I think most of us are pretty good at the problem-focused task. We are good at volunteering data, deciphering data for others that do not understand it and the rest comes from staff, such as medical data. However, unlike the outside world, we do not have support groups. There are no cancer support groups, no online chat rooms or the daily support of our loved ones. This makes it difficult to get the emotional support needed to go on with life when one is faced with a physical or emotional crisis. . . .
> Quite often people in prison do not get the support they want or need. When a person is afflicted with cancer, everyone abandons them. Friends stop calling, almost as if they think cancer is contagious. To begin with, many of us are closed off emotionally, just as a coping strategy for self-preservation. This then contributes to the creation of a larger distance between an ill person and other prisoners. We see this in this very class. When was the last time you asked M. [a classmate who was diagnosed with cancer at the time], "How are you feeling today? Can I help you with anything? Do you want to talk about it?" I am just as guilty of this.
> We see M. in a good mood or putting on a brave face, okay, we can go talk to him about legal stuff or whatever, not cancer though. Let's keep that hush. Let's keep that under the table. Then if he's having a bad day, let's just avoid him today. Yet this might be when he needs it the most. Cancer is not just a day thing; it's not just during the treatment times; it's the in-between times too. (Arrowood, 2017, p. 109)

Arrowood talks about how learning new interpersonal communication skills has had far reaching effects on his interactions. It has influenced his daily life and the work he produces in various Cal State LA classes. He reflects on the value of studying interpersonal communication. He believes teaching interpersonal communication techniques to incarcerated inmates is essential, as it would teach student inmates how to change and rehabilitate themselves. Finally, he argues that in learning interpersonal communication skills inmates also learn how to view others: "This prison has made great strides in changing our normal labels of ourselves. . . . It takes us to change our view of others first, not just ourselves" (Arrowood, 2017, p. 110).

Charlie Praphatanada spent more of his adult life inside prison than outside it. After his parole, Praphatanada gave an interview to Vanessa Rancano, which was aired and published by National Public Radio (NPR). The interview took the reader through Cal State LA's prison education program and the crucial role that the program has played in the step-by-step rehabilitation of some inmates. Thus, with the help of the program, Praphatanada moved from being an inmate serving a life sentence with no possibility of parole, to a life sentence with the possibility of parole, to an expected parole term, and finally to parole and freedom. "Paraphatananda was serving a life sentence without the possibility of parole. He was also three years into a bachelor's degree program—one of 42 men participating in an experiment that tests the limits of the public university mission to spread educational opportunity far and wide." Praphatanada used the education process, and what he learned through interpersonal communication studies, to work on relationships in his life and to ultimately request parole. One of the films he watched in class was the Academy Award winning drama Paul Haggis's *Crash* (2004). *Crash* describes the confluence of racial and social tensions in Los Angeles within a group of socially and ethnically diverse people who unwillingly interact with one another through a series of car accidents and violent events. In an excerpt from his review of the movie for class, Praphatanada notes that

> Interpersonal Communication is how we form bonds with each other. Those who choose to practice Interpersonal Communication with me, have interpreted some symbols or actions that draw them to believe we have something in common. This could be a T-shirt that voices a point of view ("Trump Sucks") or some cultural symbol that is only understood by people of my own culture. Our interpersonal communications shape our identities, morals, and values. But, if we do not practice self-reflective acts, or at least become aware of who we are, and why we do the things we do, then we squander potential opportunities for new friendships, lovers, and a better understanding of ourselves. (Praphatanada, 2017, pp. 132–133)

Jeff Stein is another former inmate who used his university study to change himself and gain parole. Stein became conscious that through self-improvement he could break with the stereotypical constructs of toxic masculinity. He also learned how to teach interpersonal communication skills to other inmates, which in turn contributed to his own sense of identity and self-worth. In one of his papers, he wrote:

> It puzzles me that the study and development of quality communication skills is not strongly encouraged in school as other subjects such as math, science, or

> other "core" courses. . . . For example, I was taught to solve complicated math problems that took up the whole blackboard—yet somehow, I went through life for decades with woefully inadequate interpersonal communication skills. I can only conclude that many of my personal and interpersonal difficulties such as substance abuse, deviant behavior, and poor relationships are directly linked to my lack of situational awareness and emotional intelligence. (Stein, 2017, p. 114)

Stein believed that interpersonal communicational skills moved beyond greater awareness of his own difficulties. It also altered the nature of his relationship with others. Whereas before he was exclusively concerned with winning every argument and every conflict, now he no longer thinks so:

> I help others and myself to make informed decisions instead of stubbornly clinging to old, worn-out positions out of pride and selfishness. . . . When I was younger, I had no definitive conflict orientation. I was all over the place. Sometimes I would achieve a "win-win" with a conflict partner, but it was rarely a decided goal on my part. Often, I would damage the relationship at least temporarily over a relatively trivial disagreement-and more than half the time I was the problem not the other party. . . . Over time this led to resentment that manifested itself in many areas of my life that were unhealthy. In addition, I harmed others around me in various ways that they did not deserve; I lied when they deserved the truth, I was an addict when they needed me at my best, and I was selfish when they needed me to be considerate of their feelings. By making a conscious, informed decision to always find a win-win outcome, I will be a blessing to others who really need me to be at my best. (Stein, 2017, p. 115)

WHY A STUDY OF COMMUNICATION INFORMED BY DRAMA THERAPY?

On a very general level, the goal in incorporating Narradrama into a course curriculum is to use the drama process to achieve deeper learning processes that can also serve as a healing and therapeutic experience in a prison setting. Classroom activities begin with instructions and discussions, but as their instructor, I encourage students to create short scripts, roles, vignettes, and to sculpt poses and stage scenes that can demonstrate concepts. This is a deeply collaborative and engaging approach that provides a multisensory context for participants to not only tell their stories but also to enact and rehearse them by calling on other students to participate.

In my rhetoric classes, both on campus and in prison, I ground this work in Kenneth Burke's (2018) "theory of symbolic action" and in its insistence that language is dramatistic. Burke deploys the imagery of a theatrical stage to depict our mental processes. I point out that Burke's (2018) Pentadic method can be embodied in the form of theatrical staging. Each rhetor is a director whose motivations can be theorized by the ways in which they foreground or background different elements of a rhetorical act.

By connecting communication theories (in this specific case, Burke's dramatism) to drama therapy exercises, students can intentionally work with role play in setting goals and solving problems while exploring and expressing feelings. At times, this leads to experiencing the temporary liberating effects of catharsis. Through these class exercises and performances, students can externalize inner experience with more depth and breadth as they explore concepts in interpersonal communication and build better relationship skills. Here, the students created a performative response to a documentary they saw in class:

> *One Student:* At the end of my sentence I will know what it feels like to serve more time in prison than I have lived outside of prison. (He stands to speak and anyone who has served more time in, than outside, at the end of their sentence raises their hand.)
>
> *Another Student:* When you feel that you do not have an opportunity to better yourself, you feel as if you have fallen into hopelessness. . . . (First student makes his way to his seat, slumping hopelessly in it.)
>
> *All the Actors/Students*: I am still a HUMAN BEING.

In order to use drama exercises and techniques in educational settings, I often have to prepare myself and my students to take play seriously. I begin with a discussion of John Huizinga (2014) who theorized play as a free and meaningful human activity that humans and other species engage in *for its own sake*. Just as the term rhetoric may first conjure images of empty verbiage, so too *play* has the unfortunate connotation of something not important. It takes some reorientation and disorientation of existing values to see the activity of play (both simple playfulness and role play) as itself valuable. Building a safe space for play requires participants to embody and project roles, tell stories, take metaphors seriously, and to have empathy. Building play also requires some distancing from strict empiricism, a capability to witness, and courage to engage in performance and improvisation. Here is another excerpt from the above-mentioned play:

> *All the Actors/Students*: I am not a man who gives into his emotions.
>
> *One Student*: Doing so would be like blood in the water, sure to attract sharks. . . . No matter what I was going through, what I was feeling, I could make no outward showing. Displaying emotions equated weakness, and weakness would make me a victim. I internalized everything.

This process of turning written material into performance texts becomes a ritual practice in the classroom that enriches the learning process. Following Benjamin Bloom's (1956) taxonomy of learning processes, this approach helps students to remember, understand, apply, and analyze the key terms and concepts. The final culminating project, the performance, is then an opportunity for them to further engage in the creative process. In this way students engage theories in communication studies, performance studies, drama and theatre, psychology, and (auto)ethnography. Students apply theories of communication to topics such as recovering from addiction, dysfunctional families, disabilities, surviving abuse, and health communication.

Teaching communication courses with the added drama therapy component can greatly benefit not only individual student prisoners, but also their families and the entire communities of prison professionals struggling to restore rehabilitation programs, reduce prison populations, and, in particular, help former prisoners prepare for encounters after release where they may deal with social stigmatization, isolation, and conflict. Both inside and outside, teaching communication and incorporating drama skills is an effective way to prepare individuals to manage anxiety, depression, and addiction, among other conditions. This work can promote positive changes in mood, insight, and empathy, and also facilitate healthy relationships.

DRAMA THERAPISTS IN PRISONS

The use of drama therapy as an expressive modality is not a new phenomenon, nor has it been limited to North America. In the process of writing this chapter, I interviewed six well-known drama therapists who have worked with prisoners, some of whom have been doing this type of therapy since the early 1980s. Some have worked internationally and published articles about their findings and some have produced award-winning documentaries.

Zeina Daccache is the director of Catharsis-Lebanese Center for Drama Therapy. Her theatrical and film productions of both men and women prisoners have received international recognition and have influenced prison reform in Lebanon.[4]

Daccache (2019) is concerned with the psychological and educational barriers we create between free and incarcerated people. She argues that in completely isolating the general public from prison life, we are not just harming the prisoners, but also the general public. "Prisons are a microcosm of society. If you want to know about all the problems in your society, go live in a prison for one day. If you want to solve the problems of your society, it would be great to start in prisons." But Daccache (2016) also believes that drama therapy is an overwhelming type of profession and not every practitioner is equipped with the right personality to work with prisoners and to achieve results.

Suraya Keating (2019) agrees that the work is difficult and can be overly challenging on many levels. The ideal drama therapist, she says, must be a type of trickster: wise about the ordinary world and not just one with bookish knowledge, also someone with a great sense of humor. Keating, a California therapist and educator, has worked extensively in the California prison system over the last fifteen years. She is one of the directors of the Marin Shakespeare Program and has used theatre as a tool for the psychological transformation of incarcerated men in the San Quentin State Prison (Keating, 2019).

In Keating's view, the best drama therapists bring in a "sacred fool role." The sacred fool (or wise fool) is a common trope in world literature and appears in the works of Erasmus, Shakespeare, and Cervantes. It is the clownish character who originally comes across as a buffoon and idiot, but later emerges as the beholder of great wisdom for those around them. The wise fool often mocks the erudite person who lacks common wisdom. Keating ties this type of trickster drama therapist to Jungian psychology. In Jung's classic works (1991), the trickster plays a key role in revealing the shadow parts of an individual, the unconscious part of personality. While the shadow often holds the negative aspects of personality or culture, it may also contain positive aspects, ones that a traumatized person with low self-esteem and severe anxiety may not dare acknowledge. Keating believes that a drama therapist should play a trickster role and bring out the shadow segments of an inmate's life into light, but do so in a humorous way that both heals and educates the patient:

> We [drama therapists] bring this capacity to go into the dark and light, and work in this playful way to dive deep into our psyches of what needs to be healed. I think that ability, the play and the depth, is really needed in our prisons which are such heavy, depressing places. The gift of lightness is very much needed. . . . Not the fluffy lightness, but lightness with awareness. I think we have the ability to really transform with our skills in that way. (Keating, 2019)

A clinical psychologist with traditional training is precisely the kind of erudite person that stands against the wise fool/trickster therapist. Often, they do not understand the world of the prisoners and their dilemmas. John Bergman is a British-American drama therapist and theatre director, who has had over thirty-seven years' experience with prisoners and prison officers in various nations, especially Australia. He is the recipient of a 2005 Research Award from the North American Drama Therapy Association. He points out that most prisoners abhor talk therapy. In fact, to them "a clinical psychologist is the enemy" because if the prisoner opens up his soul to the therapist, and inadvertently talks about his desire to harm others, the therapist might decide he has no choice but to report what he has heard to the warden, in which case the prisoner might be further punished by the prison authorities (Bergman, 2019). In addition, Bergman believes most prisoners have never had the opportunity to be self-reflexive: "many of these guys have lost or have never created contemplative techniques to engage with things that word therapy really demands." As a result, the way to reach them is not through talk therapy but through other methods of therapy such as drama therapy, art therapy, music therapy, and action therapies that are deeply engaging. Hence in his view, "Drama therapists, amongst action therapists and experiential therapists, are the ones that can most accurately, most sensitively and most successfully engage with battered people" (Bergman, 2019).

Armand Volkas (2019), Linda Gregoric-Cook (2019), Ellen Williams (2019), and Stephanie Wichmann (2019) all explore the manner in which the prisoners (and even the guards) experience change as a result of drama therapy. Volkas is an Associate Professor in Counseling Psychology at the California Institute for Integral Studies. His parents survived the Holocaust and fought in the French Resistance. Volkas has brought together children of Holocaust survivors with children of Nazi perpetrators, using drama therapy and expressive arts therapies for such intercultural reconciliation. Ellen Williams is a Professor of Expressive Arts at Rutgers University and a long-time practitioner of drama therapy in the New York and New Jersey prison systems. Stephanie Wichmann, a Clinical Social Worker in Portland, Oregon, is a drama therapist with a professional theatre and comedy background who conducts workshops with incarcerated youths on the West Coast on humor, healing, and creativity, cultivating resiliency through the dramatic arts. Together, these three therapists have accumulated a vast trove of information on using drama therapy as an educational and healing tool.

Volkas believes the problem is that "inmates are living dysfunctional life scripts" (Volkas, 2019). Drama therapy helps the prisoner uncover the narratives by which they have lived their lives unconsciously. Some narratives are those about which the prisoner has had no choice and has been told to follow compulsively. Others are narratives that the prisoner might have the option to make a choice. An example of a compulsive narrative is the case where a prisoner enters the prison yard and is told by a fellow inmate that he must hang out only with people of his own race and perhaps his gang affiliation. This may be for his own protection, but it is not of his choice. At the same time, the prisoner might decide to make new choices such as providing support and comfort when another prisoner outside his immediate orbit becomes sick, providing the kind of nurturance that a family member might provide. In the late 1990s, in response to politicians who labeled prisoners *incorrigible*, suggesting that they could not be reformed, some prisoners in Lancaster, California (where I have conducted drama therapy) and elsewhere helped create the foundations for new education programs. A group of prisoners contacted local colleges and asked to take correspondence courses (MacDonald and Williams, 2019). These are the types of actions that drama therapists such as Volkas call "re-scripting" and believe have the potential to change the prisoner while they are incarcerated. Here drama therapy is aiding the prisoner to explore other possibilities through the world of imagination. In Volkas' view, "drama therapy has the power to engage people down to the nervous system. It is one of the most powerful interventions we can have to help incarcerated people change their lives and make new choices. I think the idea of a life-script is a useful idea. We change the script through drama therapy" (Volkas, 2019).

Ellen Williams also believes that drama therapy can open the door to lifelong traumas and help heal them. Prisoners become mere numbers in prison, they are labeled, and are devalued on a daily basis. Drama therapy says, "We know you are a person with a soul and uniqueness. You may be a number in here, but you are not a number to me" (Williams, 2019). In this way, drama therapy gives the prisoners a sense of their own self-worth. It becomes a way to promote self-worth in a system that does not value it.

Finally, Stephanie Wichmann believes drama therapy not only helps heal the prisoners and creates an opportunity for them to seek education to reform themselves, it also helps change the guards and thus contributes to a different climate within prisons:

> I'm talking about the guards too. Guards see the work and realize that two people who were not talking for months are now doing a mirror exercise together. That would not be able to happen if you go into a room with a solo therapist, but being in a group allows you to see so much more perspective. You get to see creativity, collaboration and ultimately their soul. That is the power of a drama therapist; we take old stories and make them new again. We can learn somebody's stories, and what brought them here, and what their visions and dreams are for the future. We can laugh and be playful, and there is a lot of benefit in that. There is also the other side—talking about the pain and the struggle. Drama therapists are okay holding both joy and pain in the same space and making room for that. The more you can make room for both, the more people can be seen, heard and be in their authentic selves. That is why we are that and that is why we should be in more places. (Wichmann, 2019)

NARRADRAMA METHOD'S NINE STEPS

As an educator using the Narradrama method, I frequently keep a journal to document my course activities and processes. This helps me develop narrative questions that aid students externalize and develop performances. These performances then help the person change their relationship to what are often characterized as fixed and essentialized problem stories. The following is a description of the process by which I work with student prisoners to assist them in reframing their narratives and identities.[5]

Narradrama is based on a postmodern form of therapy called Narrative Therapy. It originates in the work of Michael White's (2007) *Maps of Narrative Practice*, with narrative therapists' approach the discourse on mental health with a good dose of skepticism. They consciously work to elicit an empowering experience-near language from their clients, rather than rely on the stigmatizing and disempowering discourse of experts focused narrowly on pathologies. They are informed by ideas developed by Foucault (1977) on power of discourse and Victor Turner's (1982) *From Ritual to Theatre*, and his approach to cultural ethnography of roles and rituals.[6] My courses always incorporate performance and role play as a modality, no matter how strictly theoretical or textual the course is. This has helped me a great deal in teaching in prison, and in overcoming some of the limitations.

In following this model, we begin with a general discussion of the arc of Narradrama: starting with *problem-saturated stories* that produce self-loathing, shame, stigma, and internalized oppression, and then replacing them with more affirmative alternative narratives and identities. It is a restorative justice process of moving away from fixed and essentialized identities and character traits, toward more fluid, relational, and social constructivist characteristics.

This work has had a lasting and continuing effect on students, as can be seen in 2018 when a group of students I worked with (who will speak in their own voice later in the chapter) decided to establish their own performance ensemble after the semester was over, calling it *Ubuntu Ensemble*, named after the restorative justice initiatives in South Africa after the demise of apartheid.

The overarching work, even when I insisted that they study textbooks and take multiple choice exams, involved creating a process that would invite insider knowledge (sometimes silenced) to come forth and to empower them with skills to make that insider knowledge more visible. As a result, students, time and again, chose to perform works from their repertoire when informed that they would be receiving visitors, be they media journalists or university trustees. These audiences came away deeply touched by performances they witnessed. Using a Narradrama model within the course, we sought to follow the following steps although not necessarily sequentially, nor as a hierarchical structure.

Step One: Writing prompts sought to discover new descriptions of self-identity. By rearranging the classroom space, we encouraged the creation of a preferred physical layout to change the environment. For example, we moved the tables to the side of the room and set up the chairs in a circle. This first step included a search to discover strengths, preferences, and support structures. For example, students shared their goals and visions for completing a bachelor's degree in communication. Next, we explored where students may experience themselves trapped in negative descriptions of their own identity or where they felt they were being silenced. I encouraged them to talk about where they may feel powerless and locked into a repetitive problem-saturated story, or when they may feel held back by cultural restraints. Students spoke in detail about the "obsessive ritualization of everyday life," as one student put it. Much later in the process as we delved into early childhood traumas, one student shared the following scene of his current persona going back with his childhood self to revisit a kindergarten experience:

> *Student/Actor*: This note says you can't read. Make sure your mom sees it so we can have a meeting.
>
> (The other student holds a picture of his childhood self):
>
> Dear Little Dean, today our kindergarten teacher thought something was wrong with us, because we won't read or talk in class. It's okay Little Dean, we're fine. I'll tell them that Dad died and you don't understand what that means. I'll explain to them that you found him overdosed and you're still scared.
>
> (From a drama therapy performance titled "A Fresh Start" drafted in 2018.)

Exercises like these were also followed by explorations of preferred and safe environments, descriptions of identities, and the loosening of restraints that may provide them with a foundation for future growth. Class exercises used role play and props to create a preferred environment and discover preferred self and identity as demonstrated in the above skit.

Step Two: Externalize and map the influence of *the problem.* The goal is to help experience a loosening of the problem's grip as well as to expose its effects. Sometimes this can be done by creating an external representation of *the internalized problem*. We use objects, sculptures, drawings, puppets, or masks to enact scenes with the problem. We also explore different relationships to help us remember that problem identities are not necessarily *essential* or *fixed*.

Step Three: Is to search for alternative stories and pivotal moments. Pivotal moments can be defined as turning points, moments when someone can perceive the possibility of a new life after their trauma (Gonzalez & Bosch, 2014). These stories help reveal personal strengths; they are descriptions of identity that provide hope to attain their preferred selves. Alternative stories may focus on what White (2007) called *unique outcomes*, moments when one can experience an identity change, or feel the healing of a relationship, or a moment of spiritual transformation, a possibility in the process of happening (p. 232). Class exercises may begin with objects, symbols, or art, which are further expanded into a scene (a story, poem, sculpture, or enacted song). Centered on pivotal moments, another exercise may ask students to remember and enact conversations from significant persons in their history. Here is a scene from a performance "Imagine That" drafted in 2018 where students reflected on watching a short documentary about one of their cohort and his daughter, both supporting each other to meet the challenges of being a college student:

> *One Student* (speaking about another student he has known in prison for nearly 25 years): What stood out to me was the change within him. Not the change from a teen to a forty-year-old adult, but the entire transformation he's undergone as a person, and his ability to allow that to come across through his words and actions. Knowing him, I feel conflicting emotions . . . happy to see the joy and pride he displays(s) when speaking about his daughter. . . . Saddened to reflect upon the thought that without a change in his sentence, he may never be free again.

Step Four: Work with alternative stories to expand personal agency and honor strengths and preferences. Class exercises may include creating monologues and creating masks. It is important to note that this is a process, and not everyone is ready to dive into a creative (but also vulnerable) frame of mind essential to this sort of exercise. However, having one or two willing students can have a remarkable effect on the others who may be skeptical about the role of play inside a classroom. As one student wrote in his reflections:

> Some of the friends in the cohort facilitated self-help programs on this yard. It was there that I again witnessed the effect of these drama therapy exercises: individuals who before had been reluctant to participate, were now offering valuable insights. . . . It pains me when I hear from my loved ones, knowing that they are suffering; but now, when I write them back, I feel empowered, I have a sense of purpose.

Other alternatives can include asking students to choose a moment when they made a decision they liked, or acted in a way that they preferred, or were able to access inner wisdom. To help them recall and report such a moment, they are given the option to express themselves in the frame of a reporter, or an art gallery curator, or a choreographer.

Step Five: Next is to work with students to externalize choices. We ask and explore what would be the effects of continuing with a current problem in the same trajectory. Students will then be asked to create a *double description*, a technique that compares the present course with a possible changing course. The student is asked to highlight how a problem or constraint is currently affecting their life, and then to decide on which path to take.

Enactments in the class may take the form of an imagined journey. Some students choose to create a storyboard like a comic book. This exercise also lends itself to intersectional identities which will be discussed in the next section. Other students may also join the scene in auxiliary roles that aid the protagonist or create obstacles.

Step Six: Another important step in the process is to clarify and prioritize values that may conflict with each other. During the discussions, we ask if the alternative stories reveal some taken-for-granted assumptions about norms that may cause one sadness, anxiety, or pain. How can we make preferred values more visible? We ask how can we revisit, uncover, honor, explore, and expand values that are important to us. We question how to align our ethical and moral values with personal, social, and cultural norms, especially those prevalent inside prison cultures. How can we call out practices that contradict or match our values? In addition to writing reflections, students also create *personal value collages* with drawings and objects, such as a social atom exercise that visualizes connections and relationships.

One student created a reenactment of Shakespeare's *Henry V*, act 4, scene 3, to promote their newfound identity as scholars, *as a family*. Here is a short-selected passage:

> (speaker moves back to center stage)
> Are we not family? Do we not share a collective identity? Each of us comes from disparate lands of origin and backgrounds, but do we not all bear the same identity? For certain, I speak not of the identity which has been ascribed to us, but of that identity we chose for ourselves: as scholars in pursuit of learning. Is this, then, not our collective identity? Do we not together soar like eagles, borne aloft by the wings of knowledge?
> Are we not family?

Step Seven: From there we move into expanding *possibility extensions* of personal strengths, choices, and values. This step often includes an exercise to create some distancing, and to move from a fixed viewpoint to a multistoried perspective. One class exercise has students develop and enact a dialogue with a tree, or a mythological story about a tree, then ask a series of narrative questions of the tree.

Step Eight: Is called *restory-ing* life story. Restorying is a culminating, rewarding process for participants as they assume the role of the author/director of their life story, some examples of which I cited earlier in this chapter.

Finally, in *Step Nine*, we take time to reflect and celebrate. This step is crucial to integrate, honor, and reflect on discoveries through rituals, witnessing, and other creative methods. Closures may involve rituals, drawings, letters, culminating dances, songs, murals, or other appropriate activities. At the conclusion of the work, it is important that the participant experience a culmination and celebration. Some examples are to write and/or create one-minute performances of appreciation letters to one or more of the group members. Another example is to note and reflect on a strength, new development, or special moment that they witnessed. If one wrote a letter, it is read out loud in pairs and then to the whole group. One-minute performances of letters also honor the participant and provide a closure for the process. Here is how one student reflected on the process:

> For me it was something beyond the romanticist idea of art . . . or as a refuge from alienation. Narradrama demonstrates that art can also be used to heal and make the world a better place.

Here are samples of student reflections about the ceremony where they performed "Imagine That" and "A Fresh Start":

> I must admit with each rehearsal and each story . . . simply overwhelmed my heart, bringing tears to these old Indian eyes. Each of us . . . bravely mustered internal fortitude to perform while reliving these painful events for those in attendance and for those who believe in our redemption. The plays [remind us of what it is] to be human again, contributing to society, through one's life experiences and a degree in communication studies.

> These skits were very emotional to me. I held back tears. . . . Being sentenced to Life Without the possibility of Parole is a sentence that signifies a person has no value, and will die in prison. Yet, we are staying focused on education, and pro-social activities to be the best image of ourselves.

> As the rehearsal process began, I had a feeling it would change lives. Changing lives is a primary mission of this program. . . . My own songwriting process (for "A Fresh Start") was unlike any time before. The music came to me, fueled by the moving performances and intuitive scriptwriting, as if it were composing itself.

> As we began performing this play my heart filled with joy, sorrow, and grief because I knew everything, I was experiencing at this moment made me human. . . . When thinking about education in prison it's not just a good grade, it has become life changing and empowering to remove our defects of character. Developing not only knowledge but also emotional intelligence something we lacked as individuals.

WHY AN INTERSECTIONAL AND ECOLOGICAL APPROACH

Both drama therapy and performance studies approaches involve an orientation that creates space and time for student responses and actions to explore *problem-saturated stories* and move toward *preferred* experiences. For this work to succeed in a classroom, we must encourage a playful sense of flow that is both relaxed and reflective. Although I show passion and excitement in my voice and demeanor, I proceed in a calm and welcoming way to help students activate their body's social engagement system at the same time that they stabilize their emotions. It is important to reduce the power differential between an instructor and the student. I encourage collaboration, and hold back the identity of the instructor as *the expert* in all matters in communication studies, and allow students to take the lead in presenting the material in a way that resonates with their own expertise and experience. There are times when there are setbacks, and both I and the students fall back into old patterns and forget to practice these strategies we have developed to move our lives in the direction that we desire. Over time we have developed a collaborative approach to remind each other with warmup exercises and role play activities to help get back on track. Some examples: standing in a circle playing a tag game with the words "zip, zap, zop," or mirroring each other's movements (both direct and in reverse), or counting rapidly from ten to one while moving our limbs, or improvising an imaginary scene with each person saying, "yes, and . . ." and extending the last person's claims no matter how outlandish! After three years of working with the same cohort, it is entirely possible that students can create a detailed enactment, including role assignments, staging, dialogue, and more in just ten to fifteen minutes.

In general, Narradrama's emphasis on unmasking *problem-saturated stories* that define a person's identity allows an instructor to be more proactive in encouraging students to explore the social construction of identities such as race, gender, sexuality, class, age, ethnicity, and religion. In this way, instructors become advocates for social change in providing more equitable community resources for marginalized and oppressed populations. Students who are trained to practice Narradrama engage in theoretical studies and performance activities with two paradigms that have gained prominence in contemporary social justice discourses: an ecological approach and an intersectional approach.

Intersectionality, mostly associated with the work of critical race theorist Kimberlé Williams Crenshaw (2007; 2016), addresses how people experience their identities erased as a result of being located at the intersection of two or more social systems of inequality (for example, racism and gender discrimination, or heterosexism and ageism, or class discrimination and ableism). In Narradrama classroom exercises, the instructor may ask the students to write down reflections on this erasure and then to create an *intersectional-*

ity ellipse drawing which shows an image of the experience of erasure. Small groups of students may also create a sculpture of points of intersection and give voice and shape to the intersections through interviewing, or an exercise called *doubling.*

The ecological model of development takes into account the cultural institutions and social policies that shape student-prisoners' interactions. In exploring an ecological-intersectional approach, I may ask students to identify, challenge, or resist different forms of power, privilege, and oppression they encounter. I may ask them to do a short reflection or to draw a dramatic arc using the form of a comic strip. The process begins with envisioning a protagonist who confronts a challenge or an antagonist. The protagonist may also call on other powers for help and support. Then I ask them to draw a climactic moment of dramatic resolution and the aftermath. Students will then share these images with each other as they explore patterns and common themes of their drawing. These then are developed into scenes that express their resolve to strengthen their voice and clarify their values and beliefs.

Narradrama exercises help participants to explore their identities, express those dimensions they feel may have been erased, and to create space to embody more fluid identities to which they can aspire. For example, during a discussion of the role of caregivers in health communication, students noted that lay caregivers are only identified as family members in the textbook. However, many of them shared experiences of being caregivers to each other but not recognized as such. Students then developed new scenes and enacted roles that highlighted this new identity that had been erased from their narratives for a lack of recognition. These reflective and witnessing processes, such as telling and retelling, and one-minute performance reflections, help both the instructor and the student to discern new perceptions of role.

Narradrama exercises help participants pay special attention in the interventions that develop to address the following areas:

Advocacy: In deconstructing power and the abuses of power, participants begin to recognize abuses that may be revealed through *power stories*, or through art, poetry, or sculpting. Participants create scenes, dialogues, and roles to confront the abuses. The exercise supports students to see themselves as advocates and to reinforce and strengthen their personal agency.

Diversity: Narradrama exercises help participants develop a more fluid sense of our identities and differences through externalizing fixed *problem-saturated identities* and creating a safe space to explore differences and build inclusive community.

Macroaggressions and Microaggressions: Narradrama exercises reveal how students may be the target of large-scale overt or subtle acts of aggression and disrespect directed toward those of a different race, culture, gender, religion, or sociocultural identity. Using playback and restorying techniques can help to create alternatives to these subtle and indirect discriminatory behaviors.

Resilience: Narradrama exercises such as *enacting possibility stories* and *self-identity change stories* can empower students with individual and contextual skills and abilities to overcome challenges. In these stories, participants recognize and honor their character traits, strengths, personal and cultural values and agency.

Preferred Self-definitions: Narradrama exercises can include *identity masks*, *embodied shields*, monologues, and interviews that allow students to practice and confirm their preferred identities and to move away from internalized oppressive self-definitions and descriptions based on stereotypes and prejudice, as they gain a sense of agency and control.

Social justice: In our exercises, social justice is both a process and a goal. Students work collaboratively to meet and define their needs through free-writing about relevant topics and creating performances that they then reflect on. This process is motivated by a vision of a society in which resources are equitably distributed, humans are not caged, and people are physically and psychologically safe. Restorative justice exercises may include the enactment of three images, beginning with an externalized social problem, followed by the image of a desired ideal solution, and ending with the image of a pathway to get from the problem to the solution.

For example, in one class exercise, a student recounted a traumatic experience with medical staff in excruciating detail. He described how, while shackled and in the presence of a large number of prison staff, he was told to undress and was then administered a painful procedure which involved inserting a device through his urethra into his bladder, without any pain medication. The doctor would not speak to him until late in the process, and then only to tell him to watch the video monitor. After the student completed the story, we embarked on a process of reenacting the scene, once as it actually happened, and a second time as it would happen in an ideal and just society using a textbook technique called the Teachback Method (Harrington, 2015, p. 95), in which medical providers respectfully explain and obtain consent for a procedure and ensure that the patient can explain the procedure in their own words). Students then shared examples of how after the class, they can use this in future encounters. Students expressed a sense of empowerment that they now had better skills to ask for better treatment from medical staff.

CONCLUSION

In this chapter I developed a framework to discuss what an intersectional Narradrama approach may look like. This framework in turn informs how narrative exercises and improvisations can be of help for prisoners to study interpersonal communication while building resiliency skills and social justice awareness. This work can result in participants being more present for situations that call for clarification of identities and critique of normative gender roles, particularly toxic masculinity. By combining Narradrama with teaching courses in communication studies, by using play and personal narratives, students engage in the practice of deep listening and authentic expression and gain a deeper understanding of theory not only to remember and apply course concepts, but to analyze and evaluate cultural norms that shape and reshape their identities. As a result of this work, students also gain some agency to create alternative narratives and preferred identities free from dominant pathologizing discourses. Integrating communication studies concepts and performance modalities can be a form of prison activism for empowered citizenship, and provides avenues of enlightenment and empowerment while offering powerful arguments for abolishing the dehumanizing environments created by mass incarceration and the prison industrial complex.

NOTES

1. I would like to thank and recognize the following individuals for their support, feedback, and contributions to this work: Brad Arrowood, Charlie Praphatananda, Elizabeth Malone, Janet Afary, Jeff Stein, Lee Gibson, Lena Afary, Lisa Marguerite Mora, Marianne Fritz, Pam Dunne, Sam Brawand, and Samantha J. Doran.

2. It was pioneered with the teaching of professor Bidhan Roy (2017) who has since expanded this work with the creation of Words Uncaged, a comprehensive collective effort by prisoners, family members, and community activists. Working with Words Uncaged, the Lancaster student cohort have published writings and art work that explores "how pain and trauma lead to incarceration, and how love and meaningful reflection lead to healing" (Williams et al., 2018). The Cal State LA initiative has been sustained through the directorship of Taffany Lim and the Center for Engagement, Service, and the Public Good, with the encouragement of president William Covino, and participation of faculty and administrators working to create a learning community inside prisons to both enlighten and empower, as a form of activism for engaged citizenship. During this process the university needed to create a department infrastructure, train instructors, develop sustainable funding, design courses to meet the needs of prisoners, and develop collaboration between campus and prison students. This is where the Department of Communication Studies, and its chair, Dr. David Olsen, along with the department faculty—Dr. Angela Cooke-Jackson, Dr. Nina F. O'Brien, Dr. Kamran Afary, Dr. Cynthia Wang, Dr. Gregory J. Langner, Dr. Mu Wu, Prof. Sarah Black, Prof. Tina Leisner-McDermott, Prof. Frances Chee, and Prof. Oscar Mejia—became central to this process.

3. In teaching courses on rhetorical criticism, I have also benefitted greatly from studying John M. Sloop's (1996) book titled *The cultural prison: Discourse, prisoners, and punishment* (Tuscaloosa, AL: University of Alabama Press), which provides a critical analysis of over 600 magazine articles over four decades, spanning from the 1950s to the 1990s, that document the trajectory of institutionalizing a deeper inwardization and normalizing of harsh physical incarceration, psychological repression, and punishment in the United Sates.

4. Daccache (2016) chronicles in detail how her 2012 documentary film *Scheherazade's Diary*, in Baabda Prison, featuring stories by women prisoners was influential in ratifying new legislation on domestic violence in Lebanon.

5. This section is based on a chapter that I coauthored with Pam Dunne and Pam Paulson (see Afary, Dunne, & Paulson, 2020).

6. See Julie Tilsen and David Nylund (2009) for a detailed discussion of how narrative therapy research can be contextualized within a critical cultural studies approach. Also see Julie Tilsen (2018) for narrative approach to youth work can be informed by queer theory.

REFERENCES

Afary, K. (2009). *Performance and activism: Grassroots discourse after the Los Angeles Rebellion of 1992*. Lanham, MD: Lexington Books.

Afary, K., Chee, F., & Dechaine, R. (Eds.). (2017). *Selected writings by communication studies majors at California state prison*. Los Angeles County, City of Lancaster. *Colloquy, 13*, 105–158.

Afary, K., Dunne, P., & Paulson, P. (2020). Narradrama: A narrative approach to drama therapy. In D. R. Johnson & R. Emunah (Eds.), *Current approaches in drama therapy* (3rd ed.). Springfield, IL: Charles C. Thomas.

Alexander, M. (2010). *The new Jim Crow: Mass incarceration in the age of colorblindness*. New York, NY: New Press.

American Psychological Association (APA). (2018). APA guidelines for psychological practice with boys and men. Retrieved from https://www.apa.org/about/policy/boys-men-practice-guidelines.pdf

Arrowood, B. (2017). Communicating comfort and support. *Colloquy, 13*, 109.

Baim, C. (2007). Drama in prisons. In A. Blatner & D. J. Weiner (Eds.), *Interactive and improvisational drama: Varieties of applied theatre and performance* (pp. 205–216). Lincoln, NE: iUniverse.

Behan, C. (2014). Learning to escape: Prison education, rehabilitation and the potential for transformation. *Journal of Prison Education and Reentry, 1*(1), 20–31. http://dx.doi.org/10.15845/jper.v1i1.594

Bergman, J. (2019, December 3). Drama therapy in prisons. YouTube video. 41:08. Retrieved from https://www.youtube.com/watch?v=QOMqllBfUx0

Bloom, B. (1956). *Taxonomy of educational objectives: The classification of educational goals*. New York, NY: Longman.

Bumiller, K. (2013). Transformative learning in prison and universities: Reflections on homologies of institutional power. In S. Davis & B. Roswell (Eds.), *Turning teaching inside out: A pedagogy of transformation for community-based education* (pp. 177–186). New York, NY: Palgrave Macmillan.

Burke, K. (2018). *The philosophy of literary form: Studies in symbolic action*. London: Forgotten Books.

Clements, P. (2004). The rehabilitative role of arts education in prison: Accommodation or enlightenment? *International Journal of Art & Design Education* (*JADE*), *23*(2), 169–178.

Conquergood, D. (2013). Lethal theatre: performance, punishment, and the death penalty. In E. P. Johnson (Ed.), *Cultural struggles: Performance, ethnography, parxis* (pp. 264–302). Ann Arbor, MI: University of Michigan Press.

Conrad, D. (2008). Performance ethnography. In L. Given (Ed.), *The Sage encyclopedia of qualitative research methods* (pp. 607–611). Thousand Oaks, CA: Sage.

Coogan, D. (2013). Writing your way to freedom: Autobiography as inquiry in prison writing workshops. In S. J. Harnett, E. Novek, & J. K. Wood (Eds.), *Working for justice: A handbook of prison education and activism* (pp. 60–82). Champaign, IL: University of Illinois Press.

Crenshaw, K. W. (2007). Mapping the margins: Intersectionality, identity politics and violence against women of color. In A. Bailey and C. Cuomo (Eds.), *The feminist philosophy reader* (pp. 279–309). New York, NY: McGraw-Hill.

Crenshaw, K. W. (2016, December 7). The urgency of intersectionality (TedTalk). YouTube. 2:08. Retrieved from https://www.youtube.com/watch?v=akOe5–UsQ2o

D'Orio, W. (2019, July 12). No girls, parties, cellphones: California's prison inmates are getting bachelor's degrees. Prison Education Programs. *Hechinger Report. USA Today*.

Retrieved from https://www.usatoday.com/story/news/education/2019/07/12/prison-reform-california-inmate-felon-clemency-pell-grant/1707006001/

Daccache, Z. (2016). The unheard stories of those forgotten behind bars in Lebanon. In S. Pendzik, R. Emunah, & D. Read Johnson (Eds.), *The self in performance: Autobiographical, Self-Revelatory, and Autoethnographic Forms of Therapeutic Theatre* (pp. 227–240). New York, NY: Palgrave Macmillan.

Daccache, Z. (2019). Drama therapy in prisons. YouTube video. 21:26. Retrieved from https://www.youtube.com/watch?v=6LikqZtmpsw

Davidson, H. S. (1995). Possibilities for critical pedagogy in a "total institution": An introduction. In H. S. Davidson (Ed.), *Schooling in a "total institution": Critical perspectives on prison education* (pp. 1–23). Westport, CT: Bergin & Garvey.

Davis, S. W. (2013). Inside out: The reach and limits of a prison education program. In S. Davis & B. Roswell (Eds.), *Turning teaching inside out: A pedagogy of transformation for community-based education* (pp. 165–175). New York, NY: Palgrave Macmillan.

Deal, C. E. (2014). Acting for social justice: Students, prisoners, and theatre of testimony performance. In L. R. Frey & D. L. Palmer (Eds.), *Teaching communication activism: Communication education for social justice* (pp. 435–460). New York, NY: Hampton Press.

Denzin, N. K. (2017). A manifesto for performance autoethnography. *International Review of Qualitative Research, 10*(1), 44–45.

diZerega, M. (2017). College in prison: Post-secondary education opportunities for incarcerated people. *Vera Institute of Justice.* Retrieved from https://www.vera.org/projects/college-in-prison

Dowdell, J. J. (2015, August 4). Pell grants for prisoners: Good for them, and for everyone else. *Chronicle of Higher Education.* Retrieved from http://www.chronicle.com/article/Pell-Grants-for-Prisoners-/232153?cid=megamenu

Dunne, P. (2016). Restoried Script Performance. In S. Pendzick, D. R. Johnson, & R. Emunah (Eds.), *The self in performance: Autobiographical, Self-Revelatory, and Autoethnographic Forms of Therapeutic Theatre* (pp. 141–154). New York, NY: Palgrave Macmillan.

Fennessey, S. M. (2000). *History in the spotlight: Creative drama and theatre practices for the social studies classroom*. Portsmouth, NH: Heinemann.

Fischer-Lichte, E. (2008). *The transformative power of performances: A new aesthetics*. (S. I. Jain, Trans.). New York, NY: Routledge.

Foucault, M. (1977). *Discipline and punish: The birth of the prison*. (A. Sheridan, Trans.). New York, NY: Random House. (Original work published 1975)

Foucault, M. (1990). *The history of sexuality: An introduction.* New York, NY: Vintage Books.

Freire, P. (1970). *Pedagogy of the oppressed*. (M. Bergman Ramos, Trans.). London and New York, NY: Continuum International Publishing.

Gaskew, T. (2015). Developing a prison education pedagogy. *New Directions for Community Colleges*, 170, 67–78. https://doi.org/10.1002/cc.20145

Germain, S. (2014). Prison-based education and its new pedagogical perspective. *Journal of Criminal Justice Education*, *25*(2), 196–209. https://doi.org/10.1080/10511253.2014.882962

Gibson, C. L. (2017). Poem. *Colloquy*, *13*, 108.

Goldberg, J. (2015). Pedagogy for the incarcerated: Augmenting the Socratic method in inmate rehabilitation. *Scholars' Day Review*, *3*, 35–41.

Gonzalez, T., & Bosch, J. (2014) Pivotal moments: Recognizing and embracing life-changing turning points. *Phoenix Society's Burn Support Magazine*, *3*. Retrieved from https://www.phoenix-society.org/resources/entry/pivotal-moments-recognizing-and-embracing-life-changing-turning-points

Gregoric-Cook, L. (2019, December 3). Drama therapy in prisons. YouTube video. 58:20. Retrieved from https://www.youtube.com/watch?v=8tCWCRTg1uw

Hamera, J. (2011). Performance ethnography. In N. K. Denzin & Y. S. Lincoln (Eds.), *The Sage Handbook of Qualitative Research* (pp. 359–376). Los Angeles, CA: Sage.

Harrington, N. G. (2015) *Health communication: theory, method, and application*. London: Routledge.

Hartnett, S. J., Novek, E., & Wood, J. K. (Eds.). (2013). *Working for justice: A handbook of prison education and activism*. Champaign, IL: University of Illinois Press.

Hartnett, S. J., Wood, J., & McCann, B. J. (2011). Turning silence into speech and action: Prison activism and the pedagogy of empowered citizenship. *Communication and Critical/Cultural Studies*, *8*(4), 331–352. https://doi.org/10.1080/14791420.2011.615334

Higgins, J. (2007). Sharing sociological stories: reflections on teaching sociology in prison. *International Journal of Lifelong Education*, *23*(3), 243–257. https://doi.org/10.1080/0260137042000184192

Hook, C., & Geist-Martin, P. (2018). Cultivating communities of care: A qualitative investigation of the communication of support among incarcerated woman. *Communication and Critical/Cultural Studies, 15*(2), 127–143. Retrieved from https://doi.org/10.1080/14791420.2018.1433308

Howes, L. (2017). *The mask of masculinity: How men can embrace vulnerability, create strong relationships, and live their fullest lives*. New York, NY: Random House.

Huizinga, J. (2014). *Homo Ludens: A study of the play-element in culture*. Eastford, CT: Martino Fine Books.

Jung, C. J. (1991). *The archetypes and the collective unconscious*. London: Routledge.

Keating, S. (2019). Drama therapy in prisons. Retrieved from https://www.youtube.com/watch?v=MCkSs2YHBKM

Kilgore, J. (2011). Bringing Freire behind the walls: The perils and pluses of critical pedagogy in prison education. *Radical Teacher*, *90*, 57–66. https://doi.org/10.5406/radicalteacher.90.0057

Lawston, J., & Jones, G. (2011, December 1). Critical pedagogy in prisons? A Brief Reflective Essay. *Razor Wire Women*. Retrieved from https://razorwirewomen.wordpress.com/2011/12/01/critical-pedagogy-in-prisons-a-brief-reflective-essay-by-jodie-lawston-and-gabriel-jones/

MacDonald, T., & Williams, D. (2019). *Striving for redemption*. Oakland, CA: East Oakland Times, LLC.

Madison, D. S. (2018). *Performed Ethnography & Communication: Improvisation and Embodied Experience*. New York: Routledge.

Malone, E. (2019). Scenes from the inside: Drama therapy in a maximum security prison. *Shalom: A Journal for the Practice of Reconciliation*, *39*(1), 6. http://www.canadianbic.ca/wp-content/uploads/2019/03/shalom-winter2019.pdf

McCann, B. J. (2019). Live, virtual, and spectral: Being present at the prison (tour). *Text and Performance Quarterly*, *39*(2), 95–115. https://doi.org/10.1080/10462937.2019.1598570

Meiners, E. R. (2009). Resisting civil death: Organizing for access to education in our prison. *DePaul Journal for Social Justice*, *3*(1), 79–95. https://via.library.depaul.edu/jsj/vol3/iss1/5

Paraphatananda, C. (2017). Forming social bonds, reflecting on our identities. *Colloquy*, 13, 12–133.

Platt, T. (2018). *Beyond these walls: Rethinking crime and punishment in the United States* (1st ed.). New York, NY: St Martin's Press.

Prison Communication, Research, and Education (PCARE). (2007). Fighting the prison–industrial complex: A call to communication and cultural studies scholars to change the world. *Communication and Critical/Cultural Studies, 4*(4), 402–420. http://dx.doi.org/10.1080/14791420701632956

Rafay, A. (2013). An "impossible profession"? The radical university in prison. *Radical Teacher*, *95*, 10–21. https://www.muse.jhu.edu/article/523327

Rohd, M. (1998). *Theatre for community, conflict & dialogue: The hope is vital training manual*. Portsmouth, NH: Heinemann.

Roy, B. C. (2017). Human words uncaged. *Words Uncaged 1*(1), 1–55. Retrieved from http://www.wordsuncaged.com/uploads/9/6/6/5/96657258/human-book-pages-final.pdf

Sanford, R., & Foster, J. E. (2006). Reading, writing, and prison education reform? The tricky and political process of establishing college programs for prisoners: Perspectives from program developers. *Equal Opportunities International*, *25*(7), 599–610. https://doi.org/10.1108/02610150610714411

Shailor, J. (2013). Kings, warriors, magicians, and lovers: Prison theatre and alternative performances of masculinity. In S. J. Harnett, E. Novek, & J. K. Wood (Eds.), *Working for justice: A handbook of prison education and activism* (pp. 13–38). Champaign, IL: University of Illinois Press.

Sloop, J. M. (1996). *The cultural prison: Discourse, prisoners, and punishment.* Tuscaloosa, AL: University of Alabama Press.

Solomon, D., & Theiss, J. (2013). *Interpersonal communication: Putting theory into practice.* New York, NY: Routledge.

Stein, J. (2017). Internalizing communication ethics. *Colloquy, 13*, 114.

Sternberg, P. (1998). *Theatre for conflict resolution: In the classroom and beyond.* (L. A. Barnett, Ed.). Portsmouth, NH: Heinemann.

Thomas, J. (1995). The ironies of prison education. In H. S. Davidson (Ed.), *Schooling in a "total institution": Critical perspectives on prison education* (pp. 25–41). Westport, CT: Bergin & Garvey.

Tilsen, J. (2018). *Narrative approaches to youth work: Conversational skills for a critical practice*. (1st ed.). New York, NY: Routledge.

Tilsen, J., & Nylund D. (2009). Popular culture texts and young people: Making meaning, honoring resistance, and becoming Harry Potter. *International Journal of Narrative Therapy and Community Work, 2*(1). http://2stories.com/wp-content/uploads/2011/02/2009–2–Popular-Culture-pages.pdf

Torre, M. E., & Fine, M. (2005). Bar none: Extending affirmative action to higher education in prison. *Journal of Social Issues, 61*(3), 569–594. https://doi.org/10.1111/j.1540–4560.2005.00421.x

Trounstine, J. (2008). Beyond prison education. *PMLA, 123*(3), 674–677. https://www.jstor.org/stable/25501886

Turner, V. (1982). *From ritual to theatre: The human seriousness of play*. Baltimore: PAJ Publications.

Volkas, A. (2016). Autobiographical therapeutic performance as individual therapy. In S. Pendzik, R. Emunah, & D. Read Johnson (Eds.), *The self in performance: Autobiographical, Self-Revelatory, and Autoethnographic Forms of Therapeutic Theatre* (pp. 113–128). New York, NY: Palgrave Macmillan.

White, M. (2007). *Maps of narrative practice.* New York: W.W. Norton & Co.

Wichmann, S. (2019, December 3). Drama therapy in prisons. YouTube video. 16:28. Retrieved from https://www.youtube.com/watch?v=SxbLVmnRr_Q

Widdoes, A. (2016). What prison reform looks like inside California State Prison, L.A. county. *KCET.org*. Retrieved from https://www.kcet.org/shows/departures/what-prison-reform-looks-like-inside-california-state-prison-la-county

Williams, D., Hong, J., Whitlow, D., Burnett, A., Martinez, D., Gibson, C., et al. (Eds.). (2018). *Disconnected/Reconnected: Writing from Lancaster prison.* (2nd ed.). New York: Words Uncaged.

Williams, E. (2019, December 3). Drama therapy in prisons. YouTube video. 33:43. Retrieved from https://www.youtube.com/watch?v=yo6gN4ob0As

Wright, R. (2014). Identities, education and reentry: Performative spaces and enclosures. *Journal of Prison Education & Reentry, 1*(1), 32–41. http://dx.doi.org/10.15845/jper.v1i1.609

Zoukis, C. (2014). *College for convicts: The case for higher education in American prisons*. Jefferson, NC: McFarland.

Chapter Two

More Than Human

Mady Schutzman

In speaking of expressive arts and their therapeutic potential, we may well start by describing aesthetic space. Aesthetic space is a terrain in which fiction and reality not only coexist but also cannot easily be distinguished. Broadly speaking, it is the space of play, a magical and yet common realm of experience. Gregory Bateson (1972), English anthropologist and linguist, declares in his *Steps to an Ecology of Mind* that "human beings have evolved the metaphor that is meant" (p. 183); that is, we grant, in what he calls a primary process, a truth function to representation. He goes on to speak of secondary processes of the mind by which people discriminate between the two (truth and representation), and then of a third-order function of play in which we equate and discriminate at once (p. 185). In play, participants engage their representations *as if* they are real while knowing they are not. And as we know, play has healing effects.

Brazilian theatre director and social activist Augusto Boal (1995), in his book *The Rainbow of Desire: The Boal Method of Theatre and Therapy*, was referring to aesthetic space when he spoke of *metaxis*: "the state of belonging completely and simultaneously to two different, autonomous worlds: the image of reality and the reality of the image" (p. 43). Within aesthetic space an image, any created thing for that matter, has the potential to speak for itself. Ritual objects—objects infused with sacred meaning as a result of human beings' deliberate attention and devotion (nothing is *inherently* sacred)—are good examples. Within the space of a Catholic mass, wine becomes blood; its power lies in our acceptance that it *is* blood, even as we know it *is not*. Many objects, spaces, images, and beliefs maintain their autonomous power even when removed from aesthetic space. This is the case in every culture from the prehistorical to the present; we see it in the form of talismans, keepsakes, symbols, archetypes, and myths.

I was originally asked to contribute something to this anthology based on my work with the techniques and theories of Boal, known for the participatory techniques of Theatre of the Oppressed (TO). Having recently completed a book about Boal's Joker System, *Radical Doubt: The Joker System, after Boal* (Schutzman, 2019), I was excited to pursue some of the new directions that the research suggested. Through a somewhat circuitous route—instigated, in part, by a contemporaneous study of Hopi Kachinas—I came to focus on puppets. It is not that puppets, masks, and object theatre were new to me—as a student of anthropology I had long been immersed in the innumerable ways we animate the inanimate. And, of course, when speaking of theatre and acting more generally, we are speaking in large part about *animating* one's own body to appear as someone else's. The actor on stage dons an array of movements, speech patterns, attitudes, costumes, and a willingness to be *possessed* by another, the character. Of the many theatrical modes that Boal employed consistently, I have been particularly attracted to that of replacement or intervention, which was core to his dual agenda for social healing and political change. His techniques have a carnivalesque and Brechtian quality in which actors are frequently changing roles, deepening their understanding of a scene by becoming intimate with all positions across the ethical spectrum. One might say that Boal was encouraging us to multiply ourselves, to experience the enormity of our capacity to further dialogue, empathy, resistance, community building, and healing.

So why puppetry? Whereas in acting, the site of the possession remains the actor's body, in puppetry the site is *outside* the actor's body; the thing created does not have to negotiate the body of the creator. I was excited to ruminate on why puppets emerge in just about every culture. From ancient times right on up to *Sesame Street*, people have used wood and shadows (and everything in between) to conjure monsters and gods, endearing innocents and wily tricksters, to tell the messy truth about the human condition. Things once lifeless convey wonder and anxiety, possibility and constraint, freedom and control, grandeur and denigration, delight and embarrassment, loss and renewal. Whatever the (often incongruent) pairing may be, puppets capture a strangeness, an ambivalence that brings into the lives of performers and audiences something both human and more than human.

I have written this essay without formulating a singular thesis about puppets and would caution readers from looking for one. Rather than anchoring my various thoughts in argument or in evidence, I have borrowed from the approach of Austrian-British philosopher Ludwig Wittgenstein (1969). He writes as if flowing in a river of excess, grabbing the bits he can, naming places he has been and ideas he has considered, and then suddenly turning to other unformed burgeoning concepts. He was fond of styles that capture the detours, suspensions, reversals, and inconsistencies that drive all narratives. While I have not abandoned all gestures toward narrative coherence, I invite readers to entertain something more akin to montage and assemblage, and to participate in the play space of reading and comprehending.

MULTIPLY THE SELF

Inspired by Boal's methodology whereby each actor plays multiple characters within a scene, I began to consider other realms in which the notion of self-multiplication is operative and evocative. In the following section, expansion of self is discovered in an author's approach to voice, a form of Greek dramatic dialogue, the doppelgänger effect, and the practice of ventriloquism. Puppetry reveals itself as a viable means through which to correlate these diverse phenomena.

Fernando Pessoa

Fernando Pessoa (1888–1935) was a Portuguese writer, translator, and philosopher perhaps best known for *The Book of Disquiet*, a book he wrote under the name Bernardo Soares. It consists of a series of vignettes, running from one line to five pages each, with musings and maxims on literature, politics, loneliness, dreams, and psychology. It is, by design, an incomplete book of disjointed fragments with a drifting, inconsistent logic or voice. To me, it mirrors the clatter of voices that play out in my mind every day, voices without clear origins, faces, or regularity. Some are louder and more frequent than others, some offer pleasure and others pain. But I have learned over time that in spite of all my efforts, I have little if any jurisdiction over their opinions or conduct.

Pessoa experienced himself as having no personality, a man without recognizable qualities, a chaos of moods implausible to unify into a singular identity. "I have a whole world of friends inside me," he wrote, "each with his or her own real, defined and imperfect life" (Pessoa, 2001, p. 195). For Pessoa, madness was not the failure to make sense but the attempt itself. Instead of seeking his voice, he sought his *voices*. He wrote in seventy-eight different names that he called heteronyms. Pessoa became his own pandemonium, a cacophony of tongues, flirting and cajoling himself into a state of perpetual emergence. He wrote as if he was a medium.

In imagining oneself containing a multiplicity of selves, in allowing contradictions to coexist, Pessoa found infinite space to create. Sadness could exist alongside joy, pessimism alongside youthful idealism. Even self-destruction had a place: Pessoa did not take his own life, but a number of his heteronyms did! According to British psychoanalyst Adam Phillips (2001) in *Promises, Promises: Essays on Psychoanalysis and Literature*, Pessoa was "always at the point of disappearing from himself" (p. 118), and that is the way he liked it.

What excites me about Pessoa excites me about puppets. Puppets present the opportunity to elude the illusion of unity and consistency. Suddenly, there is an invitation to give voice to any number of repressed or desired identities, memories, fantasies, and aspects of ourselves that we harbor in shame or fear and do not know how to move from inside out. Sometimes it is not until we are asked to give a voice to a doll, a family relic, or a deceased beloved that we tap the sundry community of real and imagined entities that live within us.

In a May 17, 2019, interview on NPR, author Stephen McCauley tells listeners that his books are about everyday events, trivial stuff, no crises, no death or trauma, nothing even particularly dramatic. But several years ago, when asked to write under a pen name, to his surprise he found himself writing characters who jump out of windows, audition for Beyoncé videos, obsess over their bodies, break rules, and get into lots and lots of trouble. Under his pen name the worlds he created were unsettling, bizarre, and haunting . . . even to him.

Stichomythia

Alfred Francis Kreymborg (1883–1966) was an American poet, novelist, and playwright. In the early 1900s, at the beginnings of modern American drama, he, along with several others writers of his time, were moving away from realism and toward expressionism. Kreymborg's approach involved the use of an ancient form of Greek dialogue called *stichomythia* in which single lines of verse or parts of lines are spoken by alternate speakers. The sense of a unified character was disrupted and what was conjured instead was a chorus, a discordant and self-contradicting voice that belonged to everyone and no one in particular. He used this technique most notably in his puppet-inspired plays *Manikin and Minikin* (1918) and *Lima Beans* (1925). In *Manikin and Minikin*, two automatons experiencing agonizing paralysis rhythmically perform their love-hate relationship in the style of a musical duet. For *Lima Beans*, actors were asked to move like marionettes to highlight the play's abstraction, and stichomythia was employed to highlight the play's ritualistic function. In combination, human relationships were represented as a form of mystical mechanics that conjured a whole greater than the sum of its parts. A space more than human (Kreymborg, 1926).[1]

Doppelgängers

The word *doppelgänger* is German for "double walker," a shadow self that is thought to accompany every person. Traditionally, the doppelgänger was considered either a harbinger of death or a form of self-divination. Many well-known figures including French novelist Guy de Maupassant, German poet Johann Wolfgang von Goethe, and English poets John Donne and Percy Bysshe Shelley claim to have seen their doppelgängers (Little, 2017). Whatever suspicions these authors may have had about the boundaries of themselves—suspicions that inspired visions of a double inhabiting the same streets and breathing the same air as them—they are perhaps the same suspicions that inspire all representational art. The puppet, a material prosthetic voice, captures the human being as both a physical and an imagined thing. It seems to say: dear human being, you are an entity living always in the shadow of death, and yet when you die, you will not die absolutely. The puppet, like the doppelgänger, remains. I am reminded of a line in Philip Roth's (1995) novel, *Sabbath's Theater* in which the title character, a puppeteer, bemoans the loss of his first wife: "If Nikki had been a puppet, she might still be alive" (p. 245).

A Very Brief History of Ventriloquism

Before ventriloquism was a form of entertainment, it was a religious practice. Its origins go as far back as the Bible, Isaiah 29:4: "Then deep from the earth you shall speak, from low in the dust your words shall come; your voice shall come from the ground like the voice of a ghost, and your speech shall whisper out of the dust" (Barton, 2019, p. 103). The grumblings that emerged from the earth were signs of a deceased or heavenly presence, an elder or a god sending messages to the living. Even grumblings of the stomach were taken to have a similar source and the ventriloquist (*venter,* to speak + *loqi*, from the stomach)—the one hosting these indecipherable messages—would interpret them for others. Among the Greeks, the practice was called *gastromancy*. Ventriloquists were mediums, able to speak to the dead and foretell the future.

Eurycles, of fifth century B.C. Greece, was an Athenian prophet known to cast out evil spirits; he was also one of the most successful early gastromancers. His ability to throw his voice—to make it appear as if it originated from another source—greatly enhanced his credibility. (It is disturbing but interesting to note that in the Middle Ages, women who did this were thrown into dungeons and burned as witches.) By the nineteenth century, as spiritualism gave way to stage magic and escapology in Europe and the United States, ventriloquism lost its mystical trappings. But in other parts of the world—such as among the Zulu, Inuit, and Maori—ventriloquism continues to be used for religious and ritual purposes. In Maori country in New Zealand, for instance, the common Maori hen, or *weka*, produces a peculiar thumping or thwacking call that comes from anywhere except where the bird actually is; wekas throw their voice. Maori priests, healers, and navigators learned the art of ventriloquism from the Maori hen in order to deliver wise council to their people as if through the wafting voice of ancestral spirits. The practice goes on today. Among the Zulu, the practice is even part of everyday life. Frequently, after two natives meet, say on a country road, and exchange the usual niceties, they continue to speak to each other while walking away. Even at long distances they can still hear each other.

The Dummy Roundtable

In March 2018, I hosted a roundtable discussion with four ventriloquist dummies in Los Angeles. In attendance were Markey Doodles, Darlene Hollywood, Squeaker Kelly, and Roscoe (a.k.a. Wood from the Hood). I asked their accompanying ventriloquists to please remain silent during the conversation; that is, to not speak as themselves. We sat in a circle and talked for nearly two hours. I asked the dummies a number of questions about love, relationships, partnering, friends (imaginary and otherwise), fears, everyday preoccupations, and the current political climate. "What are your pastimes?" "Are you in a relationship right now?" "What makes you sad?" "Do you have any advice for me about love?"

Before parting ways, I posed one final question: "Where do you see yourself five years from now?" Markey Doodles, the youngest of the group, did not hesitate to answer: "I'd really like to be a person by then." I found it fascinating that Markey Doodles, like the Tin Man nearly eighty years earlier, longs for what humanity has to offer while we humans are every day converting ourselves into automata at furious rates. But on second thought, I realized that human beings and their doubles want similar things: to experience that fertile and ambivalent state that hovers between dead and alive, material and ethereal, passive and willful, real and dreamed. The more I study puppets, the more I find it instructive and healthy to consider people, objects, animals, and the natural and fabricated worlds as sharing some DNA and reflecting our assorted strengths and shortcomings back to each other in a porous feedback loop.

Red

When I left Los Angeles to do field research for this essay, I considered my home relatively puppetless and dummyless. I had a small collection of masks from Mexico and Bali, a handful of dolls (bought and homemade), and a large soft-sculpture frog that I made at a residency years ago. My travels took me to the U.S. southwest (where I saw thousands of Hopi and Zuni Kachina dolls) and Mexico City (to the Museo Nacional de Antropologia and its comprehensive array of prehistoric figurines). From Mexico City I traveled the canals of Xochimilco to visit La Isla de las Muñecas, or The Island of the Dolls. The island is full of decaying and broken figures—hanging from trees, floating in swamp grass, posted like sentries on fences—all gathered by

Xochimilco native Don Julian Barrera following the tragic drowning of a young girl on the surrounding lake sometime in the mid-twentieth century. Barrera considered The Island of the Dolls a tribute to dead children and a way to appease their spirits.

My final trip was to the University of British Columbia Museum of Anthropology in Vancouver to view an exhibit of puppets from around the world. When I returned home, there was a package waiting for me. Inside was a figure, accompanied by a letter:

Dear Ms. Schutzman,

Nice to meet you.

I was recently abandoned after a dispute with my former owner, which resulted in my jaw being broken. I was subsequently put up for sale and your "friend" purchased me—this was for a sum I found phenomenally insulting. I believe your "friend" intended me as some kind of gift, though I hope you can see how perverse this is.

There are a few things I feel I should make clear to ensure that our relationship does not sour. *Accommodations*: I prefer to sleep in a size-appropriate bed. You may have one custom made if you are unable to find an existing one. Please note that cribs, children's beds, and doll beds are not sufficient. Same situation with my chair—nothing infantilizing or intended for toys. When travelling with me I prefer to have my own seat. This applies to trains, planes, and automobiles. The fact that I have been sent in a cardboard box is perhaps the most demoralizing experience of my entire life and I have been around for a very long time. *Medical needs*: I will need a full medical examination to assess my present health condition. You will need to assume responsibility for all costs incurred and I require right of refusal for any doctor you choose. *Cohabitation*: I lead a solitary and somewhat monastic life. I prefer not to be spoken to and insist on not being touched outside of the necessary situations, i.e., bed to chair, chair to bed, transport, etc.

In conclusion, I think you will find that I am a pleasant, lovable, easy going, low maintenance, co-operative, and empathetic companion. I know that you will embrace my good nature and reciprocate my kindness.

I hope this works out,

Best,
Red

I recognized Red immediately as a Danny-O'Day ventriloquist figure, a replica of the *real* Danny-O'Day I grew up with on TV. I cannot explain how urgently I felt the need to take care of Red, to follow the dictates outlined in this letter. I felt a calling; something was at stake, but what? I dropped everything I was doing and searched the house, closets, garage, and then a small downstairs studio where I found an upholstered ottoman with matching pillow—the perfect bed! I dragged it upstairs immediately and placed it under a low window with a lovely view of the garden. Red's jaw flapped open with each handling, his mouth unleashing a rash of expletives. I placed a beautiful buckwheat-filled zafu on a wicker chair to make Red's special chair and moved it into the living room facing the piano. For the next few days, I moved him delicately from bed to chair, chair to bed, as instructed. Nothing else. We did not speak a word.

It was evident that I had accepted without reservation my role in Red's play exactly as he defined it. Actually, it was more as if I had been cast in a spell than a play. I was frantic to accommodate Red, his eyes always askance but his demands direct. The scribbled letter, the hard body, the floppy jaw were as captivating as they were comedic. Kenneth Gross (2011), author of *Puppet: An Essay on Uncanny Life*, writes that puppets serve as a means to repair a loss. What loss, I began to wonder, was Red repairing for me?

After a few days of searching unsuccessfully for dummy repair shops in Los Angeles, I turned to YouTube where I discovered a manic but knowledgeable twelve year old who knew how to doctor a Danny O'Day dummy jaw (a rather common disfunction, I learned). I listened and watched closely. To fix Red's jaw not only would I have to handle him against his explicit wishes, I would have to take his head off! For the forty minutes it took to follow the meandering instructions, I experienced physical angst (*Hurry up or Red will die on the operating table*). At the same time, in full accordance with Bateson's notion of third order play, I was well aware that inanimate objects endure (painlessly) all kinds of violence, decapitation included. (*Whatever you do and no matter how long it takes, Red is not suffering.)*

As it turned out, the whole surgical drama was a gift to me, a return to a childlike sensibility that had been long lost and now returned with a ferocious persistence. I knew I was a wiser person for it; in accepting unreason, I was restoring a part of myself.

The Universality of Puppets

Vietnamese water puppets, Wayang Kulit shadow puppets of Bali and Java, nesting dolls of Ukraine, voodoo dolls of the Caribbean, Tholu Bommalata leather puppets of Andhra Pradesh, Portugal's marionetas, the Budaixi puppets of China, Rukada string puppets of Sri Lanka, Guignol of France, Punch and Judy in the United Kingdom, ventriloquist dummies in England and the United States; the list is endless. There is not a culture on the face of the planet that does not indulge in some form of puppetry for purposes of entertainment, traditional storytelling, cultural preservation, religious orthodoxy, acts of resistance, communication with ancestors, and/or philosophical reflection on the mysteries of life and death. What is this human need, manifesting across the globe and through millennia, for a material thing, an object, to become a vehicle for the human voice?

By the time I arrived home from my travels, I understood that I had been living with hundreds of puppets, or rather puppets-in-waiting: previously neglected housemates, things that speak to me now (maybe they always had) in both faint and vivid voices and insinuate so many other places and people. Three smiling ceramic mice with hands raised above their heads. Two painted square cows standing with indignant stares in a meadow in Poland or Ukraine. A carved wooden head from Haiti. A little toy truck with chipped green paint unearthed in the Mojave desert. A Zuni badger, Oaxacan tiger, and Punjab rooster. My mother's wool coat that has been hanging in my closet since 2001.

It was so darn noisy when I got home!

EXERCISE

Make a puppet of:

- a fragile thing, something that isn't going to last much longer
- some part of yourself in need of resurrection
- a tattoo (already on your body, or one you want to get)
- a scar
- a place where you like to hide
- a perceived enemy
- something that always finds you, sticks to you like a leech, will not leave you alone
- a secret
- a deceased relative
- a problem (is it speechless? despondent? outraged? courageous? comical?)

TO BE *AND* NOT TO BE, THAT IS THE ANSWER!

The puppet is a translator between being and not-being. By way of our intimacies with various material things—particularly in lending our voices to what would otherwise be lifeless—human beings and things become inextricably linked. This is an opportunity, not a problem to be solved. But what kinds of opportunities are afforded us, and in what ways do they challenge us?

The Never Occluded Puppeteer

Bruce Schwartz worked extensively as a solo experimental puppeteer during the 1970s and 1980s, performing mostly in the United States but trained in Bunraku in Japan. In a 1983 interview with C. Lee Jenner, Schwartz was asked why he elects to remain visible when he performs with his puppets. He explains that this visibility—of his body and the mechanics of puppetry—stresses that the puppet is not alive, and yet his theory is that audiences will naturally shift their attention from him to something far more compelling—the puppet. He recognizes the paradox: "I'm asking people to come into my fantasies with me by cutting me out" (Schwartz, et al., 1983, p. 106).

Schwartz gets at something core to puppetry; that is, its magical capacity to bring into relief (and into question) the binary of mind and matter, play and display. The boundaries between these pairs are revealed to be false and recast as ever shifting, if not completely absent. Performers and audience are invited into a threshold space where we meet a limit or a contradiction that necessitates a new, more expansive way of thinking, whether we are fully aware of it or not.

The Bergen Family

Candice Bergen (1984), the daughter of the famous ventriloquist Edgar Bergen, writes in her autobiography *Knock Wood* that through most of her childhood she was jealous of Charlie McCarthy, her father's favorite dummy. Charlie went everywhere with them and got the lion's share of her father's attention both on and off the stage. But Candice was by no means excluded:

> My dad would sit [Charlie] on one knee and me on the other and he'd put a hand on both of our necks and when he squeezed my neck, I'd move my mouth, and when he squeezed Charlie's neck, he'd move his. As Charlie and I yammered away at each other across my father, mouths flapping soundlessly, behind us, smiling politely, sat my Dad, happily speaking for both of us. (Bergen, 1984, p. 17)

For all intents and purposes, Charlie and Candice were siblings with equal claims to Edgar's lap. On the one hand, through Edgar's voice, Charlie came to life (and often stole the show). On the other hand (or *knee*), Candice surrendered her voice to her father and gained, through some inexplicable alchemy, with Edgar as interlocutor, the voice of Charlie. Together, all three created a circuitry of interdependency, as if they shared genes across wood and flesh.

The Masks of Nina Conti

We human beings pursue and flee from the mechanical rigidity of things. We gather things (self-powered and not) because to some extent they relieve us of physical labor and allow us more freedom. At the same time, they disappear us, extract some agency and then appoint us as their servile caretakers. Our newfound *freedom* is tied to these things that, in a way, represent our extinction. In this existential human-cyborg affair, the prosthetic becomes more and less than what it replaces; the human being, too, becomes more and less than what it previously was.

The recent work of ventriloquist Nina Conti illustrates the tragic humor of this dilemma, and casts light on why puppetry has been so culturally significant around the world for centuries. Conti has built an array of half masks—prosthetic jowls and mouths of different shapes and expressions—each rigged with a pulley that Conti controls. They hang like fractured faces on a clothes line that she rolls onto stage. Then Conti calls up an innocent dupe from the audience, straps onto them a mask of her choice, and with strings in hand begins a conversation . . . well, of course, Conti speaks for herself *and* the astonished volunteer who adjusts and responds extemporaneously as Conti's voice emanates through their flapping prosthetic mouth.

As previously mentioned, when we create a puppet we create something that possesses its own body, its own site of attention. We know it is an extension of a human being but it reads as autonomous, and herein lies some of its magic. In the case of Conti, however, this sovereign thing fuses with another human body and foregrounds clearly the existential questions that permeate our human relationship with materiality. With tremendous compassion and wit, Conti appropriates her subject's voice. In turn, the half-human/half-puppet creature exposes the messy line between aliveness and numbness that we humans navigate every day. In her unsuspecting volunteers, we witness a wide range of reactions: stunned hesitation followed by hesitant compliance, awkward discomfort followed by resistance (which Nina brilliantly toys with and adapts to), exaggerated disbelief, painful surrender, and often a riotous mix of all the above. Some volunteers so fully acquiesce to Conti's projection onto them that even Conti is forced to keep up with their improvisation. Other times, in spite of their body language, she gets them to perform something they clearly do not want to perform. Conti may be pulling the strings but anything can and does happen.

In the end—no matter what unfolds—Conti, wooden mask, and human volunteer share lines of force, lines of life. While we see the apparatus of illusion in Conti's hands, we are transfixed by the mask itself, moving with mechanical rigidity yet serving as a link between two human beings on stage. The mask here is a translator; it generates a third space between submission and control, presence and absence, visibility and erasure, as well as between the actual people who occupy these positions. This in turn intimates all the thorny political and social circumstances (regarding race, class, gender, etc.) in which these terms have consequence. Conti's act is painfully funny. We laugh at the hijacked person on stage who desperately tries to negotiate the theft of their voice. We laugh because the act so cleverly reveals the stakes of either shirking or abusing the gift and privilege of agency, stakes that we all—not only Conti and the brave dupe on stage—must negotiate.

The Encuentro Altar, Mexico City, 2019

In June 2019, I went to Mexico City to attend *The Encuentro*, a conference sponsored by the Hemispheric Institute of Performance and Politics, New York University. I participated in a workgroup that focused on climate change, particularly how performance artists might address this current crisis. We had been instructed to bring something to the first session that represented our relationship with the natural world, with the "more than human" world. One by one, each participant shared a brief story about the object they brought and then placed it on a table to create an assemblage, or what the conveners called an "altar." In the end, this altar was composed of seeds, two cell phones, a Zuni badger fetish, a rubber ducky, a piece of obsidian from an Anasazi site in New Mexico, gardening gloves, plastic water bottle, plastic necklace, a small spade fashioned from melted down guns, a golem figure, two passports, a chunk of compost, and four cardboard horseshoe crabs.

These objects formed a strange community of dislocated ghosts displaying a past and a future, a legacy and a prophecy. They formed a seemingly sacred, more than human community overflowing with unresolved conflicts.

Childhood Puppet, Adulthood Puppet

Every child with a doll or a toy learns willy-nilly to speak the universal language of Puppet. Sometimes, even a found object or ragged old blanket will begin to teach the language: *move me, speak for me, listen to me, believe in me, hold me*. Early Puppet revolves around "me" almost exclusively, allowing the young speaker an opportunity to grasp the grammar of self-involvement.[2]

Adults learn Puppet, too, from a different set of toys. And when they do, it is no longer lessons about the self alone. Now it is about ideology, philosophy, semantics, and the social body. Like all languages, Puppet evolves with such complexity that before long speakers are at risk of considerable misunderstandings. In Puppet, we grow confounded not only by *what* is being said but by *who* is speaking as well.

Dust, crystals, coffee grounds, tea leaves, dirt, metals, stones, cards, brains of sacrificed goats. All these prognosticators speak a dialect of Puppet.

For centuries we have summoned their wisdom, listened to what they have to say. Currently, there are innumerable objects not only around us but *within* us ushering in new tongues. Now that we are cyborgs—hosts to untold techno-parasites and microplastics, viruses and bacteria that have altered our genomes—we must master these new tongues in order to even speak to ourselves!

HEARING VOICES, SEEING GHOSTS, EXPERIENCING NOISE: HEALING *MADNESS*

Illusion and magic (or art) are integral to systems of religion, philosophy, healing, pedagogy, and cultural politics; in large part, they drive and formulate our beliefs. At the same time, they introduce indeterminate spaces that require us to reconsider the very meaning of truth, reality, and knowledge. In the following section, we consider how puppets and disembodied voices accompany circumstances of trauma, death, mental illness, and political oppression.

Magical Thinking in the Face of Trauma

In his review essay "Ministry of Apparitions," Malcolm Gaskill (2019) states that magical objects tend to flourish at times of war, physical and mental stress, trauma, and death. It is no surprise that we carry about amulets, rabbits' feet, and any number of charms for luck, fortune, health, or protection: it is precisely because we believe that their materiality is infused with spirit that they help us survive a trial or loss of some kind.

An interesting historical case is Ouija, or the talking board. Following mass deaths in the U.S. Civil War, spiritualism exploded across America and mediums began to employ various means to accommodate the widespread desire to communicate with the dead. With so many bodies unrecovered, devices such as the Ouija board gave people an outlet for contact and closure. With fingers hovering delicately over a planchette, which was placed on a board inscribed with letters and numbers, the dead spelled out the answers to the burning questions of their grieving relatives. While the Ouija board was not trademarked until 1890, its use had been a phenomenon since the end of the war. Just as in religious and divinatory ventriloquism, the Ouija enlisted the deceased to guide the living through hard times (McRobbie, 2013).

Gaskill (2019) discusses the resurgence of magical thinking during and after World War I: "After 1918 magic was no longer just an emanation from the cosmos, but something inside the self, closer to the unconscious and subconscious states around which psychology and psychiatry would build new ways of understanding how people survive" (p. 21).[3] At many different moments in history marked by widespread calamity or trauma, affected people experience the manifestation of another presence or voice that accompanies them, supports them. It is as if human beings spontaneously create companions in times of dire need who will stand by them, talk to them, guide them, and alleviate their fear and loneliness.

An exemplary case is that of *South! The Story of Shackleton's Last Expedition, 1914–1917*, Ernest Shackleton's (2017) epic tale of survival after the sinking of his ship *The Endurance* in Antarctic waters in 1915. Near death from exhaustion and hunger, Shackleton and two of his companions trekked across South Georgia Island to a whaling station where they found salvation. "During that long and racking march of thirty-six hours over the unnamed mountains and glaciers of South Georgia," wrote Shackleton in his memoir, "it seemed to me often that we were four, not three" (p. 173). Somewhat embarrassed by the phenomenon and its potential meaning, Shackleton did not share the experience with his companions until years later at which point he learned that each of the other two felt the presence of someone trekking with them as well.

The phenomenon has since been widely reported and given the name the *third man factor.* The people who appear tend to be loved ones, some alive and some dead. They always provide comfort, advice, or just company; there are no accounts of alarm or disorientation when they appear. In some instances, those in distress reach out to the presence as if they are suffering the same grim circumstances. Frank Smythe, for example, offered half of his mint cake to the presence who appeared to him while in distress on Mt. Everest (Geiger, 2009, pp. 47–48). In almost all recorded cases of the phenomenon, the ghostly presence disappears as soon as *real* help arrives.

Hearing voices is not always a pathology. As many as 80% of people who have lost a loved one report hearing, seeing, or feeling them in the months after their death. Creating puppets may serve as an act of healing at such times of hardship, a way to negotiate feelings with those deceased presences. Actually, creating puppets with whom we can talk, find comfort, and express emotions may serve as a preemptive act *at any time* in our lives: a chance to offset stress or loneliness before it becomes unmanageable or life-threatening. A chance to use one one's voice to access other voices—ones we need to hear.

Avatar Therapy and Cop-in-the-Head

Avatar therapy was developed in 2008 by Julian Leff, a London researcher and practitioner who studied schizophrenia (Berman, 2018). Leff asked his patients to sit in front of a computer and choose an avatar—a face and a vocal timbre—to represent the distressing voices they heard in their heads. I immediately thought of Cop-in-the-Head, one of Boal's signature techniques in which a protagonist is asked to identify the voices in their head that argue persistently against doing precisely what the protagonist needs to do to overcome an oppression, exercise a right, or restore self-worth. The protagonist then casts participants in the workshop to play each of the voices and debates with each in an effort to undo their influence. Often, the protagonist makes invaluable associations between the voices in their head and the recurrent messages of actual people or cultural institutions that they had internalized (Boal, 1995).

Avatar therapy—similar to Boal's technique in its approach to voices—is a validated therapy that provides an alternative to drugs for many schizophrenic patients. A therapist guides the experience from another room: at first, a recorded voice—eerily robotic and disembodied—expresses judgmental and disparaging comments toward the client watching the selected avatar on a computer screen. The therapist coaches the patient on how to respond, urging them to argue back and defend themselves, to use their voice to withstand them. In subsequent sessions, the therapist records a more sympathetic computerized voice—more respectful and conversant—as reinforcement for the patient's courage. Avatar therapy refutes much of the thinking and practices of institutionalized medicine, which does not recommend treating voices as people; that is, naming them or interacting with them. Leff points out, however, that we engage regularly and intimately with unreal voices in cartoons, musical lyrics heard over the radio, video games, and fictional films (Berman, 2018). We willfully suspend disbelief and grant a truth function to representation. In doing so, we take a necessary step toward play, as outlined by Bateson (1972); that is, an ability to engage and suspect "unreality" at once (p. 185).

Avatar therapy has reinforced the conviction that voices are not the problem. The problem is how people react to them. Psychotic continuum theory focuses on hallucination-like events experienced by the non-clinical population. Research efforts indicate a wide range of auditory *disorders* from otherwise healthy individuals to those diagnosed with schizophrenia, as well as a wide spectrum of resilience. What of artists and writers who circulate routinely within a culture of fantasy and illusion? Tanya Luhrmann (2018), a psychological anthropologist who studies how culture shapes psychotic experiences, is a proponent of avatar therapy and gives credence to a person's *reaction* to a voice rather than its mere occurrence. She recounts that when a group of writers attending a conference in Vancouver, Canada were asked whether they heard the voices of their characters, one quarter said that they hear them as clearly as if they were in the room. Are the voices of *madness* the very same as the voices of creativity? In large measure, she answers, it really does not matter.[4]

Noise: From Punch to Politics

To investigate puppets throughout history is also to study voice itself: the linguistics of voice, the metaphysics of voice, the relation between voice and body, the politics of voice. Such a history reveals innumerable instances of puppets speaking not in human-like voices but rather in shrieks, childlike bleats, and tongues unfamiliar or barely comprehensible. These voices are wistful, rhythmic, guttural, untamed, and amorphous. They are more or less human.

A classic example is the voice of the puppet Punch from sixteenth-century Italian *commedia dell'arte*. Speaking of Punch's words, Gross (2011) writes:

> When we can understand them, [they] are full of the broken matter of language: bad puns, malapropisms, nonsense words, and jingling rhymes: what meaning they have is always tentative, always in negotiation. . . . This disordered speech makes music along with the percussive sounds of Punch's stick with which he both dances and kills other puppets; it accomplishes the music of his wooden head itself knocked rhythmically against the stage. (Gross, 2011, pp. 69–70)

The voice of Punch reflects the voice of carnival, the masses filling the streets and marketplaces, speaking in rich, noisy, vernacular idioms that parody and mock the bosses and kings. The visceral noise explodes everyday order and delivers instead a grotesque and festive insurgency. Punch and carnival are mouthpieces of embodied resistance; they speak as the underbelly, the endangered, even the not-yet-born.

I thought of Punch while attending a panel titled "Sonodystopia" at the *Encuentro* in Mexico City. The presenters asked the audience to consider noise in relation to trauma, political displacement, and colonization, to understand it as an interior soundscape that resulted from life at the margins. They spoke of noise as an unstable aural terrain bursting from generations of forced silence. The presenters were from Ecuador, Mexico, and Costa Rica, and to demonstrate the concrete roots of noise they detailed, one after the other, the devastation of specific landscapes: thousands of miles of invasive railroad tracks, the widespread planting of coffee, sugar, and pineapple, the impacts of corrupt global money. They spoke of refugees, immigrants, and women who remain unseen and unheard, and yet live and breathe a Punch-like chaos, the convulsive effects of unrestrained and irresponsible *progress*.

It is worth noting that puppet theatre (extending well beyond Punch and his unintelligible screams) has allowed artists in many different historical contexts to take up a repertory of otherwise forbidden works. Players in Tudor England were able to perform with puppets the Medieval Passion plays that Protestant authorities had banned for human actors. African people have animated objects to express their experiences ever since arriving in America, despite the prohibition by slaveholders on performing narratives with African-centered worldviews. In the 1614 play *Bartholomew Fair*, Ben Jonson used puppets to portray pickpockets and bullies, prostitutes and drunkards, as a way to critique political and religious conflicts in London society in Jacobean England. At many moments in European history, puppetry, like carnival, was blamed for inciting revolutions, and subsequently banned. England, Germany, Portugal, and France had laws criminalizing puppeteers at various times. The history of puppet theatre is, in part, a history of resistance. Through the medium we are encouraged (and provided with the tools) to embrace our monsters, our dysfunctional bodies and communities, our crises and nightmares, all we find alien and threatening. The medium, in fact, welcomes expressions of darker, dirtier, and imperfect versions of life, ones that disrupt naïve and heroic myths that do not do justice to the complexity of our lived lives.[5]

EXERCISE

Make a puppet out of:

- a found object that you treasure without knowing exactly why
- something or someone that you feel you must protect
- the gestures your hand makes when you are angry
- a creature in a nightmare that you have had
- a childhood possession that you won't give away
- a device or machine that controls you
- an obsession
- a guilty pleasure
- a confession
- noise

PUPPET POWER, OR HOW PUPPETS (RE)ANIMATE HUMANS

In talking puppetry, we tend to focus on the innumerable ways in which a human being can animate an inanimate thing. Perhaps less considered are the many ways that the puppet animates the human being. What are some of the capacities that puppets possess and, in turn, awaken in their puppeteers?

The Power of Scale

Puppets, thankfully, can violate the laws of scale. Mice can be the size of elephants, a human hand can cup the entire Milky Way, the tip of an iceberg can emerge as the flowing hair of an elderly woman. A puppet of a human being can have several heads, the body of a huge tree or a sinking boat, and arms that extend like slithering snakes or bolts of lightning. In playing with scale, the puppet can make an impossible image concrete, thus expanding our horizons of the possible. Put another way, in making something incredible, we change the laws of truth.

To play with scale is also to play with boundaries and restraints. When we point to what is inconceivable we are also pointing to our perceived limitations. The out-of-scale puppet instigates a dialogue between one's constraints and one's desires. Can I be more than I thought I could be? Are my perceived limitations valid? What do I have to do to find out? Somewhere across the broad spectrum of what the puppet displays for us, from practical to miraculous, we locate ourselves as thinkers and makers, critics and dreamers. What part do we play, or want to play, in revising the real?

The Power of Reuse: The Case of Peter Brook and the Boot

English theatre director Peter Brook spent much of his career working with diverse communities around the world. He used objects to bridge the language and culture gap. In one of his well-documented trips to Africa, Brook started an exercise by placing a boot in the center of a large circle of participants. He picked it up, performatively transformed it into a pillow, and then passed it along. As it went around the circle, each person used it differently: it became a book, a soccer ball, a burning coal, a hat, a mirror. Objects are given meaning by those who handle them.

It is not uncommon for artists, therapists, teachers, and builders to reuse objects to create new forms. This creative reuse, or *making do*, encapsulates the gift of the puppet; that is, to put an object into motion, to make observable, and to extend, a life that we did not know it had.

Through Brook's collective play, each person animates (gives new meaning) to this thing we call a "boot." At the same time, the boot-in-motion gives us animators something back. It exposes and exercises our human capacity to adapt, to be resourceful and flexible. The boot is a connective device, it links the participants to one another through the practice of versatility. It generates a realm beyond any one language, interpretation, or purpose. This realm is the very measure of community.

The Power of Artifice, or Innocence at a Distance

German poet and dramatist Heinrich von Kleist (1777–1811) argued, perhaps ironically, that a disjunction between mind and body is precisely what makes puppet theatre more capable than live theatre to convey the art of living. The fact that the puppet's voice appears at a distance from the producer is what lends the puppet its peculiar power (Shershow, 1995). Puppeteer Schwartz shares the sentiment: "You see, puppets have no egos. They can become emblems of heightened or extreme emotional states: passion, rage, sorrow . . . that real actors could never get away with" (Schwartz et al., 1983, p. 106). But it is not only distance that creates the magic. It is also a chock full innocence that seems to come with the puppet's presence. For Kleist, the puppet is a thing that is always itself, a pure surface, an artifice that contains its own integrity, and therein lies its enchantment. Puppeteer Janie Geiser explains that even when the puppet lies, mocks, or acts with violence, "we find that we can't really blame it. We can't blame a piece of wood. And so its actions bear a kind of incontrovertible truth" (Geiser, cited in Gross, 2011, p. 141). It is this combination of distance and innocence that gives intimacy and interiority to the human words that emerge from the puppet's mouth.

During the 2018 roundtable that I conducted with the Los Angeles dummies and their ventriloquists, I learned that two of the teams conducted community work with youth, one on cyber-bullying and the other on sex education. I was told that when they sat around and talked, the youth would pay far more attention to what the dummies had to say than the ventriloquists.

The Power of Disenchantment: The Case of the Hopi Kachinas

For people of the Hopi nation, disillusionment has long been a vital ingredient in the initiation of Hopi children of the Kachina cult into adulthood and a meaningful religious life. Up until the time that children are ten years old, Kachinas are superhuman visitors, not unlike Santa Claus or the Tooth Fairy among many North American children. These Kachinas, always masked, arrive at the opening of Hopi ceremonies and enthrall the crowd, particularly the youth, heightening a sense of unity between the human world, the natural world, and the spirits. The children grow up entirely enchanted by the Kachinas; from the time they are infants they are surrounded not only by ceremonial Kachinas but also by carved kachina dolls that embody the union between spiritual and secular life. Interestingly, in the Hopi language, the word *kachina* means both doll and spirit.

As with all Hopi rites, the Kachinas arrive for the initiation service dancing and exciting the crowd. But soon afterward, the children are separated out and, according to some accounts, forced to undergo a physically harrowing experience—a forewarning about a quintessential secret they are about to learn and are obliged to keep, or else. Disoriented and frightened, they are brought to a ceremonial space into which the adored and respected Kachinas file in. To the youth's great dismay and surprise, the Kachinas remove their masks and there, standing before them, are their uncles and fathers, older siblings and cousins—their holy, superhuman world brutally recast as mere imposture. Kachinas, it turns out, are not real gods as they had previously believed. And that is not all. What is particularly remarkable is that these disillusioned, angry, resentful, and shocked youngsters are now required to imitate their deceitful elders; that is, in order to enter adulthood as defined by the community, they must now don the masks of the Kachinas and betray all those younger than them. They must enchant (deceive) others.

In the rite, the wondrous innocence conveyed by a puppet (or mask) that exists apart from ourselves is shattered, and the loss is irreversible. Sam Gill (1996) calls it the death of naïve realism. It is on this note of discord and loss that the ritual ends. How does this disenchantment function as an initiation into religion? And why is it so invaluable? For the Hopi, adult religious life must begin in a state of radical doubt and skepticism. Each child must search out their own criteria for a meaningful existence, to find their own new position (the old having been destroyed) within the social cosmology. Gill (1996) explains that "religion springs from the unique human capacity to create dimensions of reality that are beyond the material, beyond the obvious, beyond even human existence" (p. 236). The state of crisis that the children experience is not confined to the rite but rather indicates a state that the youth are obliged to respect and protect for the remainder of their adult lives. To be inducted into a religious life is to accept the perplexity of reality. Through sustained inquiry, creativity, wonderment, and painful wrestling with meaning-making, each member of the community defines what they want the *real* world to be.[6]

What I find instructive in the Kachina initiation story resonates with the lessons of puppetry. Immersive enchantment and critical thinking are each other's best friends; in fact, the paradox is the very fabric of evolution. The young Hopi initiate learns that to be a responsible and contributing member of society, they must wear a mask. They must believe fully in who they become when they wear that mask, and yet remain suspicious of masks. The puppet, too, is a container of these teachings; it serves a human need to shape-shift without shirking the responsibilities and accountabilities accordant with each shape. Puppets are threshold objects that know how to traverse the enchantment/disenchantment divide.

I recently went to an exhibit at the Getty Museum titled *Monumentality*. Tucked away in a corner glass frame, I read the etymology of the title word: from Latin *monumentum*, literally something that reminds us of a person, event, historical moment. There was also mention of the word *numen*, or divine spirit, situated right there in the center of *monumentum*. A monument, then, is a material thing that is filled with light and ineffability. It is something we can touch with our hands but it contains something "out of our hands." Gross (2011) describes puppets as "oddly clairvoyant in their muteness" (p. 14).

The Power to Destroy

We are all as vulnerable as a puppet.

One might say that we humans imagine and create because of a sense of inadequacy, and that the puppet (or mask, totem, sacred object, etc.) is an addendum or a salve, an attempt to remedy the sense of imperfection. Human vulnerability, however, is forever. In giving it physical form we do not change this fact but, rather, come to own it. In owning it, we also have the opportunity to *destroy* it. The ability to playfully destroy a replication of one's pain or shortcomings is potentially quite recuperative.

To convey this recuperative capacity, I will share a personal story about the sad fate of a deck of tarot cards. I do not use tarot cards to read the future, I think of them as a junction of art, analytic diagrams, meditation, systems theory, and oracular wisdom. Tarot images meld with what we project onto them; the card is merely the site upon which we attempt to make sense of our own confused desires and fears.

It happened many years ago. I pulled out a tarot deck, shuffled, and laid out the cards as I contemplated a tough circumstance at work, one which left me feeling humiliated and powerless. Before me was a complex message to be decoded. The card occupying the destiny position was *Death* featuring a skeleton wielding a sickle with dead and dying bodies scattered at its feet. I did not know then what I know now about *Death*, how its meaning suggests a letting go of expectation or habit, a surrender to change. On that day, all I felt was exasperation over this damning judgment from the divining spirits. To my great surprise, I responded furiously and impulsively. I grabbed a book of matches, picked up the *Death* card, and held a flame to it. Ironically, the card was laminated and while it slowly browned it would not burn. *First condemned, and now mocked!* I thought to myself. My determination to retaliate was only further incited. I dropped the card and match and searched for a pair of scissors. Without hesitation I cut the card into four parts, and then with a rush of exhilaration I cut every one of the seventy-two cards into pieces. I did so with some panic, as if I might be apprehended by the tarot police and hanged for blasphemy. But the exhilaration and pleasure were overwhelming. Enraged by the message, I was destroying the messenger!

Reading the cards, as well as cutting them up, did not solve my problem at work. I never expected it to. In using them, however, my humiliation and frustration found lodging in a material form, in this case laminated card stock painted with provocative images. I am quite certain that if *Death* had not appeared, I would have found another card to inspire me to do damage, to express my frustration. The cards were my puppets and my collaborators: *Let me infuriate you*, they seemed to say. *I am here today so that you can kill me!*

Like an urn filled with a loved one's ashes set upon the fireplace mantel, I placed the dead and silenced tarot deck in a cookie tin and set it upon a bookshelf in my Los Angeles apartment. There it sat for years, a bit like a lifeless sock gathering dust on the bedroom floor after the puppeteer's hand had departed. To this day, I chuckle over the *madness* in my play, but I also acknowledge the sense of triumph that these material things afforded me, that is, the ability to mutilate them. Years later, I scotch-taped all those cards back together, and while they remain far too floppy to use, they are monumental harbingers—all the more precious for their visible wounds.

CONCLUSION

The puppet is an object fabricated with an intention in mind: to create a vehicle for a voice, image, emotion, or fantasy that needs to be expressed and shared. Many art forms do this, serving as a medium between conscious and unconscious information. The puppet is somewhat unique in that it combines performative tropes (acting, embodiment, presence, and live voice) with properties of the plastic arts (anything constructed from tangible materials such as glass, textiles, metal, clay, wood, stone, etc.). The puppet is a medium between material and immaterial, inanimate and animate, the given and the imagined. It does not regard these pairs as binaries but rather indulges their intimacies and congruences. The puppet is a translator, and in keeping with all translation, the participating parties are transformed. Translation entails a reframing across difference. In animating a physical thing—turning a physical object into a puppet—a metamorphosis occurs that changes both the material animated and the person who animates.

When we look through our homes and offices, in our drawers and closets, our back pockets and purses, we find objects infused with messages and memories: they carry the voices and stories of mentors, friends, truth-tellers, deceivers, and protectors, alive and dead. At some point, these everyday objects came to be more than themselves, infused with context and meaning. In the study of puppets, I have been reminded of this extraordinary capacity to move anything out of paralysis into movement. (Interestingly, in Shakespeare's day, a puppet show was called a *motion*.) Every lifeless object now reminds me of its latent potential to move, and, more importantly, that this vitalizing power resides in myself. In moving the object, *I* move; in animating the object, I remake *myself*.

In today's technologically-driven climate, it is worth asking who is moving whom. We have invested the objects around us with so much agency that they seem to move without us. In fact, our devices and brands have garnered a life so fluent and formidable in contemporary Western culture that we just might be the lifeless puppets in *their* lively hands. I am thinking drones, timepieces, cell phones, the most trendy jeans or video game, the indispensable doll or action figure born of a holiday blockbuster, each with their own loud ideological voice. Are we turning to these things to give us back some of our lost vitality and meaning? Are we imitating what we own, what seems to own us? I wonder if we can engage these puppets-run-amok in a conversation about the terms of "co-animation." (Of course, this is already going on in face-recognition research, artificial intelligence [AI] think tanks, robotics labs, and many other professional arenas.) Puppetry seems a promising vehicle for listening to these characters who are indisputable parts of our culture and our nature. We might learn a great deal about how they intend to invigorate and/or aggravate human prospects. And we might learn a great deal what these intentions really mean to us.

I would like to conclude by returning to Augusto Boal and to a Cop-in-the-Head scene that I facilitated in July 2019 with graduate students in Santa Barbara, California. I offer it here because my understanding of this technique was recast when a student employed the apparatus of puppetry to move herself through a dilemma. (It is possible that I was now seeing everything through the lens of puppetry!) The student—I will call her Deidre—volunteered a story: she wanted to overcome her habit of "behaving deplorably towards men" who came into the retail store in which she worked. She attributed this behavior to traumatic experiences in her past when she had been violated by men whom she had trusted. As the exercise prescribes, she first identified the voices in her head that advocate the very behavior she wanted to change: *do not drop your guard, your distrust and behavior is warranted, you need to protect herself, you are too weak and too tired to fend off any more harm*. She then cast people in the workshop to embody each of these voices, the cops-in-her-head, and proceeded to debate each of them, one at a time. She argued on behalf of her desired behavior, wanting to access some grace in the face of random men who came into the store showing no obvious sign of disrespect or aggression. By the end of the debate, Deidre identified two "cops" whose voices were most compelling and obstructive—*you are too weak to defend yourself* and *danger is everywhere and unpredictable*—ones that she could not get out of her head.

It was in the next stage of the exercise that I recognized how Deidre employed the tools of puppetry. We went back to the original scene in which Deidre was rude and snarky to her male customers. But now Deidre could alter the original scene and act differently. It was an opportunity to see if the debates with the cops created a space for change, an opportunity to act on her stated desire not to prejudge her male customers. Deidre brought the two loudest cops into the scene with her. She placed them at arm's length, a guiding hand on each of their backs as if they were shields. As we ran the scene, she moved them around like two protective life-sized puppets; they were extensions of herself, she controlled them. As she walked through aesthetic space—the imaginary retail store in which she worked—she tentatively, but pleasantly, invited the male customers to check out the merchandise.

Boal's (1995) work foregrounds the necessity to bring forth that which has been institutionally shamed, marginalized, and silenced. So much of the recuperative work we do through the arts—Boal's Theatre of the Oppressed being only one oeuvre among so many—requires that we deal with the associative feelings of lack, loss, and emptiness. Puppetry is a fertile terrain for transforming these absences into presences, presences that can then be handled, scripted, revised, embraced, forgiven, eviscerated, and even destroyed. The capacity to multiply ourselves—or, more accurately, to stage playfully the motley family of voices that each of us harbor—is one of the most healing potentials of puppetry, an art form accessible to all of us at any time.[7]

NOTES

1. For purposes of this essay I am not attending to significant differences between automatons, hand puppets, marionettes, shadow puppets, ventriloquists dummies, avatars, dolls, etc. Rather, I am seeking to capture the uncanny and therapeutic power that they all deliver in capturing something "more than human."

2. I refer readers to the work of English pediatrician and psychoanalyst Donald W. Winnicott (1953), Transitional objects and transitional phenomena: A study of the first not-me possession, *International Journal of Psychoanalysis*, *34*(2), 89–97, particularly his discussion of transitional objects: security blankets, stuffed animals, dolls, and favorite toys that stand in for the mother-child bond.

3. This coincides with the development and spread of Freudian psychology. It is interesting to note that the consulting room in which Freud treated his patients was cluttered with figurines—diminutive statues of gods, mythological characters, iconic religious heroes, and animal-shaped idols of antiquity. Supposedly, the figurines—collective, mystical entities that had to be reckoned with on any path toward healing—linked Freud to the psyches of his patients and vice versa. While his premise may have sway, in her *Gone Primitive: Savage Intellects, Modern Lives*, Marianna Torgovnick (1990) has written an insightful essay, "Entering Freud's Study," condemning Freud's perception of the figurines as "primitive," and himself as the civilized "puppeteer" who translates them for his patients (London and Chicago, IL: University of Chicago Press), pp. 194–209.

4. For those interested in the long debated relationship between madness and creativity, I refer readers to Luis Sass (2017), *Madness and modernism: Insanity in the light of art, literature, and thought* (rev. ed.) (Oxford, UK: Oxford University Press).

5. I write this essay at the height of national corruption, distrust, and despair during the Trump administration when more and more U.S. citizens (and many others across the globe) are suffering the plague of mystification and delusion. I wonder if long-standing narratives of naïve and/or heroic resolution will lose some of their authority—for better or worse.

6. There are other interesting examples of disenchantment and disillusionment as key progenitors of belief formation within ritual settings. This can be found in the Wiradthuri tribe's Broken Bullroarer ceremony (Australia) and the Killing of Kavula rite among the Ndembu (Africa). See Sam Gill (1996), Disenchantment: A religious abduction, in R. L. Grimes (Ed.), *Readings in ritual studies* (Upper Saddle River, NJ: Prentice Hall), pp. 230–239.

7. I would like to particularly credit Kenneth Gross and his 2011 book, *Puppet: An Essay on Uncanny Life* (Chicago, IL: University of Chicago Press), for inspiring many ideas for this essay. I recommend it to anyone interested in the history, scholarship, and poetics of puppetry.

REFERENCES

Barton, J. (2019). *A history of the Bible: The story of the world's most influential book.* New York, NY: Viking Press.

Bateson, G. (1972). A theory of play and fantasy (1955). In *Steps to an ecology of mind: Collected essays in anthropology, psychiatry, evolution, and epistemology* (pp. 178–193). New York, NY: Ballantine Books.

Bergen, C. (1984). *Knock wood.* New York, NY: Simon and Schuster.

Berman, P. (2018). Julian Leff: Changing the face of schizophrenia treatment. *The Lancet, Psychiatry, 5*(4), 302. https://doi.org/10.1016/S2215–0366(18)30105–6

Boal, A. (1995). *The rainbow of desire: The Boal method of theatre and therapy* (A. Jackson, Trans.). London and New York, NY: Routledge.

Gaskill, M. (2019, July 4). Ministry of apparitions. [Review of the book *A supernatural war: Magic, divination and faith during the first world war*, by O. Davies]. *London Review of Books*, *41*(13), 19–21.

Geiger, J. (2009). *The third man factor: Surviving the impossible*. New York, NY: Weinstein Books.

Gill, S. D. (1996). Disenchantment: A religious abduction. In R. L. Grimes (Ed.), *Readings in ritual studies* (pp. 230–239). Upper Saddle River, NJ: Prentice Hall.

Gross, K. (2011). *Puppet: An essay on uncanny life.* Chicago, IL: University of Chicago Press.

Kreymborg, A. (1926). *Puppet plays.* New York, NY: Samuel French.

Little, T. (2017, November 6). Tracing the development of the doppelgänger. *Atlas Obscura*. https://www.atlasobscura.com/articles/history-doppelganger

Luhrmann, T. M. (2018, June). The sound of madness: Can we treat psychosis by listening to the voices in our heads? *Harper's Magazine*. Retrieved from https://harpers.org/archive/2018/06/the-sound-of-madness/

McRobbie, L. R. (2013, October 27). The strange and mysterious history of the Ouija board. *Smithsonian.* Retrieved from https://www.smithsonianmag.com/history/the-strange-and-mysterious-history-of-the-ouija-board-5860627/

Pessoa, F. (2001). *The book of disquiet.* R. Zenith (Ed. and Trans.). New York, NY: Penguin Classic.

Phillips, A. (2001). Pessoa's appearances. In *Promises, promises: Essays on psychoanalysis and literature* (pp. 113–124). New York, NY: Basic Books.

Roth, P. (1995). *Sabbath's theater.* New York, NY: Houghton Mifflin Company.

Sass, L. (2017). *Madness and modernism: Insanity in the light of art, literature, and thought* (Revised ed.). Oxford, UK: Oxford University Press.

Schutzman, M. (2019). *Radical doubt: The Joker System, after Boal*. London and New York, NY: Routledge.

Schwartz, B. D., Skipitares, T., Taymor, J., & Jenner, C. L. (1983). Interview: Working with puppets. *Performing Arts Journal*, *7*(1), 103–116. https://www.muse.jhu.edu/article/655456

Shackleton, E. (2017). *South! The story of Shackleton's last expedition, 1914–1917* (1920). Milano: American History Classics.

Shershow, S. C. (1995). *Puppets and popular culture*. Ithaca, NY, and London: Cornell University Press.

Torgovnick, M. (1990). Entering Freud's study. In *Gone primitive: Savage intellects, modern lives* (pp. 194–209). London and Chicago, IL: University of Chicago Press.

Wittgenstein, L. (1969). *On certainty.* New York, NY: Harper and Row.

Winnicott, D. W. (1953). Transitional objects and transitional phenomena: A study of the first not-me possession. *International Journal of Psychoanalysis*, *34*(2), 89–97. https://doi.org/10.4324/9780429475931-14

Chapter Three

Theatre for Revolution or Theatre for Healing?

Forum Theatre with LGBT2SIQ+ and Other Targeted Communities

Jessica Bleuer

Teacher: Please submit your assignments here. Thank you.

Students begin dropping assignments on teacher's desk.

Teacher: Today we are going to start the class with some group work. Let's start by splitting the class in two. . . . Guys on the left side, girls on the right.

Students get up and start grouping. Trans Male Student (Sam) hesitates and decides to move towards the "guy side." Other students start teasing Sam.

John (*Cisgendered male student*): Wrong side girlie!

All students laugh.

Teacher: Okay, okay, stop joking around. And Sam, get back over there (points to the girls' side).

Sam turns bright red, hesitates, and runs out of the class.

The above scenario is a role play devised for a larger advocacy project aimed at reducing microaggressions on campus.[1] The project, titled Safer Spaces, used Forum Theatre, a Theatre of the Oppressed method, to illustrate transphobic microaggressions that commonly occur in educational settings. Augusto Boal (1979), the founder of Theatre of the Oppressed, often spoke of his work as both a "rehearsal for revolution" (p. 122) and "rehearsals for healing" (quoted in Schutzman, 1994, p. 138).

There is a scarcity of scholarly research on the impacts of the Theatre of the Oppressed with Queer spectrum and Trans spectrum issues (Moreno, 2018). This chapter will reflect on fifteen years of Forum Theatre facilitation with Lesbian, Gay, Bisexual, Trans, Two-Spirited, Intersex, Queer, and additional sexual orientations (LGBT2SIQ+), Gender Non-Conforming (GNC), and other targeted communities. Forum Theatre is one of the principal techniques of the Theatre of the Oppressed that aims to make visible and minimize oppression, while developing tools for relational healing and revolution.

Theatre of the Oppressed (TO), originally conceived in 1964 during a brutal dictatorship in Brazil, used the term "revolution" to describe the overturn of an entire social system. The Forum Theatre workshops discussed in this chapter take place in a very different social context, that of numerous Canadian cities between 2004 and 2019, and the term "revolution" here will thus refer to smaller changes to social systems, broadly including any reform leading to systemic social change. Further specificity will be left to the particularities and goals of each project.

This chapter will address Forum Theatre's potential to advance both systems change and also the relational well-being of Forum Theatre participants. A critical incident technique (CIT) approach, outlined by Loretta Woolsey (1986), is used to reflect on fifteen years of my practice as a Forum Theatre practitioner to explore the question: What are some of the tensions that may impede Forum Theatre from addressing health equity issues with LGBT2SIQ+, GNC, and other marginalized communities?

LITERATURE REVIEW: HEALTH EQUITY

The World Health Organization states that "the root causes of health inequities are to be found in the social, economic, and political mechanisms" (quoted in Solar & Irwin, 2007, p. 67). Health equity describes how discrimination and prejudice create divergent health outcomes between different cultural groups. The term "minority stress" (Meyer, 1995, 2003) has put words to what marginalized communities have always known; discrimination and inequity are bad for one's health. The minority stress model explains that stigma and prejudice experienced by LGBT2SIQ+ communities, along with perceived rejection, concealment, and internalized homophobia, negatively impact individuals' mental health and well-being (Meyer, 1995, 2003).

Research shows that in the LGBT2SIQ+ community, Lesbian, Gay, and Bisexual populations have poorer general health, more suicidal ideation (Conron, Mimiaga, & Landers, 2010), and more mental health diagnoses than their heterosexual counterparts (Cochran, 2001). Research findings also document poorer general health (Fredriksen-Goldsen et al., 2011) and higher levels of psychological distress (Fredriksen-Goldsen et al., 2014) among Transgender individuals.

Forum Theatre descriptions in this chapter will focus on daily manifestations of inequity, sometimes referred to as microaggressions. Microaggressions are understood as prejudicial attitudes that manifest in daily insults and denigrating behavior toward members from minority groups (Sue, 2010). Research has shown a correlation between microaggressions against LGBT2SIQ+ people and psychological distress (Nadal, Skolnik, & Wong, 2012; Nadal et al., 2011; Robinson & Rubin, 2016; Seelman, Woodford, & Nicolazzo, 2017; Wright & Wegner, 2012). Multiple studies have found positive correlations between homonegative and transphobic microaggressions and post-traumatic stress disorder (PTSD) symptoms (Nadal et al., 2011; Robinson & Rubin, 2016), anxiety, (Nadal et al., 2011; Seelman, Woodford, & Nicolazzo, 2017), depression (Nadal et al., 2011), and poor self-esteem (Meyer, 1995; Seelman, Woodford, & Nicolazzo, 2017; Wright & Wegner, 2012). While oppression and discrimination accounts for many of these poor health outcomes, it is important to note that these systemic factors are often ignored and LGBT2SIQ+ and GNC communities are commonly pathologized.

Theatre of the Oppressed Healing and Revolution

Theatre of the Oppressed is a method used both for personal and relational healing and for larger systemic change.

Revolution

Jan Cohen-Cruz (2006) speaks to the depathologizing nature of TO, which when done well rejects the focus on personal limitations to instead embrace storytelling that highlights systemic injustice. It promotes consciousness raising and awareness of systemic inequity (Burns et al., 2015; Day, 2002; Sanders, 2004) and has been used to address homophobia (Francis, 2013; Iverson & Seher, 2014; Thompson & Santiago-Jirau, 2011), transphobia (Kelly-Golfman, 2019; Thompson & Santiago-Jirau, 2011), and numerous additional inequities. TO has also demonstrated its capacity to incite attitudinal change about racism (Sanders, 2004), bullying (Houston et al., 2001), behavioral change with regard to sexual assault bystander interventions (Ahrens, Rich, & Ullman, 2011), and social policy and legal change, contributing to the adoption notably of seven laws in Rio de Janeiro, Brazil (Boal, 1998).

Founder Boal (1979) is known for saying, "perhaps the theatre is not revolutionary itself; but have no doubts, it is a rehearsal of revolution!" (p. 122).

Healing

In addition to its revolutionary capacities, Boal (1979) has also described his work as a tool for healing, and Forum Theatre is well recognized and utilized as a public health intervention responsible for health-based behavioral change (Warheit, 2017). Forum Theatre addresses diverse health issues and research has shown its capacity to reduce stress (Yuksek, 2018), increase self-confidence (Moreno, 2018; Saeed, 2015; Sullivan et al., 2008; Yuksek, 2018), and develop feelings of self-efficacy (Sullivan et al., 2008) and empowerment (Karabekir, 2004) among its participants. Forum Theatre has also improved health care, by working with health service students and professionals to address stigma faced by mental health service users (Wilson, 2013) and the prejudice experienced by LGBT2SIQ+ people accessing assisted reproductive technologies (ART) (Tarasoff et al., 2014).

Forum Theatre further contributes to well-being by building communities of people who are connected through similar lived experiences (Cohen-Cruz, 2006; Erel, Reynolds, & Kaptani, 2017; Saeed, 2015) and who can help each other practice responses to oppressive situations (Erel, Reynolds, & Kaptani, 2017). Using theatrical scenarios, Forum Theatre recreates life-like situations of unresolved oppressions. Participants are then invited to practice how to address the oppression by role playing potential resolutions. By role playing a situation repeatedly, participants have the opportunity to develop a multi-faceted understanding of the conflict and are thereby more likely to discover an improved outcome (Boal, 2002). In a study about TO effectiveness with LGBT2SIQ+ communities, Lorena Moreno (2018) found that "eighty-eight percent of participants agreed that TO had helped them to gain courage to face oppressions they experience in their everyday lives" (p. 218). These spaces reduce feelings of isolation (Erel, Reynolds, & Kaptani, 2017), support minoritized individuals to learn about their identities (McClimens & Scott, 2007; Sanders, 2004), and address internalized oppression (Burns et al., 2015).

Theoretically, Forum Theatre has the capacity to contribute toward health equity by addressing social isolation, experiences of exclusion, discrimination, historical trauma, lack of coping skills, and other Government of Canada (2019) health factors identified to negatively impact the health of LGBT2SIQ+ and other targeted communities. However, due to Forum Theatre's relational and spontaneous nature, Forum Theatre's outcomes cannot be easily controlled or predetermined. Healing and emancipatory goals are not always met.

METHODOLOGY

My discomfort with the collateral damage that frequently results from Forum Theatre work has motivated me to review the last fifteen years of my Forum Theatre practice. As someone who has been involved in Forum Theatre for the past two decades, I believe in the power of the method and have witnessed its multiple benefits, supporting both individual and community well-being, while also advocating for systemic change: both healing and revolution. This research is based on the belief that Forum Theatre has the potential to support health equity by addressing certain social determinants of health such as coping skills, social isolation, exclusion, discrimination, and historical trauma.

As discussed earlier, this study was developed by using a self-administered version of the qualitative research method known as the CIT (Woolsey, 1986) to explore the tensions that may impede Forum Theatre from supporting health equity with LGBT2SIQ+, GNC, and other marginalized communities. "Critical incidents are short case studies or vignettes depicting a cross-cultural interaction and potential misunderstandings between culturally different individuals" (Dela Cruz et al., 2006, p. 120).

Although I began practicing TO when I studied with Boal twenty years ago, data was drawn from eight Forum Theatre workshops that I facilitated over the last fifteen years. These workshops were initially selected by memory, as workshops that had left me feeling unsettled and concerned for the welfare of one or more participants.

The selection criteria for workshops included:

1. the Forum Theatre theme addressed one or more Government of Canada (2019) defined social determinants of health (social status; employment and working conditions; education and literacy; childhood experiences; physical environments; social supports and coping skills; healthy behaviors; access to health services; social exclusion; experiences of discrimination; historical trauma; gender; culture; and race);
2. a critical incident occurred during the Forum Theatre process, where I perceived and or/ participants confirmed that the personal cost or risks taken by participants was too high; or
3. the ideas shared during the Forum Theatre workshop were in some way problematic vis-à-vis equity goals; and
4. I had a sharp memory of the workshop and access to post-workshop journals.

The referred-to journals are post-workshop reflections where I describe the scenarios and interventions presented, my perceptions, audience feedback, observed participant affect, and my own feelings about the work. My journals often contain ruminations about perceived successes and dissatisfactions, and I noted events or processes that made me concerned for a participant's well-being, as well as any equity issues that I perceive to have been poorly or insufficiently addressed.

Data was also created from the self-administered CIT interviews I conducted, using typical CIT questions: What happened? With whom did it happen? What did the parties concerned feel? What were the consequences immediately and longer term (if I know them)? How did the participants cope (Chell, 2004, p. 49)? I also added: What did I feel? What where the challenges? What, if anything, would I do differently?

Both journals and CIT interviews were analyzed for thematic content using the social determinants of health as a frame of reference. The journals were mined with the following question in mind: What tensions or limitations emerged that were not in the service of either health equity and/or general equity? Because I did not interview workshop participants, the data collected and analyzed relied solely on my perceptions as the Forum Theatre workshop facilitator. After highlighting all the relevant content, I inductively formulated categories, and the main themes that emerged from these categories are discussed in detail below.

The Process

Eight Forum Theatre workshops were analyzed. Half of the workshops focused on topics of homophobia and transphobia and the other half included topics of colonization, the Israeli/Palestinian conflict, racism, and ableism. All of the workshops addressed social exclusion, and how the Forum Theatre itself engages social supports and coping skills (all determinants of health).

SNAPSHOTS FROM FORUM THEATRE WORK

The vignettes below will illustrate unsettling experiences and reflections that have emerged from the last fifteen years of my practice as a Forum Theatre facilitator.

Workshop One: Transphobia

The Safer Spaces Forum Theatre vignette at the beginning of the chapter was performed for a 200-person audience on a college campus. The vignettes were constructed through focus groups in which students, staff, and faculty shared microaggressions they had experienced on campus. Composite and anonymized theatrical vignettes of real experiences were then shared with audience members who volunteered to act out the scenes.

Boal's Forum Theatre invites audience members to leave their traditional role of spectator, and become spect-actors (Boal, 1998, p. 52) who embody the role of the protagonist to offer new actions that address the oppression. Many current TO practitioners diverge from the replace-the-protagonist only rule, and during the Safer Spaces project, the majority of spect-actors chose to embody the role of the teacher who perpetrated the initial microaggression in the scene (first, by assuming that all her students identified on a gender binary, and second, by not addressing the transphobia/cisgenderism that ensued). By taking the place of the teacher, students were able to give their teachers practical ideas about more inclusive pedagogy. One spect-actor who took the role of the teacher offered this solution: "Okay class, if your last name starts with A to M form a group on the left side of the room, and if your last name starts with N to Z form a group on the right side of the room." Another spect-actor playing the teacher: "I will give you each a number—if your number is even, go to the left corner of the room, and if your number is odd, go to the right corner of the room." While their strategies succeeded in avoiding the original microaggression, they did not address the core conflict of cisgenderism and the invisibility of Trans and GNC identities in the classroom.

Later in the workshop, a student spect-actor chose a different strategy: replacing the student experiencing the transphobia, the spect-actor stood up for themselves and said "I am not a girl," and proceeded to stay on the side of the room that represented their male gender identity. I will not assume the actual gender identity of the student who did this intervention, but let us imagine, for the purpose of analyzing the efficacy of the Forum Theatre structure, that this student identifies as a Trans male (the same identity role played on stage). In this case, the intervention that confronted transphobia has the potential to be empowering for both the spect-actor and other Trans and GNC audience members. Of course, the empowerment potential of this intervention is affected by its general audience reception; audience reactions of indifference, disdain and further ridicule will have a very different impact than reactions of validation, affirmation, and celebration.

Now, again for the purpose of exploring Forum Theatre's structural limitations, let us suppose that the spect-actor who intervened identifies as cisgendered. What are the implications of a cisgendered person inhabiting the role of someone who is Trans and giving suggestions to Trans and GNC people? Without the lived experience and a lack of understanding of the power dynamics at play, their proposed intervention risks being ignorant, insensitive, and/or irrelevant. And regardless of the sensitivity and the feasibility or success of the proposed intervention, the impact of having a person from a dominant group tell a person from a targeted group how to cope with their oppression must be considered. A cisgendered person does not run the same real-life or actual in-the-moment vulnerability and risk as a Trans person does trying out the same intervention. How can a cisgendered person know what a Trans person needs in this scenario? And what is the lived experience, identity, and knowledge of the Forum Theatre facilitator to facilitate these complex dynamics?

Joker (Boal, 1979), the TO term for the Forum Theatre facilitator, will be used from here onward. The Joker's role is to facilitate the Forum Theatre structure, guiding participants to support the storyteller otherwise referred to in Forum Theatre language as protagonist (Boal, 2002) in finding ways to cope with or overturn (when possible) their oppression.

I acknowledge that "There is no transhistorical culture-free, disinterested way of knowing" (Lather, 2004, p. 207). As the Joker of the Safer Spaces Forum Theatre, it is important to locate some of the many ways that my own knowledge has been shaped. As a Latina-Canadian-Jewish, Queer, middle income, highly educated, neurotypical, able-bodied, cisgendered woman in my late thirties (at the time of this workshop), how do I work across difference and make appropriate facilitation decisions that mitigate risks and vulnerability for Trans and Gender-Diverse individuals? How do I as a cisgendered person know what is needed? These considerations speak to the power dynamics inherent in representation, a topic that will be discussed in further detail in the results section.

Workshop Two: Cisgenderism

Take-Two was a Forum Theatre project that took place in a university setting. The project aimed at supporting educators in understanding how to address typical microaggressions that occur in classroom settings. The vignettes for this project were created by speaking to students from different cultural groups about their experiences of microaggressions on campus. Unlike the previous Safer Spaces project, these workshop participants were comprised solely of educators. Also dissimilar to the previous forum, Take-Two's theatrical vignettes were prepared by professional actors who had prepared the scenes in advance.

> *Sam* (*student*): I can't keep track of the of "he" and "sirs" and "man" and "brother" and other gendered terms I get called regularly. Each one is like an unintentional punch in the gut. I am not these things. I have had classmates use words like "normal" or "regular" to refer to cisgendered people, implying that my gender is not normal. Gender is not a binary where the only choices are "men" and "women," but many teachers force us into these categories without realizing it. Some of my classes are in buildings that don't have gender inclusive washrooms, making me choose between genders that I am not.

Professor: I hope everyone did their readings this week. It will be a hard class to keep up with if you have not. Okay, let's see. Triple question: What was Mead's main argument about sexuality in this chapter? And also what were Friedman's following critiques? And then, what were the critiques of those critiques?

(*Two students, Sam and Karen, raise their hands.*)

Sam: Mead was ahead of her time, acknowledging publicly that sexuality is fluid, that while we may all have preferences, all people can have relationships with people from different genders (*she described gender on a binary*), and her ethnographic research backed this up, showing that before marriage, women had sex with women and men had sex with men (*again describing gender on a binary*). Friedman's critique was that Mead is biased, he did not find the same thing when he came to Samoa years later, and he felt that Mead's bias is because she herself was a Lesbian (*laugh out loud*)* and therefore she saw in others what she lived herself. Friedman was critiqued because of his homophobia, suggesting that a *Lesbian researcher* cannot be objective. Mead did not self-identify as Lesbian, by the way. Friedman was then again critiqued because he went to Samoa after Christian missionaries were there for many decades, effectively changing the culture in many ways, especially indoctrinating people in Western homophobic heterosexist forms of sexuality; i.e. love should be between a man and a woman.

Professor: Nice synthesis Sam. . . . Karen, you also had your hand up, would you add anything to what he said?

Karen: (*awkward silence*) Umm. . . . Yeah I think they got it all, but umm Sam goes by "they."

Professor: They?

(*Professor is confused. Sam feels put on the spot to explain their gender identity. Does so briefly.*)

Professor: Thank you for explaining, so just to make sure I have this right, Sam, your preferred pronouns are "they"?

Sam nods. (*it is clear they feel put off by the question*)

Professor: (*sincerely*) I learn something new every day. I learn so much from you students. Thank you.

After class:

Professor: Sam, can I talk to you for a moment? (*Sam walks up to the teacher.*)

Professor: Sam, thank you for telling me today. You know, I'm not too aware of . . . (*searches her mind for the proper words*) . . . Trans and Gender Non-Conforming community, so you can be my teacher.

This scenario reflects the misgendering and outing that many GNC students experience by their professors and well-intentioned fellow students. Workshop participants in Take-Two engaged in many promising interventions that acknowledged more inclusive pedagogy. For instance, one spect-actor playing the professor in the scene shared their pronouns and invited students to share theirs. Another spect-actor professor sent an email inviting students to share anything that would be important for professors to know about them, including their gender pronouns.

However, a number of proposed interventions also showed resistance toward inclusion. One professor in the audience protested that the microaggressions were not intentional and that professors should not be held accountable or expected to know their students' gender pronouns. Another professor engaged in a further microaggression during their intervention. Without breaking the role play, the actors remained in character and did an excellent job in addressing the new microaggression; however, a comment from a participant in a post-workshop feedback indicated that they found the audience members' microaggression demoralizing and would have felt more supported if I, the facilitator, had explicitly called out the microaggression. Jokering (Boal, 1979) requires an enormous level of presence and also the ability to respond spontaneously to the unfolding content. There are times when the Joker needs to respond to further oppression emerging from spect-actors. Is it enough to facilitate the actors in responding to ignorant ideas through the Forum Theatre method? It appears that some participants would have felt more supported had the Joker addressed the emerging microaggressions directly, further making visible the oppression.

"While Theatre of the Oppressed is usually utilised in support of politically progressive agendas, the work participants initiate and the choices they make do not automatically orient towards social justice" (Snyder-Young, 2011, p. 30). As described in the workshop above, not all participants or interventions will be made in the service of equity. As Dani Snyder-Young (2011) reflects, "who decides how the lines between oppressor and oppressed are drawn? What happens when one community of spect-actors defines their own 'liberation' in ways oppressing another?" (p. 32), and perhaps even more importantly, when this happens, and it frequently does, do all audience members feel sufficiently supported by how the Joker responds?

A similar phenomenon occurred in Workshop Three.

Workshop Three: Creating Our Families

The following Forum Theatre project, Creating Our Families, took place in various ART clinics as well as an LGBT2SIQ+ community center. I was hired to create a research dissemination strategy for a qualitative research study about the experiences of Queer and Trans peoples accessing ART. Using the interview transcript, I created Forum Theatre pieces to illustrate the microaggressions experienced by LGBT2SIQ+ clients. In order to give back to the research informants who shared their stories, the Forum Theatre was presented at a well-established LGBT2SIQ+ community center. As cited in Using Theatre to Disseminate LGBT People's Experiences with Assisted Human Reproduction Services (2019), after participating in the Forum Theatre, one community member commented, "The forum theatre experience gave me a feeling of hope. . . . I learned that the research hadn't just ended up in a journal I would never read. I actually saw my story and many other Queer and Trans stories out there in a real way" (par. 6).

Attempting to influence structural change, the research was also presented in different ART clinics, giving staff an opportunity to practice doing better. Medical and administrative employees shared their enthusiasm for the work, claiming, "This presentation highlighted practical ways in which we can make ART services truly accessible to the LGBTQ community" and "The changes that can be made at the health care levels to improve patient welfare are small but have a big impact" (Tarasoff et al., 2014, p. 139). Tarasoff et al. (2014) speak to the effectiveness of the workshop that encouraged medical staff "to rethink previously held assumptions about LGBTQ people and their ART service needs" (p. 139).

The following feedback from a service provider further illustrates consciousness raising in action: "I have to admit, I had my doubts about a performance-based workshop, but it was incredibly effective. As far as we have come with people of the LGBTQ community having access to ARTs, the experiences as performed in the workshop were shocking, eye-opening and traumatic. From the things that we can easily remedy to be more sensitive, such as offering genderless bathrooms, to the way consent forms are drafted making assumptions as to gender and sexuality, this presentation highlighted practical ways in which we can make ART services truly accessible to the LGBTQ community" (Cohen, 2012). As evidenced by participant feedback, the workshops seemed to create both possibilities for healing and advocacy/conscientization.

Despite the workshops' success, it is important to draw attention to a challenge that occurred during one of the presentations. One of the Forum Theatre actors who identifies as belonging to a LGBT2SIQ+ community described the emotional burden of replaying oppressive situations and contending with prejudicial strategies offered by ART staff. Although this is always an anticipated risk of any Forum Theatre project, anticipating the risk is not enough to prevent what this actor framed as injury. Repeating traumatic situations evokes real feelings and experiences of harm. This is problematic for a theatre that intends to promote healing and social change. What responsibility does the Forum Theatre team have toward the actors and the audience members who may feel further impacted by potential prejudices presented by the spect-actors?

Berenice Fisher (1994) explains, "Theatre of the Oppressed assumes that someone—the group using the technique or the person introducing it—has a fairly developed consciousness. Without such consciousness, Theatre of the Oppressed runs the risk of reproducing rather than representing oppression" (p. 190). I did not Joker this particular workshop; however, similar to the one I did facilitate, a participant, this time one of the actors, felt that the Joker did not do enough to address the oppression occurring in the moment. Given the prevalence of microaggressions, and the complexity in responding to them artfully in the moment, Jokers would do well to think about what can be added to the Forum Theatre structure or its facilitation that might better attend to participants' needs post-microaggression.

Some brief descriptions about the additional analyzed Forum Theatre workshops are included below.

Workshop Four: Homophobia, Setting; a Forum Theatre Facilitator Training

A Lesbian participant shared a story about how her partner coped with homophobia. Interventions from heterosexual spect-actors centered on the Lesbian partner's anger and not the injustice of homophobia.

Workshop Five: Israeli/Palestinian Conflict, Setting; a Youth Peace Camp

Israeli and Palestinian workshop participants share their respective experiences of the Israeli/Palestinian conflict. In an attempt to stand in solidarity, a six-foot-tall male Israeli spect-actor took the place of a four-foot-tall Palestinian woman who had shared a story where she had been spat on by an Israeli soldier. The Israeli spect-actor proposed an intervention where he told the offending Israeli soldier about his rights and that he would be reporting his unethical and unprofessional behavior. Gender, height, ethnicity, and the social context of war were not adequately taken into account with the proposed intervention, and the Palestinian participants quickly pointed out the infeasibility of the presented solution. An important process of conscientization was occurring where Israeli participants were learning about injustices that as pre-military youth they had not imagined possible. Unfortunately, despite the Palestinian participants denouncing the intervention as unrealistic and the informative discussion that ensued, the Palestinian woman left the workshop upset with the intervention, feeling that it was implied that she could have acted more courageously in the moment.

Workshop Six: Colonization, Setting; a Youth Social Justice Retreat

A First Nations student was suspended after becoming violent with a classmate who had killed a spider. Interventions by settler spect-actors revolved around the First Nations student's anger, neglecting the cultural context, and ridiculing the First Nations student's insistence that the spider was an important character in the story and must be personified by an actor. Further detail will be provided in the analysis below.

Workshop Seven: Racism, Setting; a University Conference

A group composed of white European-ancestry graduate students engaged in Forum Theatre where one graduate student shared a story about being bullied by another graduate student in his research laboratory. The bully's cultural background was not initially revealed. Close to the end of the workshop, when it was revealed that the bully was of Latin American origin, an intervention that was thought to be successful by the general group was proposed by a white European ancestry spect-actor. The intervention proposed relied on stereotypes about Latin American people, collapsing all Latin American cultures together and making multiple assumptions about the Latin American student's intentions.

Workshop Eight: Ableism, Setting; a Peace Education Conference

A caregiver of a young woman with cerebral palsy asked for support in addressing the multiple forms of ableism her client experienced on a regular basis. Some interventions located the young woman's mother as one of her oppressors. One of the audience members whom I had a personal relationship with left the workshop early, visibly upset. In debriefing with her afterward, I learned about her family background, where her sister had a debilitating disease similar to cerebral palsy and that she felt that the audience members were being invalidating and ignorant of the hardship of a parent raising a child with disabilities, who faces stigma and financial and time limitations.

Emerging Categories and Themes

As I reviewed these workshops, the following salient categories and themes emerged: (1) *Equity concepts* of power, positionality, working across difference, representation, invisibility, absence, and silence; (2) *Emotional states* included anger, shame, vulnerability; (4) Forum Theatre *Structural components* included heterogeneous groups versus homogeneous groups, spontaneous versus prepared forums, and aesthetic distance; and (5) *Health equity* concepts of safety, coping, social isolation, and discrimination.

RESULTS

Can Forum Theatre deliver what Boal and his enthusiasts say that it can, that is, both revolution and healing? The review of eight workshops has revealed that three main tensions interfere with health equity potential: Excessive Vulnerability; Heterogeneous Structures; and a poorly managed Larger Equity Goals Versus Individual Well-Being Tensions.

Tension One: Excessive Vulnerability

One theme that seemed to connect across all categories was that of vulnerability. I need to clarify that as a therapist and educator by profession, I do not believe that individual or systemic change can happen without a certain degree of vulnerability. I understand vulnerability and discomfort to be natural and inevitable parts of healing and learning. The vulnerability that I am concerned about here is of a different stripe, an unrewarded one that is not in the service of healing and equity, but rather to its detriment. I am referring to an excessive vulnerability that is often accompanied by shame and/or victim-blaming.

At the heart of TO work is the principle that we are all experts of our own lives and that people should speak for themselves. I do not wish to speak for my workshop participants nor could I accurately assume their perspectives, which would be as diverse as the individuals with whom I have had the honor to work. Rather, I approach the topic of vulnerability from my perspective as a Joker who strives to facilitate Forum Theatres that contribute toward the justice and healing for those involved.

Vulnerability is intrinsic to the Forum Theatre structure: the vulnerability of offering a sensitive part of one's life story and risking that it may not be understood; the vulnerability of working across difference with people from diverse positionalities and access to power; and the vulnerability of further exposing oneself to ignorance regarding one's lived experience but also potentially to further ridicule, social exclusion, and prejudice. Also inherent to the Forum Theatre structure is a frequent storyteller experience of feeling discomfort when others offer suggestions of how individuals could have behaved differently at the time. Defensiveness and embarrassment are common results of this structural element. The potential for these vulnerabilities is present in each forum.

A Joker committed to their workshop participants' well-being can address vulnerabilities both pre-emptively and as they emerge. However, when the workshop is large, such as the 200+ person Safer Spaces workshop, it is difficult to address the multiple simultaneous and unnoticed vulnerabilities that occur. How did the spect-actor who offered the intervention confronting transphobia feel during and after the workshop? Was it a positive experience for them? And what is the experience of the other GNC and Trans people in the audience who may be holding their breath to see how fellow classmates respond to the scenario? Vulnerability runs through each scenario.

The spect-actors in Workshops Four (addressing homophobia) and Six (addressing colonization) seemed to use the Forum Theatre structure to socialize and even to ridicule the storytellers. In Workshop Four, the spect-actors, who were largely heterosexual, presented solutions that attempted to bypass and ignore the resentment resulting from experienced homophobia, and modeled a softened expression of anger. The proposed interventions felt like judgments on how the protagonist's partner expressed anger and there were efforts to socialize what spect-actors felt to be more socially appropriate expressions of emotion. For example, one spect-actor suggested that the partner should take meditation classes to control her anger, while another one suggested therapy, and a third spect-actor role played the scene speaking calmly, showing no sign of hurt or of anger at the homophobic aggression. Rather than situating homophobia as the antagonist in the situation, the proposed interventions located the protagonist's partner as the problem.

As the Joker, I uncomfortably watched this scenario unfold, while also perceiving the protagonist's discomfort. I hoped that the Forum Theatre structure could rectify the unfolding situation and I used a Forum Theatre convention of asking the storyteller whether the solutions presented were "magical," a term used to describe the viability of a solution. While the storyteller expressed discontent with the proposed solutions, she was not able to, or did not feel safe enough to express her discomfort publicly. Later, the storyteller privately expressed that the Forum Theatre process was a shaming one that minimized and made invisible her experience of homophobia. With her consent, I stepped outside the traditional Forum Theatre structure and facilitated a discussion with workshop participants the following day, naming some of the processes that had occurred and pointing out the tendency and frequency with which Forum Theatre's structure could invite oppressive dynamics of socializing and inadvertently shaming the other.

Similarly, socialization processes occurred in Workshop Six when the Indigenous protagonist insisted that one of the spect-actors impersonate a spider. The spect-actors, who were largely settlers, joked around and did not take the impersonation of the spider seriously. The spect-actors in the scene and the other audience members found the protagonist's insistence in honoring the spider's life humorous. There was a clear absence of effective cross-cultural communication. The Forum Theatre furthered the violence that was originally experienced by the protagonist by not acknowledging his cultural values and ridiculing him in his attempts to express his holistic view of the world and the importance of all living beings. To little avail, I reminded the youth participants many times that their role as allies required them to attempt to understand the protagonist's desires so as to act in solidarity with him. In a post-workshop check-in with the protagonist, he expressed to me that the Forum Theatre experience helped him concretize and name the xenophobia and colonizing attitudes that he had been a recipient of throughout the whole social justice retreat.

In both Workshops Four and Six, the proposed interventions did not feel like attempts to stand in solidarity with the protagonists, but rather they seemed to be exercises in telling them how to act in accordance with dominant values and behaviors. Working across difference creates opportunities for cultural exchange and understanding. And in post-workshop discussion, some participants did self-report the Forum Theatre's role in furthering their understanding of the impacts of homophobia and ethnocentrism. While these examples demonstrate Forum Theatre's potential for sensitization, or conscientization, as the Joker during these workshops, I ask myself what is the personal cost of revolution? And, is it too high?

Tension Two: Heterogeneous Structure

As seen in the examples above, particular Forum Theatre structures contribute to vulnerability. Working with groups that share many of the same cultural identifiers is certainly different than working across difference. Perhaps the most pronounced form of vulnerability arising from Forum Theatres Four through Eight was due to interventions being proposed by people from vastly different positionalities. Different lived experiences, access to power, and cultural realities risk interventions not being useful at best and replicating violence at worst.

Fisher (1994) maintains that Forum Theatre works best in groups with a high degree of homogeneity, creating opportunities for spect-actors to culturally identify with the protagonist. Moreover, Moreno's (2018) Forum Theatre research with LGBT2SIQ+ communities shows that the courage to face oppression increases in the presence of other Queer-spectrum or Trans-spectrum youth. There are important benefits in engaging in same community Forum Theatre work. However, Younghee Lee (2015) points out that due to intersectionality and the multicultural societies in which most practitioners work, working within one homogeneous community is impossible.

Thinking about representation is essential when engaging in equity work. Workshops Seven (addressing bullying) and Eight (addressing ableism), for example, evoked a vulnerability exacerbated due to absence of representation. Workshop Seven attempted to engage solutions of cross-cultural communication without having sufficient cross-cultural representation. The workshop took place at a university where workshop participants were predominantly white, and involved discussions about a perceived bully who came from an unidentified Latin American culture. Stereotypes and assumptions were used in the interventions proposed. As the only Latinx person present, I seemed to be the only person bothered by the solutions presented. As the Joker in this situation, I was in a unique position of power that enabled me to take time from the workshop's traditional structure to address my discomfort. This experience made visible the challenge of accurate representation, which is impossible when there is only one participant of a particular cultural background. Of additional concern, had I not been present, the emerging stereotypes would not have been confronted, and a new set of microaggressions would have been left invisible and silent.

Workshop Eight employed a similar dilemma of absence of representation in that people with cerebral palsy and other visible debilitating health conditions were not present among workshop participants. Family caregivers for people with disabilities were also seemingly absent. The only known family caregiver present did not feel safe enough to share her dissenting opinion and thus remained silent, only sharing her experience with me after the workshop. If it had not been for our personal relationship, and the participant's courage to share with me afterward, I would never have learned about this participant's negative experience. Lee (2015) speaks to how linguistic and cultural barriers can contribute to silence in Forum Theatre, and calls for Jokers to facilitate more dialogue about the challenges in crossing identity. How might the Forum Theatre structure and facilitation style expand to create more safety to invite dissenting voices to participate? In the deficits of representation and the silences of unsafety, enormous wisdom is lost, detrimental to both equity and the participants' well-being.

Tension Three: Larger Equity Goals versus Individual Well-Being

While working across cultures evokes important challenges, it also creates necessary spaces for conscientization and equity work. Workshop Two (Take-Two) and Workshop Three (Creating Our Families) were carefully constructed to engage people in positions of power. The goal of both these workshops was to help participants learn about the inequitable systems in which they were participating, and to practice behavioral change that would carry into the classroom and into ART clinics. A tension between well-being and larger equity goals is illustrated in Workshop Three. In addition to successfully meeting systemic change objectives (as indicated by participants who self-reported change in knowledge, attitude, and projected behavior), one of the actors described their experience of the workshop as injurious. The actor reported feelings of anger and of hurt as she recounted the intolerability of reliving microaggressions produced by medical staff members' prejudicial interventions.

The question remains, is the personal cost of "revolution" too high? A Lesbian participant leaves a Forum Theatre feeling judgment by heterosexual participants; a Palestinian woman feels belittled and judged by the presentation of unviable solutions toward her oppression; a First Nations youth is maligned and ridiculed for his values; the absence of representation contributes to stereotypes of Latinx people; and a workshop participant leaves feeling angry and silenced by judgmental propositions about family caregivers. None of these encounters seem to promote these particular participants' well-being. While working with diverse groups of people creates important opportunities for social change, conscientization, and sensitizing people in power to do better, also needed are intentional structures that adequately address the inherent power dynamics of the work. Otherwise, these workshops risk reproducing the same microaggressions or violence that negatively impacted participants' well-being in the first place.

Mady Schutzman (1994) notes that Forum Theatre often focuses on the emotional personal nature of stories being told with less or no time focused on the systemic injustice(s) at the root of the problem. I argue that this individualized focus is not only problematic for larger revolutionary goals, but also problematic for the participants' well-being, because not acknowledging power, positionality, working across difference, representation, invisibility, absence, and silences that are ubiquitous within Forum Theatre processes negatively impacts the well-being of the most vulnerable participants.

DISCUSSION

Forum Theatre has a great potential to address injustices that are detrimental to minoritized peoples' health. Forum Theatre uses storytelling to address real-life experiences of social exclusion, discrimination, and historical trauma (social determinants of health); and in the process, it addresses further social determinants of health by reducing social isolation (Erel, Reynolds, & Kaptani, 2017), building community (Cohen-Cruz, 2006; Erel, Reynolds, & Kaptani, 2017; Saeed, 2015), and improving coping skills, helping Queer-spectrum and Trans-spectrum youth learn how to address oppression (Moreno, 2018).

What conditions need to be put in place to obtain such worthy benefits? Jokers describe creating a sense of safety among participants to be a primordial task of the Forum Theatre (Moreno, 2018). It is this sense of safety that allows for the conditions necessary for behavioral and attitudinal change (Somers, 2008). However, within society's inequitable structures, the full achievement of safety is likely not feasible. As recounted above, participants in these eight workshops expressed feeling judged, misunderstood, hurt, and angry due to microaggressive events that took place during the Forum Theatre process. Furthermore, judgment and perceived rejection are elements of minority stress that negatively impact LGBT2SIQ+ individuals' well-being. A natural tension seems to arise between the structures that lend themselves to potential, larger systemic change (heterogeneous workshops that work across difference) and more homogeneous structures that potentially limit microaggressive exposure to targeted participants.

My concern is for both the well-being of individuals risking their vulnerability in the Forum Theatre space as well as the enhancement of Forum Theatre's possibilities for furthering health equity. What are the optimal conditions for a change that is both systemic and that takes the individual well-being of its participants under consideration?

RECOMMENDATIONS FOR JOKERS

I have put together a list of recommendations that I believe would have been helpful to my younger, less experienced, Joker self. Although the Joker can never control the relational outcome of Forum Theatre, in hindsight, I believe that had I known then what I know now, I might have left these eight workshops feeling more satisfied with Forum Theatre's contribution toward health equity. Expanding the Critical Social Consciousness Guidelines created for Ethnodramatherapy (Snow & Bleuer, 2020, forthcoming), the following recommendations modify this model: (1) Analyze Power and Assess Relational Risks and Benefits; (2) Share Power by Engaging the Conditions for Authentic Collaboration; and (3) Design Ethnodramatherapy Projects to Engage the Most Systemic Change Possible, to create a new frame adapted for Jokers concerned with both healing and systemic transformation:

"1–Analyze power" (Snow & Bleuer, 2020). Jokers should take time to recognize and address equity concerns of *representation* (who is in the room), *absence* (who is missing from the room), *positionality* (how do our intersecting cultural identities and lived experiences prepare us to understand ourselves and the other), *working across difference* (what tools do we have to work with our differences), *silence* (what realities may impede participation), *invisibility* (who and what are we ignoring), and the concept that relates to all of the above concepts, *power* (how do all these pieces fit together to address the dynamic in the room, who benefits and who is targeted by the Forum Theatre work).

It is important to consider the different ways in which the Forum Theatre structure changes the above questions about power. This chapter has already shared some of the challenges of working in heterogeneous environments, where the spect-actor offering a solution may hold different lived experiences than the protagonist with whom they are meant to stand in solidarity with. And what of the Joker's lived experience limitations? Schutzman (1994) points out that "Boal and many North American practitioners of TO are working with groups to which they themselves do not belong, and thus represent, ironically, the very element of oppression the exclusion of which the group is founded upon" (p. 141). How then can a Joker effectively work across difference and power?

Power dynamics change with different spect-actor configurations. Consider Take-Two (university professors as allies addressing microaggressions experienced by their students) and Creating Our Families (assisted reproductive technologies staff addressing their own workplace microaggressions against their clients) as two examples of Forum Theatres where spect-actors aspired to be allies on a particular topic. Returning to the questions of representation, positionality and working across difference is the concern that the protagonist is not present in the room to share their perspectives about whether or not the spect-actors are engaging effectively as allies.

It seems inadequate to rely on the traditional Forum Theatre structure to rectify power imbalances within the work. When done with heterogeneous groups, the Forum Theatre structure will naturally prioritize conscientization and the learning of the oppressor or bystander instead of the vulnerability of person who has courageously shared their story. Moreover it is not enough to just name the oppression, as was seen in the Israeli Palestinian workshop, where a frank discussion did not help the storyteller feel well with the process.

The multiple power dynamics that exist when both oppressed and oppressor are present may very well exacerbate minority stress, enhancing social isolation, fear of rejection and/or actual rejection and discrimination, perpetuating the very violence Forum Theatre seeks to address. Exposing participants to the factors that make up minority stress will not always be worth the revolution. There will be occasions when it would be conducive for the healing of targeted communities to work among themselves without the presence of the dominant other. It can be restorative and empowering to connect with community on issues of shared social discrimination, without needing to explain, defend, and justify what one knows and has lived to be true.

"2–Share power by engaging the conditions for authentic collaboration" (Snow & Bleuer, 2020). Cross-cultural spaces are emotionally laborious and vulnerable for those who share their stories, and the embodied nature of

Forum Theatre where the storyteller physically exposes their vulnerability in front of an audience adds multiple additional layers of susceptibility that necessitate informed consent. Jokers must find ways to elucidate the potential risks inherent in the work. As Joker David Diamond (1994) puts it, "the richest and most productive way to work with oppressed groups is to help them find their own voice, not to speak for them" (p. 35). Participants should be informed about the limitations, vulnerability, and potential tensions that may arise in Forum Theatre work. Sharing the knowledge about potential cost of participating is not only respectful, but it also fundamental to sharing power.

Authentic collaboration can be furthered through the use of theatre. If Theatre of the Oppressed is a tool for revolution, then its techniques should be used to explore the inequity that causes excessive vulnerability in the work. Aesthetic distance is an artistic process that Bleuer, Chin, and Sakamoto (2018) found could be useful when working towards equity. Aesthetic distance refers to using artistic processes to help people access all of their resources both cognitive and emotional (Landy, 1983, 1996). Some theatre processes elicit emotional connection while others promote rationalization and intellectualization. Aesthetic distance seeks to find a balance that mitigates vulnerability thereby creating conditions that are optimal for learning and change. Finding aesthetic balance can enhance fuller participation by supporting participants to remain emotionally present for this challenging work.

Using theatre to illuminate unspoken dynamics can also enhance participation. Creating theatrical images that concretize the challenges of representation, positionality, absence, and silence can better prepare a group to share power and address complex group dynamics that impact participants' emotional safety. Boal (2002) states, "Images are polysemic—they can have many meanings" (p. 139). Perception is also polysemic and deeply contingent on context and positionality. Images have great potential to invite and contain diverse and divergent perspectives, elucidating and creating room for different positions and lived experiences.

Perhaps the Israeli/Palestinian workshop would have had a different outcome had it been pre-empted with image theatre work about the meta-process of engaging Forum Theatre between Israeli and Palestinian youth. Might some meta image theatre have changed the colonizing attitudes of the youth in the social justice retreat? Perhaps addressing representation, positionality, and absence would have helped university conference workshop participants tread more cautiously around stereotyping cultures that were not well represented in the room. And similarly, might this structural addition to Forum Theatre work create more safety to invite the dissenting voice of the caregiver who was upset with what she perceived to be an unjust representation of a character with whom she identified?

"3–Design projects to engage the most systemic change possible" (Snow & Bleuer, 2020). Take-Two, Creating Our Families, and Safer Spaces make design decisions about who to invite so as to engage the most systemic change possible. Take-Two and Creating Our Families focused on spect-actors in positions of power to make a difference regarding classroom-based microaggressions and prejudice and discrimination experienced by LGBT2SIQ+ assisted reproductive technology users. Safer Spaces followed the Forum Theatre process with a Legislative Theatre process (Boal, 1998) that asks participants questions about what laws or policies should be put in place to address the injustices explored through the Forum Theatre work. Safer Spaces participants shared important ideas about policy change that were then shared with the college administration.

Adding to the Original Critical Social Consciousness Guidelines created for Ethnodramatherapy (Snow & Bleuer, 2020), is a fourth element that supports Forum Theatre work.

4–Learn about the mental health impacts of microaggressions and trauma. With the exception of the Safer Spaces Forum Theatre and the Take-Two Forum Theatre, the other Forum Theatre workshops took place prior to me becoming a therapist and engaging in doctoral work on microaggressions. In my training as a therapist I learned about how nervous systems respond to feeling judged and rejected. I also learned about the emotional impacts of trauma. During my doctoral work I studied the mental health impact of microaggressions. As a result of this learning, my Joker work has shifted dramatically, giving me tools to address participant well-being.

Responding to trauma stories and the health and well-being impacts of microaggressions is challenging. The traditional Forum Theatre does not adequately address the emotions that accompany the traumas lived by storytellers. Moreover, given the prevalence of microaggressions that occur during the Forum Theatre process and the complexity in responding to them artfully, Jokers would do well to learn more about the impact of microaggressions on health and well-being. Image theatre work can pre-emptively warm-up a group to possible nervous system reactions that may be activated throughout the workshop (fight, flight, and freeze). Anticipating defensiveness and the ways our bodies respond to protect us from stress may support participants in experiencing more control and understanding of their bodies and emotions during the workshop, which may in turn contribute to participant well-being.

CONCLUSION

Forum Theatre is seemingly both a great health promotion intervention (Warheit, 2017) and a risky vulnerable endeavor that demands a great deal from its participants. Are revolution and individual well-being mutually exclusive? Or, can we have both revolution and healing? Schutzman (1994) explores the space where activist and therapeutic agendas coincide, saying, "In fact, they necessarily redefine each other . . . politics and therapy once again implicate each other as inseparable, interwoven threads within the social fabric" (p. 148). Health equity requires a focus on both the larger systemic inequalities and the smaller relational injustices that make up these systems, both revolution and healing.

There will be occasions when it will be conducive for the healing of targeted communities to work among themselves without the presence of the dominant other. The multiple power dynamics that exist in the presence of both the oppressed and the oppressor may very well exacerbate minority stress, and thereby enhance social isolation, the fear of rejection and/or actual rejection and discrimination, perpetuating the very violence Forum Theatre seeks to address. Exposing participants to the factors that make up minority stress will not always be worth the revolution. Rather, it could be more restorative and empowering to connect with community on shared injustices, without needing to explain, defend, and justify what one knows and has lived to be true.

Under other conditions, and with informed consent, collaborative cross-cultural Forum Theatre spaces have great social change potential. There are great benefits from spaces where communities can learn from each other, fumble, make mistakes, and grow together. Storytelling about injustice promotes learning about inequity, and hopefully increases empathy (Frederick, 1995; Keehn, 2015) and motivates people to take action.

For these benefits to be felt, the Forum Theatre process must attune to its participants. In therapy, the process of attunement refers to an "affective state" (Beauregard & Long, 2019, p. 128) where clients feel deeply understood by their therapist. Forum Theatre that promotes well-being amongst its participants requires an attunement, where those risking the most in the process by sharing their vulnerable stories feel understood, valued, and validated by the audience members who participate in seeking solutions. The Forum Theatre scenarios shared above highlight examples of misattunement between Forum Theatre participants. Positive attunement has many benefits including the regulation of one's nervous system, and this is of particular relevance for Queer, Trans, and Gender Non-Conforming people who have experienced repetitive relational traumas rooted in transphobia and homophobia.

When the right systemic elements are in place, and both Joker and spect-actors have explicitly considered and played with power, positionality, working across difference, representation, invisibility, absence, and silence, Forum Theatre has the capacity to attune more consistently, becoming a meaningful advocate for health equity. When successful, Forum Theatre has been shown to change inner and outer realities—supporting LGBT2SIQ+ people to learn about their identities (McClimens & Scott, 2007; Sanders, 2004), address internalized oppression (Burns et al., 2015), build the courage to face everyday oppression (Moreno, 2018), and change policy and law (Boal, 1998). For LGBT2SIQ+ people whose identities have been discriminated against, invisibilized, and subjected to other forms of heteronormativity, becoming the director of one's own story and confronting oppressive actions in front of a captive audience has great self-efficacy and empowerment potential. When inequitable systems marginalize, invisiblize, and enact violence on LGBT2SIQ+ and other targeted communities, TO tools can create spaces that fight back. The challenge is to design Forum Theatre spaces that create opportunities for personal empowerment while maximizing potential for larger systemic change. Analyzing power, enhancing the possibility for authentic collaboration among all stakeholders, and working in trauma- and microaggression-informed ways will strengthen Forum Theatre designs and the possibility of achieving aspirations of both healing and revolution. Boal (1992) believed that human beings have the power to change the world, explaining, "Theatre can help us build our future, rather than just waiting for it" (p. xxxi). What Forum Theatre project might you design to create healing and revolution in your community?

NOTE

1. A special thank you for the generous support and critical eye of my friend and first reader, Marjan.

REFERENCES

Ahrens, C. E., Rich, M. D., & Ullman, J. B. (2011). Rehearsing for real life: The impact of the InterACT sexual assault prevention program on self-reported likelihood of engaging in bystander interventions. *Violence Against Women*, *17*(6), 760–776. https://doi.org/10.1177/1077801211410212

Boal, A. (1979). *Theatre of the Oppressed* (C. A. McBride & M.-O. L. McBride, Trans.). New York, NY: Urizen Books.

Boal. A. (1992). Games for acors and non-actors. London and New York: Routledge.

Boal, A. (1998). *Legislative theatre: Using performance to make politics.* New York, NY: Routledge.

Boal, A. (2002). *Games for actors and non-actors* (2nd ed., A. Jackson, Trans.). New York, NY: Routledge.

Burns, M. A., Beti, B. N., Okuto, M. E., Muwanguzi, D., & Sanyu, L. (2015). Forum theatre for conflict transformation in east Africa: The domain of the possible. *African Conflict & Peacebuilding Review*, *1*(5), 136–151. http://www.jstor.org/stable/10.2979/africonfpeacrevi.5.1.136

Chell, E. (2004). Critical incident technique. In C. Cassell & G. Symon (Eds.), *Essential guide to qualitative methods in organizational research* (pp. 45–60). Thousand Oaks, CA: Sage.

Cochran, S. D. (2001). Emerging issues in research on lesbians' and gay men's mental health: Does sexual orientation really matter? *American Psychologist*, *56*(11), 931–947. https://doi.org/10.1037/0003–066x.56.11.931

Cohen, S. R. (2012, June 29). In honour of pride week—Assisted reproductive technologies (ARTs) and the LGBTQ community. *Fertility Law Canada*. Retrieved from http://www.fertilitylawcanada.com/fertility-law-canada-blog/in-honour-of-pride-week-assisted-reproductive-technologies-arts-and-the-lgbtq-community

Cohen-Cruz, J. (2006). Storytelling. Redefining the private: From personal storytelling to political act. In J. Cohen-Cruz & M. Schutzman (Eds.), *A Boal companion: Dialogues on theatre and cultural politics* (pp. 103–113). New York, NY: Routledge.

Conron, K. J., Mimiaga, M. J., & Landers, S. J. (2010). A population-based study of sexual orientation identity and gender differences in adult health. *American Journal of Public Health*, *100*(10), 1953–1960. https://doi.org/10.2105/AJPH.2009.174169

Day, L. (2002). "Putting yourself in other people's shoes": The use of forum theatre to explore refugee and homeless issues in schools. *Journal of Moral Education*, *31*(1), 21–34. https://doi.org/10.1080/03057240120111418

Dela Cruz, K. C. K., Salzman, M. B., Brislin, R., & Losch, N. (2006). Hawaiian attributional perspectives on intercultural interactions in higher education: Development of an intercultural sensitizer. *International Journal of Intercultural Relations*, *30*(1), 119–140. https://doi.org/10.1016/j.ijintrel.2005.08.008

Diamond, D. (1994). Out of the silence: Headlines theatre and power plays. In M. Schutzman & J. Cohen-Cruz (Eds.), *Playing Boal: Theatre, therapy and activism* (pp. 35–52). New York, NY: Routledge.

Erel, U., Reynolds, T., & Kaptani, I. (2017). Participatory theatre for transformative social research. *Qualitative Research*, *17*(3), 302–312. https://doi.org/10.1177%2F1468794117696029

Fisher, B. (1994). Feminist acts: Women, pedagogy, and Theatre of the Oppressed. In M. Schutzman & J. Cohen-Cruz (Eds.), *Playing Boal: Theatre, therapy and activism* (pp. 185–197). New York, NY: Routledge.

Francis, D. (2013). "You know the homophobic stuff is not in me, like us, it's out there": Using participatory theatre to challenge heterosexism and heteronormativity in a South African school. *South African Journal of Education*, *33*(4), 1–14. http://www.scielo.org.za/scielo.php?script=sci_arttext&pid=S0256–01002013000400011

Frederick, P. (1995). Walking on eggs: Mastering the dreaded diversity discussion. *College Teaching*, *43*(3), 83–92. https://eric.ed.gov/?id=EJ513728

Fredriksen-Goldsen, K. I., Cook-Daniels, L., Kim, H.-J., Erosheva, E. A., Emlet, C. A., Hoy-Ellis, C. P., Goldsen, J., & Muraco, A. (2014). The physical and mental health of transgender older adults: An at-risk and underserved population. *Gerontologist*, *54*(3), 488–500. https://doi.org/10.1093/geront/gnt021

Fredriksen-Goldsen, K. I., Kim, H.-J., Emlet, C. A., Muraco, A., Erosheva, E. A., Hoy-Ellis, C. P., Goldsen, J., & Petry, H. (2011). The aging and health report: Disparities and resilience among lesbian, gay, bisexual, and transgender older adults. *National LGBT Health and Aging Center*. Seattle, WA: Institute for Multigenerational Health. Retrieved from https://www.familleslgbt.org/1463149763/Fredriksen-Goldsen%202011.pdf

Government of Canada. (2019). Social determinants of health and health inequalities. Retrieved from https://www.canada.ca/en/public-health/services/health-promotion/population-health/what-determines-health.html

Houston, S., Magill, T., McCollum, M., & Spratt, T. (2001). Developing creative solutions to the problems of children and their families: Communicative reason and the use of forum theatre. *Child & Family Social Work*, *6*(4), 285–293. https://doi.org/10.1046/j.1365–2206.2001.00219.x

Iverson, S. V., & Seher, C. (2014). Using theatre to change attitudes toward lesbian, gay, and bisexual students. *Journal of LGBT Youth*, *11*(1), 40–61. https://doi.org/10.1080/19361653.2014.840765

Karabekir, J. (2004). *Performance as a strategy for women's liberation: The practices of Theatre of the Oppressed in okmeydan social centre*. Master's thesis, Boğaziçi University.

Retrieved from https://www.academia.edu/293014/Performance_As_a_Strategy_for_Womens_Liberation_The_Practices_of_the_Theatre_of_the_Oppressed_In_Okmeydan%C4%B1_Social_Center

Keehn, M. G. (2015). "When you tell a personal story, I kind of perk up a little bit more": An examination of student learning from listening to personal stories in two social diversity courses. *Equity & Excellence in Education*, *48*(3), 373–391. https://doi.org/10.1080/10665684.2015.1056712

Kelly-Golfman, R. (2019). Watch act vote: The impact of Theatre of the Oppressed NYC legislative theatre on New York City policy and civic engagement. *Theatre of the Oppressed* (version 1.2, pp. 1–32). Retrieved from https://d3n8a8pro7vhmx.cloudfront.net/tonyc/pages/53/attachments/original/1518111556/LegislativeTheatre_Report_02.01_Screen.pdf?1518111556

Landy, R. J. (1983). The use of distancing in drama therapy. *Arts in Psychotherapy*, *10*(3), 175–185. https://psycnet.apa.org/doi/10.1016/0197–4556(83)90006–0

Landy, R. J. (1996). *Essays in drama therapy: The Double Life*. London, UK: Jessica Kingsley.

Lather, P. (2004). Critical inquiry in qualitative research: Feminist and poststructural perspectives: Science "after truth." In K. B. deMarrais & S. D. Lapan (Eds.), *Foundations for research: Methods of inquiry in education and the social sciences* (pp. 203–215). Mahwah, NJ: Lawrence Erlbaum Associates.

Lee, Y. (2015). Theatre for the less oppressed than I: Reconsidering Augusto Boal's concept of spect-actor. *Theatre Research International*, *40*(2), 156–169. https://doi.org/10.1017/S0307883315000036

McClimens, A., & Scott, R. (2007). Lights, camera, education! The potentials of forum theatre in a learning disability nursing program. *Nurse Education Today*, *27*(3), 203–209. https://www.ncbi.nlm.nih.gov/pubmed/16790301

Meyer, I. H. (1995). Minority stress and mental health in gay men. *Journal of Health and Social Behaviour, 36*, 38–56. https://www.ncbi.nlm.nih.gov/pubmed/7738327

Meyer, I. H. (2003). Prejudice as stress: Conceptual and measurement problems. *American Journal of Public Health*, *93*, 262–265. https://www.ncbi.nlm.nih.gov/pubmed/7738327

Moreno, L. O. (2018). Fighting LGBTQ oppression through theater: A mixed methods study of the impacts of theatre of the oppressed with queer-spectrum and trans-spectrum individuals (Doctoral dissertation). Available from ProQuest Dissertations Publishing (10816071).

Nadal, K. L., Skolnik, A., & Wong, Y. (2012). Interpersonal and systemic microaggressions toward transgender people: Implications for counseling. *Journal of LGBT Issues in Counseling*, *6*(1), 55–82. https://psycnet.apa.org/doi/10.1080/15538605.2012.648583

Nadal, K. L., Wong, Y., Issa, M.-A., Meterko, V., Leon, J., & Wideman, M. (2011). Sexual orientation microaggressions: Processes and coping mechanisms for lesbian, gay, and bisexual individuals. *Journal of LGBTQ Issues in Counseling*, *5*(1), 21–46. https://psycnet.apa.org/doi/10.1080/15538605.2011.554606

Robinson, J. L., & Rubin, L. J. (2016). Homonegative microaggressions and posttraumatic stress symptoms. *Journal of Gay & Lesbian Mental Health, 20*(1), 57–69. https://psycnet.apa.org/doi/10.1080/19359705.2015.1066729

Saeed, H. (2015). Empowering unheard voices through "Theatre of the Oppressed": Reflections on the legislative theatre project for women in Afghanistan—notes from the field. *Journal of Human Rights Practice*, *7*(2), 299–236. https://doi.org/10.1093/jhuman%2Fhuu028

Sanders, M. (2004). Urban odyssey: Theatre of the Oppressed and talented minority youth. *Journal for the Education of the Gifted*, *28*(2), 218–241. https://doi.org/10.1177%2F016235320402800205

Schutzman, M. (1990). Activism, therapy, or nostalgia? Theatre of the Oppressed in NYC. *Drama Review*, *34*(3), 77–83.

Schutzman, M. (1994). Brechtian Shamanism: The political therapy of Augusto Boal. In M. Schutzman & J. Cohen-Cruz (Eds.), *Playing Boal: Theatre, therapy and activism* (pp. 137–155). New York, NY: Routledge.

Seelman, K. L., Woodford, M. R., & Nicolazzo, Z. (2017). Victimization and microaggressions targeting LGBTQ college students: Gender identity as a moderator of psychological distress.

Journal of Ethnic & Cultural Diversity in Social Work, 26(1–2), 112–125. https://psycnet.apa.org/doi/10.1080/15313204.2016.1263816

Snow, S., & Bleuer, J. (2020, forthcoming). Ethnodramatherapy. In R. Emunah & D. R. Johnson (Eds.), *Current Approaches in Drama Therapy*. Springfield, IL: Charles C. Thomas.

Snyder-Young, D. (2011). Rehearsals for revolution? Theatre of the Oppressed, dominant discourses, and democratic tensions. *Applied Theatre and Performance, 16*(1), 29–45. https://doi.org/10.1080/13569783.2011.541600

Solar, O., & Irwin, A. (2007). A conceptual framework for action on the social determinants of health. Discussion paper for the Commission on Social Determinants of Health. Retrieved from http://www.who.int/social_determinants/resources/csdh_framework_action_05_07.pdf

Somers, J. W. (2008). Interactive theatre: Drama as social intervention. *Music and Arts in Action, 1*(1), 61–86. https://musicandartsinaction.net/index.php/maia/article/view/interactivetheatre

Sue, D. W. (Ed.). (2010). *Microaggressions and marginality: Manifestation, dynamics, and impact.* Hoboken, NJ: John Wiley & Sons.

Sullivan, J., Petronella, S., Brooks, E., Murillo, M., Primeau, L., & Ward, J. (2008). Theatre of the Oppressed and environmental justice communities: A transformational therapy for the body politic. *Journal of Health Psychology, 13*(2), 166–179. https://doi.org/10.1177/1359105307086710

Tarasoff, L. A., Epstein, R., Green, D. C., Anderson, S., & Ross, L. E. (2014). Using interactive theatre to help fertility providers better understand sexual and gender minority patients. *Medical Humanities, 40*(2), 136–141. http://dx.doi.org/10.1136/medhum-2014–010516

Thompson, L., & Santiago-Jirau, A. (2011). Performing truth: Queer youth and the transformative Power of theatre of the oppressed. In Toby Emert and Ellie Friedland (Eds.), *"Come closer": Critical perspectives in the theatre of the oppressed* (pp. 97–108). New York, NY: Peter Lang.

Using Theatre to Disseminate LGBT People's Experiences with Assisted Human Reproduction Services (2019). Researching for LGBTQ2S+ Health. Retrieved from https://lgbtqhealth.ca/projects/usingtheatre.php

Yuksek, C. (2018). Dealing with stress using social theatre techniques with young Syrian students adapting to a new educational system in Turkey: A case study. *Intervention, 16*(2), 175–180. http://www.interventionjournal.org/article.asp?issn=1571–8883;year=2018;volume=16;issue=2;spage=175;epage=180;aulast=Yuksek

Warheit, E. J. (2017). *Forum theatre as theatre for development in East Africa* (Unpublished doctoral dissertation). University of Maryland, College Park. Retrieved from https://drum.lib.umd.edu/bitstream/handle/1903/20379/Warheit_umd_0117E_18614.pdf?sequence=1&isAllowed=y

Wilson, J. J. (2013). Let's all play "Stigma"! Learning together using forum theatre in collaboration with mental health service users and nurse lecturers. *Working Papers in Health Sciences, 1*(4). Retrieved from https://pdfs.semanticscholar.org/c541/bab7148c3c3e3a10261c3c54c92519dd89c8.pdf

Woolsey, L. K. (1986). The critical incident technique: An innovative qualitative method of research. *Canadian Journal of Counselling, 20*(4), 242–254. https://cjc-rcc.ucalgary.ca/article/view/59733

Wright, A. J., & Wegner, R. T. (2012). Homonegative microaggressions and their impact on LGB individuals: A measure validity study. *Journal of LGBT Issues in Counseling, 6*(1), 34–54. https://psycnet.apa.org/doi/10.1080/15538605.2012.648578

Chapter Four

Two Snapshots

Staging Image Theatre as a Healing Art

Bonny McDonald

> Four white teenagers look bored: yawning, falling asleep, looking at their watches. Four Black teenagers look absorbed: faces filled with pride, leading toward the speaker, giving the teenagers pointed looks of disapproval.—February 2010, Plaquemine, Louisiana

> A room full of college students stand slumped against one another, heads lolling, eyelids half closed, open mouths aimed at the floor.—January 2017, Louisiana State University

The above are descriptions of "snapshots" fixed in my memory from two Image Theatre (IT) workshops I led in two different contexts. IT is an introductory part of Brazilian theatre theorist-practitioner Augusto Boal's (1985) *Theatre of the Oppressed* system, a set of techniques and exercises inspired by Paolo Freire's (1970) work in *Pedagogy of the Oppressed*, which endorses learning as collaborative process and reimagines drama as participatory theatre. Most often deployed as a warm up to Boal's other more well-known techniques within the *Theatre of the Oppressed* system, IT has gotten relatively short shrift in scholarly work. I have experimented with isolating and modifying the method with a large variety of participants and contexts, from youth calling out bullying, to performance artists critiquing environmental practices, to adults reflecting on substance abuse, and others. The form facilitates group consideration of participants' perceived personal stressors and/or community struggles. As in other *Theatre of the Oppressed* work, participants begin by making kinesthetic images of their everyday difficulties, and these artifacts of personal or community stress serve as the primary content of the workshop-based practice. It is not a method exclusively for performers or theatre classrooms: the method works as beautifully in a middle school history classroom as it does in a critical theory graduate seminar, with an adult dialogue on local environmental concerns, or myriad other contexts. After working with the form primarily in the U.S. South for about ten years, I remain fascinated with the infinite variations of IT as a method for healing community dialogue.

I have made one significant departure from the way Boal imagined IT: using the form as a staging device rather than as participatory theatre in its own right. In typical IT practice, there is no audience: group members all make images of their day to day struggles, the images are next considered by the group, and then the images are understood to have done their job. However, my own practice leads me to ask, "what if we turned those images into a work of art designed to be shared beyond the participant group workshop setting?" After doing just that many times over in experiments using IT to make a final artistic product for an audience, I have begun to ask several additional questions: What are strategies for engaging group IT work as a therapeutic practice? How can we move groups from images and into productive dialogue about social stressors and shared solutions? What are ways that we can expand the reach of Boal's participatory theatre tools without compromising IT's commitment to embodied and local knowledges? How can IT be used in different curriculums to increase student engagement, critical consciousness raising, or both?

Critical performance pedagogue Elyse Lamm Pineau (2002) has differentiated between engaging the "body-as-a-medium-for-learning" and the "body-on-display" in order to understand performance pedagogy as a method of learning separate from staging an aesthetic performance (p. 50). This distinction remains useful; however, in my practice I have found that the aims of democratic liberatory pedagogy can be served by the dynamics possible when we move intentionally from what Pineau calls "the rigorous, systematic, exploration-through-enactment of real and imagined experience in which learning occurs through sensory awareness and kinesthetic engagement" (p. 50) toward the display of bodies in an aesthetic performance. Using IT as a staging tool combines these two modes: the nonverbal, kinesthetic, intuitive exploration of social stressors with the verbal, analytical, purposeful clarification of those stressors. In this combination, I have found the form to have a therapeutic effect on groups of all sorts.

While I am not a licensed therapist and do not claim to be, I proffer this method as a valuable tool for individual and group healing, for the ways it draws directly on what Judith Aron Rubin (2016) in her introduction to *Approaches to Art Therapy: Theory and Technique* and other expressive arts therapists posit as the foundational elements of meaning-making within the healing practice. According to Rubin, the first element involves symbolizing (creating art) and the second involves seeing (what happens when we consider and show the final product) (p. 17). Similar to the way that visual art invites the *putting down on paper* of our symbolic struggles, IT provides a structure of expression in which to make visible the symbolic aspects of our inner worlds in tandem with others' inner worlds and experiences. Affirming this interpretation of how IT functions, Warren Linds (2006) has asserted that Boal's image methods' "structured language serves as a bridge between the image of the world and the world of the image. The image as symbol requires us to make a leap both into it and out of it. Simultaneously, individual experience gets subsumed into the collective through the collaborative forming and reforming of the image" (p. 119). IT is an expressive art practice that uses the body as the primary medium for these processes, calling on a group to craft symbols of their struggles with their own and other bodies, and to see what they have created with the help of a group of invested participants. Drawing on IT as both process and product elicits group investment and serves both of these foundational elements of therapeutic art (the symbolic and the seen).

I set out in this essay to reflect on two images (and the processes around them) that stand out to me from my own work with IT for the way they illustrate the healing potential of the form. I also consider ways of using IT to stage a finalized work of group performance art that can have therapeutic value that goes beyond using the method only as a participatory workshop tool. The first is a Black History Month presentation at a racially tense high school; the second is a group performance in a performance composition class at Louisiana State University (LSU) where I teach in the Communication Studies department. Both took place in and around south Louisiana in educational settings. Both involved modifications to Boal's IT methods to generate scripts including, in the first case, building performance text directly from the descriptive step of IT, and in the second, incorporating group-guided writing prompts into IT work. I have used each of these two modifications in a variety of settings since these initial discoveries and I have since named them: The Group Describes Itself and The Statue Garden Speaks (McDonald, 2016).

I want to share these practices in the spirit of those practitioner-scholars who aim to modify Boal's exercises in order to invite their constituents into critical dialogue and collaborative problem-solving within historical and ideological contexts, rather than simply staying in a personal narrative mode (Schutzman, 1994). One such practitioner-scholar, Leigh Anne Howard (2004), encourages these modifications of the form, noting that many practitioners "have not followed Boal's lead to communicate their own experiences and adaptations. Many practitioners seem more willing to follow his method like a template rather than molding the techniques to meet the particular needs of their personal or social situations" (p. 218). Indeed, she argues that failing to modify *Theatre of the Oppressed* methods undermines the spirit of Boal's participatory, democratic objectives (Howard, 2004). I have found that moving from the symbolic, kinesthetic IT workshop mode into the process of staging an aesthetic performance to be seen asks participants to make choices about what they care about and how they might name and express their concerns to others outside the group. Seeking clarity on what a group wants to express to an audience can lead groups into broader, contextual examinations of what are initially personal images. In this work, groups have elected to call on interviews, each other, and even academic research to clarify their personal discoveries in IT practice. I have found that recognizing one's personal battles as an expression of broader social norms, systems, and problems can serve a healing function.

Of course, IT is not a magic bullet. I have had my share of challenges in this work: people walking out, tears, anger about interpretations of images, and uncomfortable conversations that I struggled to manage. I have retooled and gone back to the drawing board many times in my pursuit of designing workshops that help participants to think through their own positionality or to solve a problem that a group presents while maintaining a safe space. I will continue to write and speak about my challenges in this work, but here I want to share two modifications of IT that worked well for participants, according to those participants, audiences, and me. By mining the process around two key images closely, I aim to share some idiosyncrasies of my practice, since I have learned most about Boal's methods, and IT in particular, by observing critical pedagogy and performance practitioners at work. As a practitioner and educator, I value *teacher talk* and avidly collect it from my teacher-mentors in conversation and observation. Therefore, I rely on thick descriptions of what happened in these workshops to demystify the practice for anyone who might want to launch similar IT experiments in their own communities or classrooms. In response to scholarly calls for comprehensive examples of how Boal's method can function as a healing practice, I include descriptions of techniques along with verbal prompts that I use in workshops. I offer my reflections for fellow critical performance pedagogues, Boal-based practitioners, group facilitators, and teachers of all levels interested in creating healing spaces and fostering community dialogue.

A BRIEF OVERVIEW OF IMAGE THEATRE

While IT is a fairly straightforward set of exercises primarily detailed in Boal's (1992) book *Games for Actors and Non-Actors*, he writes that the practice contains within it the "totality of the [*Theatre of the Oppressed*] process" (p. 176). That is, a practice that oppressor/oppressed relationships are explored, exposed, and reworked via the corporeal body of the participant-actor engaged in games and exercises of the theatre. Boal (1985) calls these participants "spect-actors," his famous combination of the terms "spectator" and "actor," by which he theorizes a theatre practice that blurs the lines between actor and audience and challenges participants to use theatre as a rehearsal for reality (p. xxiv).

I have primarily used the IT games discussed in Boal's (1992) *Games for Actors and Non-Actors*. Like other *Theatre of the Oppressed* exercises, IT relies on a guiding "Joker" figure, whose role, as Francis Babbage (2004) in *Augusto Boal*, writes, "is to mediate between actors and spectators and in all ways possible assist the latter's participation within the dramatic action" (p. 143). The Joker serves as a facilitator in workshops, explaining the exercises and pushing participants to work expressively and in community. The Joker leads participants through three stages: (1) the nonverbal creation of an image out of participant bodies (their own or each other's); (2) dynamizations of those images, which are variations on the image that require participants to isolate, exaggerate, or extend static poses by layering movements, sounds, or words; and (3) a group discussion of the images (1992, pp. 174–215). The Joker guides groups through the above steps to create static and moving images of verbal prompts (usually shared concerns generated by the participants), and then to discuss what those images evoke for each participant. The images serve as artifacts that participants use as centerpieces around which they describe what they see and what memories, associations, and feelings those artifacts evoke.

Since one person's symbolic physical illustration of their personal experience of a concept may be wholly abstract to someone else, the images groups create allow for multiple interpretations, and thereby draw out and expose the wide breadth of subjectivities in the room. Boal (1992) calls this multivalent aspect of images wrought by the differing descriptions offered by participants the "multiple mirror of the gaze of others" (p. 175). One image is held up to many "mirrors"—the psyches of fellow participants—which in turn reflects back to the creator of the image many interpretations unique to observers' subjective positions. Such a reflection can reveal new insights to those who create the image, as well as to those who listen to what others see. As Adrian Jackson (1995) writes in the preface of *Rainbow of Desire*, "a group of individuals will perceive a whole range of different, but often intriguingly related, meanings within a single image, often seeing things which the sculptors had no idea were there" (p. xxiii). At the very least, the multiple mirror gaze of others shows us that we do not all see the same things—a critical takeaway in some contexts.

Scholarly discussions of IT have pointed to the sense of group identification that the method engenders thanks to its use of nonverbal invitations into potentially sensitive topics. However, once the discussion of images has occurred, the process is more or less complete. Hence, many practitioners use IT as a warm up and then move into Boal's other forms of participatory theatre in the pursuit of social justice aims. Berenice Fisher (1994) writes of her work with *Theatre of the Oppressed* and feminism is this vein, noting "the lack of pressure to verbalize afforded participants a certain measure of safety to express deep feelings they could not or did not wish to explain. Sharing these feelings through group sculptures helped build trust among participants" (pp. 192–193). I am interested in building on the trust established in kinesthetic stages of IT work to support dialogue about the places where personal stress and shared social problems meet.

SNAPSHOT ONE: THE GROUP DESCRIBES ITSELF

Several years ago, I found myself tasked with directing a segment of a Black History Month celebration for a school assembly at the school where I worked as high school theatre teacher in Plaquemine, Louisiana. The school lies on a stretch of the Mississippi River along with chemical plants, sugar cane fields, and former slave plantations. Sensitive to the historical racial inequity in the community, the school's leaders worked to maintain a fifty-to-fifty Black-to-white racial student ratio that reflected the demographics of the area. While the school generally maintained a peaceful atmosphere, white supremacist attitudes became apparent in classrooms during discussions about race, certain political figures, and perhaps most evidently during Black History Month when a significant number of white students broadcasted a lack of interest in Black history while Black students defended its importance. The lead organizer this year was a colleague who discussed the need to make sure the event was as student-led as possible, particularly when white teachers like me were at the helm of each department's contribution. The core group of student leaders decided to make the program a museum of sorts, where the audience would wander through the roped-off gymnasium to see various exhibits. Art students would display thematic drawings, and media students would make videos splicing present and past. I was tasked with contributing a few *skits* from my theatre classes.

I called for interested participants. In our first meeting, I simply opened the floor for thoughts and ideas, and Black students in attendance made it clear they wanted this year's assembly to be "good." Specifically, something different from, as one junior called it, "the-Rosa-Parks-play-then-Maya-Angelo-poem-then-I-Have-a-Dream routine." We discussed the fact that though those stories and texts were certainly important, repeating them in nearly identical ways in the school's Black History Month program implied that they were the only exemplars of Black history worth mentioning. One junior said, "I hear a lot of the white kids at school saying stuff like, why is it always Black history? I think the 'why' should be a big part of this."

I knew I needed to facilitate a process that would help the group address both the big picture, "why Black history?" question, as well as the highly localized concerns of these students. I wanted to foster students' thinking about their own experiences at the school as text in its own right. Knowing the participatory form of IT could mitigate the uneven power relations of a director who sets out to make a show from participants' experiences, I suggested we make a skit starting with an image, a snapshot of sorts, of "students at the typical Black History Month assembly at [our school]." The group eagerly agreed. Because we had to get a performance together quickly and because they had so many thoughts about what was going on during the typical Black History Month assembly, I thereby stumbled onto a method I would return to many times again: making several images of a key concern offered by the group; landing on an especially striking image; and then building a simple performance around that still image using descriptions elicited from the group itself. Hence, I have since called the technique "The Group Describes Itself."

After a series of warm ups, we started the next meeting where we left off the first: making an image of the "typical Black History Month program at [our school]," this time with a few more white students who had been recruited to join us. I played the role of the Joker in our work, guiding the group through IT exercises with the ultimate goal of making these images into a final performance. I moved participants through steps that were an amalgam of Boal's (1992) exercises "Image of the group" and "Image of the word: illustrating a subject with your body."

In Boal's (1992) exercise "Image of the word," participants are asked to make a still pose based on a particular word or phrase, and then to show their image to the group for consideration. In this case, I asked the group to make an image out of the bodies present at "a typical Black History Month program," trying to represent either themselves or the people they see. Next, I invited all the participants, one at a time, to exit the group image and to make any adjustments to other bodies that might make the image clearer, more interesting, or closer to how they saw the problem we were exploring.

In IT practice, when no one wants to make further adjustments to an image, the Joker asks the group to describe what they see in the image. Descriptions can come from all the group members, and when the group is small, this may be the only option. With a large group, the Joker may ask half of the participants to make an image and the other half to serve as audience members and commentators, and then switch off with the same or different prompts. Following Boal (1992), I try at first to request simple, concrete descriptions of physical bodies and their positions in order to encourage careful acknowledgment of participant choices.

In the Black History Month project, some concrete descriptions were: "The white guy in the back is slumped over, not even looking at the speaker";

and "The guy in the front is leaning way back away from the speaker and looking bored." Once the group has taken time to notice the image in detail, I begin to invite participants to offer descriptions that are interpretative rather than concrete. I might ask: "So what do you think is going on in this scene?" In the Black History Month scene, interpretive descriptions of the group ran like so: "The Black guy cares but he can't concentrate because the white girl next to him is pissing him off with her attitude"; "The guy up front talking is over-doing it; he's exaggerating it all too much"; and "That's because he's trying to get these people to listen to him!" I asked the performers to try this out as a script right then. Their descriptions of each other became the text for the scene, with each actor describing themselves in third person, using the short line that was offered by someone else moments before about their own pose. The student in front of the group performing described himself: "The guy up front talking is over-doing it; he's exaggerating it all too much." The white student at the back of the group said, "The white guy in the back is slumped over," etc.

The next step of this modification gets to the *why*, as per student request. I simply asked the group: "Why does the white audience member not look at the presentation?" The group offered a few answers: "They think it's not about them"; "They think it's boring"; and "They don't get the point of this. They don't realize that a lot of Black history is left out of the curriculum." I asked the group: "Why does this make the Black guy mad at him?" Answers: "Black history is all our history"; "I listen to white history every day in history class"; and "There has been so much dishonor to my race and this is one place where my race is honored." These answers structured our second draft. I asked each person to rewrite their line including the original description and the *whys* that spoke to them—I told them to borrow anything they heard anyone else say, but to make sure they reflected on what was said in this room. I floated around and helped edit; I asked students to edit each others' lines, too. We tried it again.

In the second draft, the line the white student in the back said was, "The white guy in the back isn't listening because he thinks this isn't about him and he doesn't think about how history textbooks focus mostly on white history the rest of the year." The Black student who sat next to him said, "The Black guy who sits next to him is giving him the side eye because his ancestors went through centuries of pain and dishonor, and still stand, and this is one short hour when we acknowledge that." We added to and complicated these lines over the course of the next few meetings, sticking fairly closely to the first descriptive draft. When students made assertions like "most of history is white history," I sometimes asked, "Is this true?" or "Why is this true? How can we find out?" These questions lead the group to pursue readings and resources connected to our conversations around the script, and ultimately to use new terminology (like "eurocentrism") and to refer to local civil rights history in the final script. The performance was a hit at the "Black History Museum" school assembly. A tour guide started by offering a brief introduction about what the audience would experience in the museum and the protocol for *activating* living exhibits, which was to press an orange button (a sticker) on one of the participants' shoulders. The museum began with our talking tableaux, labeled underneath with a paper placard: "The History of the Black History Month Program at [Our School]." The tableaux set an introspective tone for the museum experience. It insisted: this history is about us, all of us.

Students reported feeling very nervous as each new group encountered the scene, and very proud in the weeks afterward, for the way this particular exhibit stoked further consideration in classrooms and hallways. The talking tableaux initiated a cross-racial conversation that simply was not happening among the student body at large. Echoing the way IT functions within a limited group of participants, the performance created an opening for the larger school community to consider a shared social stressor. And, since actors left the performance as authorities of their creative work thanks to the IT process (speaking their own lines, with an image of their own making), both white and Black participants were consistently looked to as leaders of this conversation at the school. They saw themselves as redressing a recurring wound in the school community.

Rather than the process being the product, the locus of drama as Boal (1992) imagined IT, we modified the method to make an aesthetic performance that was crafted from multiple perspectives and intended for a broader audience. In "The Group Describes Itself" skit, participants stage their multiple mirror gazes of one another within a delineated context, then offer their reflection to an implicated public. By speaking to many students' personal, isolated discomfort at this school assembly, we explored what this discomfort meant to the school community. Audience members reported both being surprised by the *realness* of the exhibit and also relating to it. However, because the performance remained in the third person descriptive mode drawn from IT practice, the image offered both participants and viewers a bit of emotional distance in order to consider a highly emotional topic.

I see this as an important offering from IT as a healing practice: it is a way to leap into a difficult conversation with a group without necessarily pointing directly to one's own experience. The images become an artifact of our mutual creation, standing ever so slightly outside ourselves so that we may reflect on what we see with a sense of safety that comes from a small, symbolic distance. But when we add words to develop the image into a performance, there is no mistaking its message, or hoping the images simply speak for themselves.

This modification is infinitely malleable: the image might become a base which breaks apart and reforms as each person tells their part; actors begin and end in a frozen tableaux, playing out a traditional scene in between; actors describe each other instead of themselves, and more. Indeed, others have probably stumbled on similar modifications, and certainly similar styles of staging a performance: a still image that talks is nothing fancy, aesthetically speaking. But asking a group to describe itself, using the IT process to generate both image and text enables a unique sense of security, ownership, and space for deep listening in conversations where those are needed most.

SNAPSHOT TWO: THE STATUE GARDEN SPEAKS

In a Performance Composition class I taught at LSU, I leaned on IT to help students explore physical expressivity and also to practice interpreting abstract images made from bodies on stage. One of our first experiments was to put together a group performance around a theme. I wanted to model a facilitative direction style before setting them off in small groups to create their own performances. IT was one of the strategies I offered for entering this sort of work. After a few Boal-inspired warm ups, I lead an exercise that I have come to call the Statue Garden, a particular way of facilitating a group in one variation of Boal's (1992) "Image of the word: illustrating a subject using other people's bodies" (p. 181). I first encountered the movement protocol in an afterschool theatre program whose teachers, I suspect, drew on Boal, but have not located a particular credit for this specific physical arrangement of bodies for the sculpting exercise Boal (1992) describes.

The exercise calls on Boal's (1992) description of the "modeling sequence," particularly "the sculptor touches the model," or "sculpting," as we called it for short (p. 136). In the classic exercise, one person is the "sculptor" and the other the "sculpture," or the "clay." The sculptor creates an image using the other person's body by physically manipulating them into a position in response to a prompt. I also always offer the option to sculpt without touching the body—a technique Boal suggests which involves keeping at least six inches away while motioning how the sculpted body should move, as if the sculpture is a marionette manipulated by the sculptor on invisible strings (p. 137). In the "Statue Garden" version of this exercise, participants arrange themselves in an inner ring and an outer ring, with sculptors on the outer ring in front of their sculpture-partners in the inner ring. This arrangement allows the sculptors to walk around the statues when the sculpting is complete, and then to compare, contrast, and discuss what they have seen. Sculptures can also turn inward toward each other to observe fellow sculptures.

I like to start this exercise with the word "Joy" as a prompt because it is positive and easy to do: most students wind up in big open postures with smiling faces and their arms up. When I ask students to describe what they see, as IT prescribes, they describe those basic elements. If I press for more details, groups often note a general physical openness, with bodies confidently taking up a lot of space, bellies showing, a lack of fear of being seen by others, and so on. Next, sculptors and statues switch positions and change roles. I like to practice the protocol again with a simple but contrasting term for the new set of sculptors ("gross" is a favorite): (1) sculpting, (2) walking around the "Sculpture Garden" to observe others, and finally (3) discussing similarities and differences. Asking "What do these statues say about how we think of this term?" can be a productive question for the group. When asked this of "gross," for example, participants often notice it is "low," "close to the ground," or "having to do with bodily orifices." Once everyone is familiar with the protocol, I ask the group what word they would like to do.

In my performance class, students were thrilled at the idea that they got to choose words for the statue game and immediately, or so I suspect, tried to push my boundaries. They chatted for only a second before many started exclaiming "Drunk!" Their tone was exuberant, daring, as if testing me: would I let them do "drunk?" I said, "Sure, we will do drunk." They were both a little surprised and also not certain I was being wise about this. I asked them to return to their two circles and get started.

There was much giggling as the students sculpted peers into poses. Laughter as shoulders were made to slump, tongues were made to hang out, eyes to roll back. People were positioned on the floor. Only one state of drunkenness was described with these bodies: what might be called "black out drunk," or something on the way to it. One woman was leaning over a toilet, with her friend holding her hair. One woman lay on the ground, eyes closed, body passive, with two others pointing at her and laughing. One student did a keg stand, while others egged him on. One student stared blankly into space. One student appeared dizzy, in a frozen pose holding her head, looking like she would soon vomit. The laughter peaked when the poses were set, then I counted down from five, asking everyone to finish their statues. Following my mentor in this work, Dr. Ruth Bowman (1997), my last step as the Joker, before participants reveal their images to each other, is to ask everyone to commit to their poses, to extend the lines of their bodies, and to turn up their expressivity a bit so that the poses are really clear, defined, precise, made for an audience to see. Finally, I prompted the group to walk around the room to observe the "Statue Garden."

The buzz of laughter began to quiet, then quiet more, into a solemn silence in the large room, with only the soft sound of feet walking around the statues. Instead of stopping in front of their original partner, the class walked around a second time, a solemn march with slow, deliberate steps. Finally, someone broke the silence: "This is really depressing. This is really what a party looks like at the end of the night, like this is a real scene I see every weekend." I asked them to back up and describe what they saw. "People so drunk they are in dangerous situations." "People who are sick." "Kids being really stupid." "People throwing up, passed out, giving each other alcohol, not in control of their bodies." "People are pushing each other to drink more." "The alcohol is in control." We were all surprised at how serious this exercise became. Someone wiped tears off of her face.

"Let's move this to the page," I said, sensing a need for reflection. The class was used to my asking them to jot down ideas, to *freewrite*, or to reflect on paper for a few minutes in response to performance exercises. But this time, since they seemed so struck by the exercise, and inspired by my giving them the freedom to choose "drunk" (despite my fleeting worries of its appropriateness for a classroom setting), I asked them to take over the prompts. It did not occur to me until later that while traditional IT work would likely not call for setting interpretive words to the practice in this way, calling on the group to guide the writing is precisely in the spirit of Boal's and Freire's fundamental assertions that groups know best how to address their own most pressing issues. In this case, I asked, "Does someone have a place for us to start, either a question, an image that stuck out, or any prompt to offer?" We quickly got into a rhythm, with students asking a new question every couple minutes. Here were some of the questions and a writing prompt:

- Why do you drink?
- How often do you drink?
- What's the worst situation you have been in while you were drunk?
- Have you been involved in hazing here at LSU?
- Write about the one with the girl on the ground.
- What kind of parent or family examples of drinking did you see as a kid?
- Write how you felt in the pose your partner put you in.

The writing session felt anything but rote. I have learned to aim for this as a facilitator in a reflective writing exercise: a soft buzz of pens moving fast on pages, a palpable focus, an urgency to record ideas. Sometimes I have great juicy questions to get pens moving; other times passing that responsibility to the group is the best path to reflecting with sincerity. I generally find the more I can let go of the reigns, the deeper students will invest in a project. In this performance classroom, some students chose to share segments after the fifteen minute writing session when I suggested this possibility. They offered thoughts on the drink-till-you-pass-out culture of tailgating at LSU, accounts of friends having their stomachs pumped after a frat party, and worse.

I asked the students to look at what they had written, pick a piece of it they would be willing to share with the class, edit it into about a one-minute chunk, and bring it back next time to try to stage it with the statue garden they had created. I challenged them to think about the still poses they had created and at some point in their writing to *nod* to the statue itself. I offered the examples of writing about their own pose, someone else's, or the group as a whole, but their creative challenge was to add at least one line that described the posed bodies, drawing on the way we describe the physical poses themselves in IT. I asked them to imagine saying their lines as they stood in their poses.

The (Drunk) Statue Garden Speaks showed up at the end of the semester for a small audience. The end result was similar aesthetically to the Black History Museum image-performance. Statues described themselves in the third person using additional texts from their quite varied personal monologues. The whole image rotated to showcase a different pair—sculptor and statue—while they spoke. I asked the groups to try out sculpting each other while one or the other partners did their monologue and they tried this in different combinations, sometimes with a third party reading the monologue while the sculpture and sculptor pair made slow moves into the final position. In one case, a male student molded a female student (without touching her, and with much gentleness) into the "passed out on the floor pose," while she narrated:

> Her head is slack and feels heavy. She can't think. She is off balance. The room is spinning. It's hilarious! (crazy fake laughter). Her "big sis" made her screwdrivers all night. She kept thinking: This is college. This is awesome. Everybody gets wasted: it's a party school. It's awesome. He was drinking beer. He seemed like a "nice" guy. She didn't know his name. It doesn't matter. She won't remember what happened. She doesn't remember what happened. Not exactly.

Watching someone sculpt a body into a position of abject drunkenness, while the statue tells a story like the one above, or of watching their father get really drunk, or getting pushed into drinking at a frat party, was painful and revealing of the ways we are *pushed* into such situations in real life. The sculpting underlined students' thinking about the relationship between peer pressure and drinking, about how culture can mold us into accepting uncomfortable norms. Students spoke about this piece at the end of the class, noting in some cases how it had made them see college drinking as a "bigger social problem" and even inspired some to drink more responsibly. I admit I have tried to recreate the same rich experience with the word "drunk" with other students, but it has never been so interesting. One cannot re-create the specific experience using participatory theatre and nor should one try. However, I have used "The Statue Garden Speaks" exercise as a performance experiment with other groups using other self-generated topics since, such as "social media," "shame," and even "traffic." To find a topic for this exercise, I have asked, "What's something that stresses a lot of folks out in here?" College drinking is not the only thing we do where we might feel forced into a social norm we are not entirely comfortable with.

Paired with a shared social stressor, the act of sculpting becomes a layered visual metaphor of our compliance with norms, institutions, spaces, and culture, and an entry point into conversation about what we lose or gain by this compliance. When statues and sculptures switch roles, further possibilities open for expressing how we might resist these pressures. In the "drunk" performance, for example, the young woman slowly got up on her feet, staring at the young man and facing him as if standing up to him. After she finished her monologue, she stood all the way up, while he backed away and walked off stage. The young woman ended by simply facing the audience, her feet firmly planted underneath her, trying to show the audience that she was now steady on her feet. Like the "Image of a group" or "Image of a word" exercise, sculpting as a participatory theatre technique generates topics, conversations, and artifacts for group consideration. Yet using the sculpting technique as a performance device has its own unique potential for helping participants and audiences to see ourselves as part of a social macrocosm, and to begin to untangle the tensions between our own needs and the social pressures which shape us.

SUGGESTIONS AND MUSINGS FOR EDUCATORS

Experimenting with IT is a risk worth taking. I encourage fellow educators across the curriculum to experiment with this dynamic form. Engaging the kinesthetic mode in the classroom infuses a discussion with new kinds of energy and investment. Even the simplest version of this work has a lot to offer a variety of classrooms or groups. A condensed exercise to test out the practice is to ask students to work in a small group (of three or four) to make a kinesthetic image in response to a shared reading or topic. Groups might make an image out of their bodies of a plant cell, a vocabulary word, characters in a novel, Abraham Lincoln's relationship to slavery, the worst problem in their city right now, the electoral college, "decolonial pedagogy," or anything else. Then, each group displays their image to the class. The class describes the image as they see it, then the image-makers may explain their image. More formal scripting could follow for a whole-class performance. The building blocks of this practice are simply space to create a symbolic image and time to allow it to be seen by others. Like other pedagogical methods, facilitators and students alike grow more comfortable and more skilled at the form as they practice it. Complex prompts or sensitive group-generated topics can be built upon the foundation of the basic Image of a Word and Statue Garden exercises. What follows are some lessons I have learned in my own ongoing experiments with IT.

First, never skip warm ups. My own use of and interest in IT broadened significantly as a doctoral student in Performance Studies at LSU under the

"Jokering" of Bowman (1997), who among other things developed my interest in using bodies as a way of complicating a text. Bowman emphasized the importance of moving through Boal's (1992) prescribed process of (1) knowing the body, (2) making the body expressive, (3) theatre as language, and (4) theatre as discourse. As such, I always move through a series of warm ups before engaging IT to foster bodily awareness, to practice defamiliarization as outlined by Boal, and to establish trust within the group. Following Bowman (1997), planning a workshop starts with thoughtfully crafting a series of warm ups to meet the needs of various groups that start with simple movement exercises designed to connect us to our bodies and senses, then games that *shake off* our everyday habitual movements, then exercises that turn our attention to the group and to making and then reading images. Warm ups can be especially important when we are using the form in a context where movement or performance is not the norm. An adult dialogue or science class might need extra encouragement and plenty of time warming up to acclimate to creative kinesthetic engagement before broaching serious topics via image-making.

Even after a thorough set of warm ups, however, making expressive images challenges participants. I have found that when groups can let go of trying to make poses that make perfect sense (even for their maker) and simply commit to whatever emerges in the initial stages of image-making, groups have better chances at evoking the multiple mirror gaze of others and moving into more profound dialogue. Often, participants hesitate to make initial images: it is vulnerable to put oneself out there, and to think beyond everyday images.

My prerogative in this phase of the practice is to encourage bold experimentation by modeling big bold choices myself and by verbally reminding participants that *anything goes*. I demonstrate what it means to exaggerate a pose and display full energy to my own warm up and other movement exercises. I repeatedly remind groups, "You don't have to know why you are choosing this image right now, just trust your instincts," or "Just go for something now and we'll think about it later." If they say, "I don't know what to do," I say: "It's okay: anything goes; why don't you express 'I don't know' if that's all you have right now. Commit to 'I don't know!'" Calling for big bodies and exaggerated images even when you have no idea what you are doing often elicits the best conversations, because the images created leave that much more room for varied interpretations by the group. And other times, finding out what you do not know or what kind of bodies share certain kinds of not-knowing is exactly the point.

Another takeaway from my experiments with IT has been to make room for thematic, pre-planned prompts offered by the Joker in addition to spontaneous participant-generated prompts. Both can support the democratic engagement and healing possibilities of IT. I consistently depart from Boal

(1992) by using specific prompts for images in themed workshops with specific conversational and/or performance goals in mind instead of calling exclusively or primarily on participant prompts. Sometimes, the pre-planned prompts function as warm ups designed to ease groups into IT. Boal often asks participants to think of an oppression they experience and then to suggest prompts for sculpting (see Boal, 1985). Although I do often encourage participants to suggest prompts once we have experimented with a few I have offered, I think it is also important to craft prompts that are carefully designed to encourage participants to interrogate themselves and to engage with complex ideas. Of course, inviting participant prompts remains an important part of the fun and the ethics of this work. Moreover, a carefully thought out series of prompts moving from the simple to the complex can set a tone for deeper engagement, including improving the quality of work when the Joker finally does turn prompting over to the participants.

In the projects I discuss here, I found the move toward a final performance product to be especially effective for using IT to host productive dialogue. Staging what we discover in the multiple mirror gaze of others invites crystallization of the symbolic matter generated by the IT process. When we make images of our struggles, as Boal (1995) notes in *Rainbow of Desire*: *The Boal Method of Theatre and Therapy*, "To our own point of view we add others, as if we were able to look at the earth from the earth, where we live, and also from the moon, the sun, a satellite or the stars. In daily life, we see the situation; on stage, we see the situation we are in" (p. 26). To this end, I have found myself encouraging departures from Boal's encouragement to describe bodies per se and to go ahead and call for interpretations in the IT process (going beyond descriptions of physical bodies) when the aim is group reflection. Instead of allowing the images to speak for themselves, I ask for clarification from participants about their understanding of images.

I often press participants for more information about their reactions to images: Why does this strike you? What does this mean to you? How exactly do you relate? Why do you think our poses are all this way (or not that way)? What does this remind you of? Do you relate to this or not? Why are so many people making this sort of image? These leading questions have sometimes led the group to call for external sources, new vocabularies, a trip to an archive, demographic maps of their cities, and even academic sources. On the one hand, when a group's goal is to create a script to go along with their images, groups themselves often call for sessions in the rehearsal process in which participants can read and discuss expert voices that directly address the questions and concerns that have arisen from the workshop process. On the other hand, the Joker can use the opportunity a performance allows to help participants articulate those feelings into broader conversations about power and powerlessness, social responsibility, or social change. Whether arising from self-generated prompts or from discovering investment in a topic thanks to a Joker's prompts, research questions that arise from the groups' scripting process feel more urgent and relevant than those posed by a teacher/facilitator without that context.

In this ongoing work, I have found that IT supports solidarity and dialogue by building trust (as others have documented), and also due to the way images invite us to step outside ourselves and reflect with others on the social world in which we are collectively implicated. In Boal's multiple mirror gaze of others, I see Freire's ideas about critical consciousness raising and the relationship between subjectivism and objectivism made concrete. In *Pedagogy of the Oppressed*, Freire (1970) writes of the radical teacher whose "subjective aspect exists only in relation to the objective aspect (the concrete reality, which is the object of analysis). Subjectivity and objectivity thus join in a dialectical unity producing knowledge in solidarity with action, and vice versa" (p. 20). The IT images are symbols of the concrete realities we analyze; our descriptions of what we see make plain the multiple subjectivities at play in our shared reality. And this is the crux of Image Theatre's power: it shows us we must discover the nature and limitations of our own subjectivities—and thereby better know the world—in community.

REFERENCES

Babbage, F. (2004). *Augusto Boal*. London, UK: Routledge.

Boal, A. (1985). *Theatre of the oppressed* (C. A. McBride & M.-O. L. McBride, Trans.). New York, NY: Theatre Communications Group.

Boal, A. (1992). *Games for actors and non-actors* (2nd ed.) (A. Jackson, Trans.). London: Routledge.

Boal, A. (1995). *Rainbow of desire: The Boal method of theatre and therapy* (A. Jackson, Trans.). London: Routledge.

Bowman, R. L. (1997). "Joking" with the classics: Using Boal's joker system in the performance classroom. *Theatre Topics*, *7*(2), 139–151.

Fisher, B. (1994). Feminist acts: Women, pedagogy, and theatre of the oppressed. In M. Schutzman & J. Cohen-Cruz (Eds.), *Playing Boal: Theatre, Therapy, Activism* (pp. 185–197). New York, NY: Routledge.

Freire, P. (1970). Preface to *Pedagogy of the oppressed* (M. Bergman Ramos, Trans.). (pp. 17–22). London: Penguin Books.

Howard, L. A. (2004). Speaking theatre/doing pedagogy: Re-visiting theatre of the oppressed. *Communication Education*, *53*(3), 217–233.

Jackson, A. (Trans.). (1995). Introduction. In A. Boal, *Rainbow of desire: The Boal method of theatre and therapy* (pp. xviii–xxvi). London: Routledge.

Linds, W. (2006). Metaxis: Dancing (in) the in-between. In J. Cohen-Cruz & M. Schutzman (Eds.), *A Boal companion: Dialogues on theatre and cultural politics* (pp. 114–124). New York, NY: Routledge.

McDonald, B. L. (2016). *After images: Using Augusto Boal's image theatre to balance artistry, analysis, and activism in the performance composition process.* PhD dissertation, Louisiana State University.

Pineau, E. L. (2002). Critical performative pedagogy: Fleshing out the politics of liberatory education. In N. Stucky & C. Wimmer (Eds.), *Teaching Performance Studies* (pp. 41–54) Carbondale, IL: Southern Illinois University Press.

Rubin, J. A. (2016) Introduction. In J. A. Rubin (Ed.), *Approaches to art therapy: Theory and technique* (3rd ed., pp. 1–15). New York: Routledge.
Schutzman, M. (1994). Brechtian Shamanism: The political therapy of Augusto Boal. In M. Schutzman & J. Cohen-Cruz (Eds.), *Playing Boal: Theatre, Therapy, Activism* (pp. 137–155). New York, NY: Routledge.

Chapter Five

Eyas on the Prize

Mapping the Relaunch of Performance at the University of Houston-Clear Lake

Andrea Baldwin

"If you do performance work, then we now have it at this institution," my future dean said to me. I was in an on-campus interview for the job I now have. The call for the position asked for a generalist to teach the required public speaking course and one writing class. My research, while grounded in teaching to the job call and core classes, is rooted in performance studies. I was told before this interview to "adjust the language" about my artistic work to anyone who may not "get" what I do. Performance studies, in the communication studies frame, is and remains the light force that consumes my professional, personal, and public life. It is the common drive to my desire to be in higher education, but it is not a common topic of study at many institutions. Words such as "theatre" get thrown into the conversation when administrators unfamiliar with what I do try to make sense of it, and while there are theatrical components, it is not entirely what I do.

I was told by my mentors to use the words "embodied learning/mentoring," which is a quick and easy way to explain the breadth of what I do. Performance studies, for me, is the frame that allows us to answer social communication questions through praxis and practice (Park-Fuller, 1994). Performance provides the means of embodying research, ultimately allowing us to make sense of our world. As I spouted my rehearsed veiled narrative, a careful verbal gymnastics routine that would reassure the administrator in front of me that what I do is practical and palpable to the heavy science, technology, engineering, and mathematics (STEM) based institution, but that I also have the ability to do what the job call asked. The dean stopped me with that statement; this is the only green light to get going, rather to find ways to bring my research and passion to this institution. I was hired only to teach public speaking and media writing, but that statement rang in my ears for the first month of my arrival at University of Houston-Clear Lake (UHCL). We now have it. And, I have got to build it.

The UHCL campus has a 500-seat theatre, called the Bayou Theater, which is the only remaining relic of the theatre and dance program that once existed there. The program was eventually absorbed into the curriculum at the main campus, leaving the UHCL campus's large proscenium stage, two dressing areas, and scene shop empty. Since the end of that program, the theatre has only been used for outside contracted performances, a few school events requiring an auditorium, and the occasional staff photo. Since the 1990s, UHCL has not had an in-house performance or any performing arts until my arrival.

In the past four years, UHCL has been able to present five productions featuring students, send two students from the university to graduate Performance Studies programs, and consistently attend performance festivals. In addition to these accomplishments, Storytelling and Oral Communication is the first performance-based class taught on this campus in twenty years. While my experience is not unique, as many of my colleagues have similarly brought performance studies/performing arts to programs that previously lacked this emphasis, it is marked through the timing of my joining this institution. I arrived at a time when the institution needed the tools of performance to help process and lend itself to a community in need of healing. For all of the work listed above, teaching the breadth of knowledge of performance, producing productions, and mentoring students are skills that would or should be found in a full program with multiple professors, but were at this time all required of one lecturer.

I am telling this story in the hopes of documenting how the return of performing arts can help students make sense of the world around them and find outlets for their feelings. Though most educators, students, and practitioners may support, in a vague, general sense, the inclusion of a performing arts component at an academic institution, it is in its absence, in STEM-focused institutions, that we truly see the detriment of what not having the performing arts can do. I encourage those who find themselves in STEM-focused institutions to become the "A" (for Arts) in those institutions, thus turning STEM into STEAM.

I was in the unique position of arriving at an institution that was undergoing a massive transition. UHCL, established in the 1970s, was a two-year, upper-level institution until 2014, when they became a four-year institution by welcoming the addition of first- and second-year students. This *downward expansion,* the term used to define the university's expansion from a two-year institution to a four-year institution, meant that the university now welcomed a larger pool of students. For some, the amenities that come with a four-year institution arrived on campus for the first time. Students were able to help pick the school colors, as well as the school mascot, settling finally on the hawk. I recall during my first year hearing stories from our charter faculty, faculty who have worked at UHCL since its inaugural year and who are baffled by the incoming freshmen coming to school in pajamas. I am amused by those faculty members' bewilderment, by the idea that something so commonplace to me as first-year students in sweatpants, would be outlandish to others. While I welcome their perspective on the makeup of the university before the arrival of first- and second-year students, I came to this institution much like those first years, bringing my own culture and ideas to remake the fabric of my university.

The hawk is native to the swamplands that surround the campus and greater Clear Lake area. In addition to sharing a backyard with NASA, UHCL sits next to Armand Bayou Nature Center, meaning members of the campus community occasionally encounter the wildlife face to face. As totemic figures, alligators were already taken by our sister campus downtown, while egrets, majestic though they are, do not evoke power. The hawk watches over all, sitting on the occasional post on a streetlight over the center of campus. As with all animals, there are stages of inception, growth, and development. Hawks of this region, like most birds of prey, hatch eggs and raise their young so they develop and grow into their full size and can care for themselves. These young hawks, called *eyas*, spend only a small amount of time in the care of their parents before they gain the strength to care for themselves. Just as hawks go through different stages of growth, this is a story about my hatching and finding independence, about enlisting students to own these steps as much as I do, and to always, above all things, give them back what was given to me. Mentorship and artistic creation are genealogical; as the mentors before me taught me and nurtured me, I hope to do the same.

As the *eyas* grows, it develops much like my institution with its new dorm on campus. We as practitioners and educators also continue to evolve. We make ways to sustain the communities we have with the ebb and flow of students, funding, and interest. In this chapter, I will document the process of growth in the institution and program I am building, starting with the recruitment of students from non-performing arts classes. Next, I will explain what it means to bring students to the experience by providing opportunities for them to have agency and ownership in the process of creating performance and to witness performance. Lastly, I narrate the experience of helping students create their own performance, and how the students and the larger community processed their feelings through performance in the aftermath of Hurricane Harvey. With these narratives, I will demonstrate how a (Performance Studies) program can be built through the participation of the community.

BUILDING AND MENTORING A PERFORMANCE PROGRAM WITH THE COMMUNITY IN MIND

My work is informed by performative pedagogical ideas that emphasize mentorship through embodiment. Since performance practitioners learn by doing, we learn to become good mentors by enacting those behaviors that once were modeled for us. To bring a performance program to life, I grounded myself in the understanding that mentorship is a genealogical performance and act. My perspective comes from an appreciation of the genealogy, or the family tree of academic life and disciplinary identity. For example, I track my own genealogy to former instructors and the institutions where I received my degrees. My identity as a teacher, artist, and scholar derives from my experiences with these instructors. I create my performative pedagogical body from their performances.

To bring the performing arts back to this university, I understood that there was no blueprint to follow. Therefore, I needed to rely on the positive and affective experiences that brought me to performance in order to encourage others to come into this world as well.

To document and discuss my own experience in this process, I turn to autoethnography as a method of presenting my narrative. Autoethnography is a form of research that uses narrative and personal reflection to connect experiences to social understanding. In the *Handbook of Autoethnography*, Stacy Holman Jones, Tony Adams, and Carolyn Ellis (2013) remind me that autoethnography comes from a place of *mimesis*; in other words, this method acts as a reflecting mirror for examining social life from the perspective of the self. Holman Jones, Adams, and Ellis (2013) write that "one characteristic that binds all autoethnographies is the use of personal experience to examine and/or critique cultural experience" (p. 22). As Heewon Chang (2008) notes in *Autoethnography as Method*, to write from the self is a personal process, and implies trust in your own body of knowledge as a credible source. This method allows me to create a living, theoretical archive of my experience. The discourse of story, given life with context and narration from the storyteller, will help paint the picture of how the creation of Performance Studies at UHCL is healing and benefiting the university, the students, and the greater Clear Lake community.

Tami Spry (2001) writes that "through performative autoethnography we write ourselves into a deeper critical understanding with others of the ways in which our lives intersect with larger sociocultural pains and privileges" (p. 59). While experience and memory are ephemeral, performative autoethnography gives a way to document these moments so that we can share our experiences with others across time. Spry reminds us that autoethnography is socially constructed to the study of collaborative knowledge and praxis (p. 52).

My use of autoethnography aligns with Spry's notion of the textualized body, which represents how, why, and what we think of particular experiences in our lives, and then how we negotiate the people in those experiences. This document is my attempt to develop not only an academic archive of how to create a space for the performing arts where one did not previously exist, but also, as Spry writes, to generate scholarship about this educational experience. The present essay serves several important functions, including verifying to administrators the importance of Performance Studies as a program or field of study to higher educational spaces, documenting the enrichment of students who participate in them, and enhancing scholarship in the field.

Elyse Pineau (1994) writes that teaching is performative, a creative, collaborative, and critical process, and one that "acknowledges that identities are always multiple, overlapping ensembles of real and possible selves who enact themselves in direct relation to the context and communities in which they perform" (p. 29). I connect to Pineau's (1994) notions of identity-making as I note my own intersections of performance and pedagogy. Each opportunity from my past molded my performative body toward my pedagogic one. A mentor once told me that to create your own teaching body, start with remembering all the best traits of your former teachers and try them on, or emulate them. Jane Gallop's (1995) *Pedagogy* refers to this process as "impersonation" (p. 8), noting that we physically and emotionally incorporate aspects of our own best teachers in shaping our pedagogical personae. I know that my own performative pedagogic body has grown and changed with each great mentor and educator I have encountered in my life.

When I arrived at UHCL, I taught four sections of public speaking, a required course that satisfies many degree requirements, often taken by many first-year students. My first step to conceiving a Performance Studies program began in those General Education public speaking classes, where I used the course's kinetic educational elements to recruit students to the storytelling class I would teach in the spring.

While public speaking focuses on the act of communication, specifically oral presentations, I would use these skills as well as teaching moments in dialogue-based discussion to enact small role play moments and even small theatre games to bring students to their feet and translate abstract concepts into hands-on experience. Not only did the students find the class, usually dreaded by many, fun, but they also found the elements of *doing* to be a break in the norm, a breath of fresh air that became a memorable experience for them. For me, as an educator, it was important to identify and recruit to my storytelling course those students who seemed especially confident in their skills or who I felt would benefit from such a course. Toward the end of the semester, I mentioned to a handful of students who fit those criteria that they should enroll in my course the following semester. While I announced and offered the opportunity to every student, I asked those who demonstrated that comfort and skill I had observed in face to face encounters. This was what my mentors had done for me in the past; when they saw I had potential, they made sure I knew it and would encourage my artistic energy.

Just as Pineau (1994) and others agree that performance functions as a dimension of pedagogy, I see mentorship as a way of marking how the educational process we share with students is passed on, both in the care we convey to our students and in the knowledge we share with them. Judith Hamera (2005) reveals the embodiment of mentorship and pedagogy as a performative space. Hamera (2005) writes that "We don't just teach or study bodies. We teach and study *as* bodies and our bodies are, in turn, literally reshaped by the 'hows' and 'wheres,' the material practices, of our pedagogy" (p. 84). Performative pedagogy illuminates the genealogical line of mentorship as a line of disciplinary history. It highlights that it is in the doing that makes us good educators.

When I was a student, I was artistically minded but did not receive any guidance or mentoring in the performing arts until late in my undergraduate career. I came to the performing arts as a first-time performer who was confident, enjoyed the work, and had little skill but was eager to learn. I realized early on in my time at UHCL that many of those students may have a similar profile. While there are students who have taken theatre and done some performance, many of them will not have had any theatre experience but may have the desire. Those mentors were encouraging of my efforts, even when my ideas and efforts may have seemed ill-conceived or less than stellar, they focused on my enthusiasm. As I recruited for my storytelling class, I chose to ask students who were also enthusiastic about theatre in person to subtextually say, "I see your energy. I see your passion. I have a place for that." This proved a successful recruitment tool for those who had time in their spring schedules for the class. However, I had many who were still on the fence about it all. They would admit that they liked the idea of performing, but asked: what would it do for their degree plans? how would they be able to work in a class that asks for so much *doing* when they must also balance their jobs and families? and most commonly, what if they're not good at it?

To this, I pulled from a mentor, who once said this to me: "Well, you will have the rest of your life and career to dedicate to yourself. However, you are running out of time and options to play, experiment, and embody theory, all of which is beneficial too. And storytelling can do that for you." This statement explains the importance of the performing arts for all students in higher learning—while education in a university setting can be designed to help students acquire a specific skill, a well-rounded experience allows the student to reimagine the world around them. It is to this statement that several students said yes, as they were saying yes to a possibility of expansion, to enrichment, and to be open to play.

RITUAL AND STORYTELLING: CREATING A *WELL*

Once students enrolled in Storytelling, I relied on what we all understand as practitioners and artists as the key to the performing arts. Once we get them comfortable, then the possibilities can open up. The plan was to teach a course that was grounded in the theoretical findings of scholars, which meant introducing those students to academic research for the first time, as well as making sure we got them *on their feet* every class period to translate theories into praxis. The theoretical grounding was important to introduce them to the larger world of scholars, many of whom are housed at schools that offer theatre programs with performance spaces, seasons of shows, and an army of student performers. I wanted them to see, above all things, that the work was accessible and that it was very real. Often, when we think of theory, we think of people, who lived long ago, to whom we have no access. It was and will always remain important to me to make sure they understand that some of the people who wrote the fancy articles they are reading were not only brilliant, but were also real human beings who they could potentially talk with. Accessibility, in this sense, opens the door of the ivory tower and opens any preconceived notions of scholarly work being beyond them, making it easier to consume.

Praxis, the effort to make theory come alive, is important as it allows students a chance to embody the theory or method firsthand. We would often re-adapt Aesop's fables with twists that reference the theory we had been reading about. These restagings would allow for more creative possibilities than what was linearly communicated. This exercise would tell me how the students were audiencing and applying the work in their everyday lives. They would pull from their experiences to recreate the Aesopian characters in their performances. Therefore, the students became comfortable in their work and became even more expressive.

Victor Turner's (1988) *The Anthropology of Performance* reminds us that "anthropological literature is full of accounts of dramatic episodes which vividly manifest the key values of specific cultures" (p. 139). These episodes Turner (1988) writes about come to fruition in the performing arts and in moments of conviction to the craft and discipline. By conviction, or rather a convicting moment, I refer to the experiences that occur in a pedagogical setting where a students is inspired to pursue knowledge or a field of study as a career choice. What calls me to conviction solicits and shakes me to action in a way that just reading or talking about my learning experiences does not.

In sum, while my students may not have access to or even the experience of the performance arts, through the conviction to the craft and the lived and shared experiences the students make in the classroom, it comes to life. This is always an eye-opening experience for first-time performers. In moments such as these, I observe that my jaded weight comes undone, and I am convicted with them again as if it were also my first experience. I am reminded of Victor Turner and Edward Bruner's (1986) *The Anthropology of Experience*, in which they make a distinction between behavior and experience. They argue:

> Experience, in our perspective, is not equivalent to the more familiar concept of behavior. The latter implies an outside observer describing someone else's actions, as if one were an audience to an event; it also implies a standardized routine that one simply goes through. An experience is more personal, as it refers to an active self, to a human being who not only engages in but shapes an action. We can have experience but we cannot have a behavior; we describe the behavior of others but we characterize our own experience. (Turner & Bruner, 1986, p. 5)

The active self, which is my own mode of being in the classroom, means that performance studies becomes a personal experience, one that requires the use of a new language to express thoughts and feelings. Students who approach performance with their active selves achieve the ability to decipher artistic work as they encounter it outside of the classroom. By the end of the semester, the students were eager to consume more performance work. And since Storytelling was the only performance-based class at UHCL, I encouraged the students to seek opportunities to perform or to witness performance.

This is where the story turns, as it no longer becomes my solo adventure to bring performance to our campus. It became the call and mission of the students, recruited from my required Public Speaking class, then again from my Storytelling course, who took up the call with me by *seeking the work*. This seeking manifested in the establishment of the UHCL Storytellers, our first student organization dedicated to talking about, doing, supporting, and witnessing performance work. It manifested, most conspicuously, in the students' desire to see more performances. For example, the students traveled with me to the Petit Jean Performance Festival. This festival is held every October at Petit Jean State Park in Arkansas. It hosts schools from across the country who come together for two days to witness invited performances brought from the attending schools, to perform either in those performances or in workshops of their own individual work, and lastly, to participate in a two-day workshop with the invited festival leader, culminating in a performance created just for the festival. As an avid attendee of the festival, I spent a great deal of time talking about the event and encouraging my students to go with me.

I repeated a mantra in my head as I worked that year—*Just get them to the mountain. You got to get them to the mountain.* It became my silent battle cry, as I knew I was one human. While I could excite the students about the work, they needed to see it, all of it. While I could take them across the Houston area to see shows, make attempts to bring scholars to talk and participate in workshops with them, we did not have the means and time to make that work. And until I had a season of multiple shows and multiple classes to help with their praxis, the festival would have to serve as a master intensive on the world of performance.

I took four students to the 2016 Petit Jean Performance Festival. We made the drive from Houston, Texas, to northern Arkansas in one long drive. The night before the festival, as schools arrive with their faculty, graduate students, and undergraduate students, I walked with my students to meet people from those programs, in particular, my own alma mater. In this special moment of genealogical performance, I witnessed my students meet my mentors, whose names they knew by the stories I told about them and by the articles they had read. The praxis that occurred in the classroom was here in the flesh. I observed my students that evening and the following morning, wide-eyed by the realization that the world I had painted for them in the classroom, of scholars who believed in performance and went to great lengths to bring it to all students, was here. This part of the conviction process is important to developing a program. For students to see and to participate in the growth of a performance program where they are enrolled gives them both investment and reification into the craft. As Turner (1982) writes in his *From Ritual to Theater: The Human Seriousness of Play*,

> An experience is never truly completed until it is "expressed" that is, until it is communicated in terms intelligible to others, linguistic or otherwise. Culture itself is the ensemble of such expressions—the experience of individuals made available to society and accessible to the sympathetic penetration of other "minds." (Tuner, 1982, p. 14)

Even before the festival started, I could see the conviction grow in my students, as they chatted with other undergrad and graduate students, as they graciously met scholars whose work they had read, as they heard the language of performers leap from the classroom and the textbook pages into real life. I watched it become deeper for them that night.

The festival has three main foci. First, a festival leader, chosen from a group of scholars, runs a two-day workshop. Second, students are broken into groups to workshop and to showcase solo work. Last, the festival showcases several invited performances, both group and solo, put on by attending universities looking for feedback. It was important for my students to see group productions, as they have only seen solo work in the classroom. There is something magical that occurs when witnessing original ensemble work that collectively demonstrates what students have learned in the classroom, as well as incorporates metatextual themes and staging. I purposely sat behind my students to witness how they processed the work. The piece they watched was called *The White Bicycle*, which discussed the phenomenon of memorial bicycles painted white to indicate where a rider was killed. It included personal, professional, and popular texts compiled and directed by Nicole Constantini, then a graduate student at Louisiana State University.

After the show, I recognized the positive processing of artistic work in their eyes, the fragmented speech that indicated, "I am still working through it, but it did something for me," and the verbal utterances of, "it was so good," "It was good," "I loved it." It was gratifying for me to see that the students were excited, but I could tell that they were also struggling to piece together what they saw, as it was unlike any traditional theatre work they had ever seen. Yet, the show still evidently moved them in a powerful way. I helped them unpack what they witnessed, asking them to indicate a particular moment that stood out to them. I then asked an important question, one that would again turn the story of progression for the UHCL performance studies program, "Do you think you could do something like that? I can help you. However, it would take time outside of the classroom to create it." I was met with a resounding "Yes!"

I then encouraged them to *seek the work* again, to ask Nicole and the cast how they created scenes that moved them, and to ask what it is like to share the stage as an ensemble. Again and again, they asked each cast of every show they saw the same questions. My students had begun the quest for their own creation, guided by me, but fueled entirely by the other students they met at the festival.

Turner (1982) also notes that not all experience is transformative, but it must be linked with performance for transformation to occur, because performers generate meaning in that process. Convicting moments and ritualistic experiences occur hand in hand because the experience and the potency of *doing* make the event transformative. In *The Ritual Process: Structure and Anti-Structure*, Turner (1969) writes, "You are moved literally by ritual, figuratively by literature. Action and intersubjectivity dominate ritual; reflection and subjectivity dominate reading. Both abound in symbols" (p. 65). Where staged performance can do the work of transformation, participating in ritual taps into a deeper connection because the body remembers by doing.

We planned to craft a show for the next Petit Jean, meaning we had a year to recruit, write, and rehearse the show. During that time, I listened, offered feedback, and engaged in their ideas as their performance experience expanded and grew. As the student organization gained steam, and I taught

Storytelling for the second time, the students were finding their own ways of *seeking the work.* As they had by now made friends with students at the larger schools with performance studies programs, they would travel to see productions in their spaces, sleeping on the couches and floors of graduate students. Each time they returned, further committed to the work of performance, their performance vocabulary and aesthetic desire grew, and they infected the new storytelling students as well with their enthusiasm. We decided to write and rehearse the show over the summer. The show would discuss what it meant to be from the suburbs of Houston, the home of many students in the class. None of them had a Houston address, but by association, they identified as Houstonians. We named the show *Well*—as a play on words, but also the opening response to the question, "but you are from Houston, right?" thus queuing the explanation of where they were actually from, with an exasperated "well."

Each week, I sent them writing prompts with metaphors alluding to how they experience the city, how they explained transportation, or what it meant to have a brown water beach. I did a combination of assigning and applying metaphors that the cast could use, mostly to inspire them and to show a format to write creative performance work. However, two of the prompts asked the student to create and develop their own metaphor in place to frame their experience. The prompts were due at the end of each week, and the students' responses were compiled into scenes by the end of the summer.

We began rehearsals on Monday, August 7, 2017, with plans to meet every Monday and Wednesday for rehearsals. On Tuesday, August 16, we began getting alerts that a storm was developing in the gulf. As a junior faculty, I never experienced hurricane preparation before, so I took the lead of others around me to *hunker down* and gather supplies. I urged the cast to do the same, all of them Houston natives. We canceled rehearsal as Hurricane Harvey moved toward the city.

WELL; HURRICANE HARVEY AND PERFORMANCE AS HEALING

While I experience performance studies programs to exist by someone *hanging a door*—the metaphor of making space when space does not exist—this situation is not common, as it takes risks. The skills to build and establish a program at an institution are not quite quantifiable, and it is frightening to create and experience something that does not have a blueprint. However, I have found in this experience that in the process of building a sustainable performing arts community, while I can get lost in the fight for space and creation, the process alone can offer a healing experience in large and small ways. In that, I found a community that was open to performance. Ultimately, performance proved to be an outlet for this community to process their emotions during the larger narrative of a natural disaster.

Spry's (2011) *Body, Paper, Stage: Writing and Performing Autoethnography* reminds me that experiences cannot be studied directly, but rather, they are mediated by language, speech, and other systems of discourse. Autoethnographers lead with their experiences and the way their bodies operate in the rituals in which they participate. Spry (2011) writes that embodied knowledge, which is the breath of the performative autoethnographer, is the somatic represented through the semantic, and this merging provides a cultural map that aids in documentation. The narratives gathered for this essay provide a living archive of the experiences of creating art during and after a natural disaster. The discourse of story, given life with context, will help paint the picture of lived experiences as I explore performance as a process of healing.

I remember waking early that Sunday morning to the sound of relentless rain on the roof, loud and heavy as if the roof would cave in at any minute. I checked to see if I had power, WiFi, and cell service. I had all three. I walked to my front door, turned the porch light on, and peered out the front window. The street I lived on was a river creeping halfway up the lawn to my house, the view barely visible through the massive downpour.

I knew I could not go back to sleep, so I turned on the television to watch nonstop coverage of Hurricane Harvey as it hit Houston. This is how the next three days would go for me, a continuous cycle of checking for power, WiFi, and cell service, and watching the news, as I could not go anywhere because of the incredibly high water. Isolated, I watched as the city seemed to swallow itself on the news.

For me, the memory of this time comes in pieces—a texted photo from a friend in Dickinson, Texas, of water that had welled up to the second story of her house; a news station flooding, and a reporter stranded on live TV, unable to go back to the studio that was now underwater; crying alone in my living room; copy/pasting the same message that I was alright to every person who tried to contact me; watching areas I frequent in the Houston area, now submerged completely; more helpless crying; and my neighborhood, while flooded, was spared.

I took breaks to check my university email. We were supposed to begin school that Monday. The barrage of frantic emails from students I had not yet met, that I would have met on Monday or Tuesday, informing me that they will try to be in class when the school opened. But they were flooded out, and their only mode of transportation was gone. They had lost everything but their phone. They are staying in a shelter but "Wanted me to know that they are taking their education seriously and didn't want me to think otherwise."

Those messages broke me. I understood what it meant for them to message me, the need to grasp at normalcy while they made sense of the loss that engulfed them. It will eternally stay with me—the memory of those messages, the sound of that unbearable rain, and the solitude of my dry apartment, fielding the inquiries form students I have not met, who had lost everything.

I kept in touch with the cast, checking in with them via text. I kept the conversations short (for fear of dying batteries and limited electricity where they were); however, I did not want to encourage any artistic work, I did not know how they felt. I was certain that after enduring the storm, they would not want to do the show at all. Then, to my surprise, in the group chat, one performer said, "y'all we have to add a scene about Harvey, this show is about the city we live in, and we are living through something right now." Enthusiastic, positive responses followed this statement, "yeah, when school opens, let's meet up to write about it!" All of this, as I found out later, while one of the performer's parents' house was being devastated by the storm.

While experience and memory are ephemeral, performative autoethnography gives a way to document these moments so that we can map our experiences with others across time. I was experiencing how this show was offering a chance to move forward, a chance to heal. As we were pulling from experience, it was personal and deep for myself and the cast.

To add this profoundly emotional event to the show was a risk. When we met again to write the following Monday, I did not know what to expect. I worried that the idea of creating so soon after the storm would be too much for the cast, or that producing a scene that was traumatic and so recent would manifest in work that was too raw to be communicated to an audience. I prepared myself for when the inspired texts, created while the storm was raging, would reveal themselves to be something too big to tackle in the short time we had to rehearse.

I sent them one last writing prompt, to be edited in rehearsal and staged. I asked them to write one to two pages about their experiences, after which I would help them stage a Meyerhold-like sequence to move their bodies with the text they created. The Meyerhold method includes the combination of movements that connect to emotional experiences. In its simplicity, it helped effectively express in body what the students were feeling at the time. I was concerned they would lose their nerve to recount this experience, so I gave the cast twenty-four hours to write. I kept asking them the same questions at every rehearsal until we traveled to the Petit Jean Performance Festival, "Do you want to do this? Do you want to perform this and travel?" The answer was always yes.

The narratives they wrote were complex, honest, and heartbreaking. One performer wrote about what it meant to help others after the storm. Another wrote about balancing concern for their home and things while caring for others who had lost everything. Another wrote about the waiting and the loss of control that comes when one is at the mercy of a storm. One student told the story of losing their family home and recounted how their parent and siblings swam to safety from the second floor of their home, but had to leave their pets, which were too frightened to swim, behind in an attic. The student narratized that while they sought shelter at one parent's house in the city, their other parent, siblings, and pets stayed behind in their house in Dickinson, Texas, a town five miles from campus. The water rose faster than the family could prepare for, and during the evacuations, their dogs, two large Great Danes, and cat were too frightened to swim to the evacuation boat. They made the decision to put the pets in the attic, and swim to safety. Upon hearing this, the performer recounted their feelings, "I cried when they told me." I quietly whispered, "I'm so sorry, you don't deserve this, I love you." Helpless to save them. It would be three whole days before we could return to the home, to get them, and they were all alive and hungry." The student then continued to recount the homes recovery in their performance, saying, "Who are you when all of your childhood photos and memories are gone? Who are you when the home you grew up in is covered in mud and all the furniture washed away by floodwater?" The performers then ended their piece by saying, "I still wipe my feet, before entering my home," a heartbreaking reminder of the familiarity of home spaces and of their absence.

We edited the scene together in a somber and quiet room, I could see the brevity of the scene for the cast. We are editing as the water is receding, and everywhere we looked, some part of the community had been touched by Harvey. Now that school was in session, the aftermath permeated every aspect of our campus lives. Students were sleeping in cars, or suddenly jumping up to leave class because they needed to help with the cleanup, or help with assessment awaiting an insurance issue for a home, or just because they were feeling overwhelmed. The cast and I tried our best to feel normal while living in chaos. We tried to use all that we were feeling in that moment, the pain, the guilt, the sadness, and confusion, and to channel it all into the scene.

We rehearsed the show, and the scene about Hurricane Harvey, often. We rehearsed while a performer nursed an injury from cleaning debris. We rehearsed through a thunderstorm, the clap of thunder and torrential downpour that momentarily knocked the lights in the building triggering a flash of memories of the not-so-distant past and terrifying the cast. During that time, we staged a movement sequence, lit only by window light as that storm blew by. In repetitive motion and silence, the cast performed a movement sequence embodying the processes of enduring the storm: a leaning in and out to represent watching television, a wiping feet motion that symbolized the natural motion before one enters a home, but still doing it even as the home is gone. We practiced the scene in that space until the darkness left, the cast moving through the sequence in silent tears.

We did a one-night-only show in the UHCL Bayou Theater on October 7, 2017, six weeks after the storm hit and one week before the Petit Jean Performance Festival. The show held great weight for me, as it was the first in-house ensemble performance at the university in thirty years. However, I also knew that the community, along with the cast, would still be fresh with the pain of Harvey. I was aware that the reception could vary, and I prepared myself as much as I could. The cast, while anxious, seemed eager to perform, and eager to showcase what they created.

As I reflect on this experience, I am aware of the work, or invisible labor, that it took to make this production happen. While all of the students took my storytelling class, which focuses on solo performance, I found much of my rehearsal time was spent educating the cast on stage mechanics, blocking, vocal projection, and lighting, all in a crash course that sat atop processing Hurricane Harvey. In the moment, it did not feel like labor. Only in retrospect can I quantify the fatigue, mentally and emotionally, that comes with producing a show like this under such adverse circumstances.

The show was well received by an audience of family members, friends, and students seeking extra credit. When the show reached the Harvey scene, as we called it, I noted the silence; all sound in the theatre ceased, only to resume again as sniffles. I realized that many in the audience were still living this experience and would go home to it after the show was over. In the end, many of those audience members would tell me that this was the first time they could process what had happened to them. Students who attended the show were asked to write papers about how the scene and the show allowed them to give shape to their feelings aroused by the disaster. This area, twenty-five miles from the city center, considered the quiet suburbs, had been given a voice to process its pain. The cast left the show elated, basking in the post-show glow that occurs. They felt comfortable and confident, and I felt we were ready to go to the festival.

We attended the 2017 Petit Jean Performance Festival to perform the show. As a long-time attendee of the festival, I knew the saying that there is "no audience like the Petit Jean audience," and it would bode well for the cast. The festival audience is made up of undergraduate and graduate students of theatre and performance studies from across the country as well as faculty and performance practitioners. When one performs for other performance people, the audience reacts well; they cheer and reward the performance with rapt attention as they know the hard work behind each play. In my final chat with the students before the show began, I reminded them to be aware of that dialogic audiencing, rather the ability to read the audience and feed off their energy; to pause for laughter before continuing, to feel the energy from the audience, to not let it consume them so much that they lose control of their work, and to, above all things, project their voices. We performed in the Petit Jean State Parks old recreation hall, a large space with wood floors and a vaulted, cathedral-like roof. In the moments before the cast took the stage, I stood back and reflected on the past two years. In those months, the university went from showing no interest in performance studies to some, from no performing arts classes to one, and from students who have never performed before to a group of four that will take the stage at a national performance festival.

Before the show began, I was allowed to say a few words on behalf of the cast to the audience. I briefly told our story, how the school had no performing arts until now, how we wrote the show over the summer, and then, when Hurricane Harvey happened, how we regrouped to add another scene about our experiences. I told the audience that the cast wanted to work through the storm and produce the show even as tragedy surrounded us. I chose to be transparent, as my own act of healing, to communicate that the arts offered an outlet for us to come together and process pain and our proximity to each other.

As a director who was already familiar with the show, I delighted anew in the nuances that come from a show going well. The small nonverbal reactions from the cast when a joke landed and they had to stay focused; the ease and comfort to play and interact with the audience that comes with the confidence that fuels performance when you are *in it*; all built up to the scene about the storm.

I understand it now as an attempt to heal when disaster strikes by forces beyond our control. There is no balm or how-to book on healing. It must come from within, and with the resources and people you find in your proximity. Our show became the balm for the cast, a way to articulate feeling as it was occurring and to process experience when words failed. In *Dramas, Fields, and Metaphors: Symbolic Action in Human Society*, Turner (1974) writes that "meaning arises when we try to put what culture and language have crystallized from the past together with what we feel, wish, and think about our present point in life" (p. 33). The performance helped crystalize the experience in a way that would help the cast move forward and make sense of the world.

This moment is significant because of the audiencing. I believe that those who practice and teach Performance understand that it is about giving students and audience members the feeling you have. Just as my mentors gave me the gift of performance to give to an audience, I am giving it to this cast. In the ways that performance has healed me and helped me process my feelings, by delivering my artistic expressions to an audience, it is now regifted to this national audience. It is a full-circle moment to give the tools I learned to my students and watch them succeed and grow.

CONCLUSION

"If you do it, we now have it" is a statement that, in all its simplicity, is a call to arms. It is saying that if you perform the steps, it exists. When my dean said this to me in my interview, I knew even at the moment that there is more to it than just the action alone. To build a performance program where there was not one means that the doing of this act needs to be *dialogic*—it needs to be in conversation and alignment with the resources already established at the institution—and it needs allies in support. Most practitioners understand that no performance or show is ever truly solo. Many hands help it, behind the scenes, to grow. It is no different when building a space to continue creating performance work. I learned that it is a negotiation of the already established and a gentle guide into the new. Many hands make light work.

Of the students who performed in *Well*, three of the four are now in graduate programs, two of them in Performance Studies programs. Since this production, our campus has put up four in-house productions featuring student writing and performers. While the group of performance-interested students waxes and wanes depending on the semester, there is slow and steady growth in Performance Studies at UHCL. The successes, however small, were always due in part to the students involved in this work as they had hands in this success every step of the way. Their investment in this work showed and continues to show the campus the importance of the performing arts. The interest stays alive and continues to grow because these students demonstrate that the arts do more than just create an aesthetic experience. The way in which performance helped the cast of *Well* and the larger university community heal after Hurricane Harvey is a prime illustration of this.

For this practitioner, to say that performance can have a transformative or healing effect on a person often means that it is difficult to find the words to communicate how to articulate what these experiences mean and how to quantify them. However, I believe we as practitioners push to find ways to give people the feeling of invincibility on stage, or of a movement of the body that gets to what the brain cannot articulate into language. To practice and to teach performance work to others is giving them the tools with which to participate in their own healing. While I may be present for a possible breakthrough, the real work comes from handing over the tools. We give freely, fully aware that some who receive will only participate for a little while, and some for a lifetime; but we continue to give, to aid in this cyclical trend of teaching, because it also provides healing for ourselves. We get as much out of giving the gift of performance as the students.

REFERENCES

Chang, H. (2008). *Autoethnography as method*. Walnut Creek, CA: Left Coast Press.

Gallop, J. (Ed.). (1995). *Pedagogy: The question of impersonation*. Bloomington, IN: Indiana University Press.

Hamera, J. (2005). Exposing the pedagogical body: Protocols and tactics. In B. K. Alexander, G. L. Anderson, & B. P. Gallegos (Eds.), *Performance theories in education: Power, pedagogy, and the politics of identity* (pp. 59–78). Mahwah, NJ: Lawrence Erlbaum Associates.

Holman Jones, S., Adams, T. E., & Ellis, C. (Eds.). (2013). *Handbook of autoethnography*. Walnut Creek, CA: Left Coast Press.

Park-Fuller, L. M. (1994). Performance as *praxis*: The intercollegiate performance festival. *Text and Performance Quarterly*, *14*(4), 330–333. https://doi.org/10.1080/10462939409366095

Pineau, E. L. (1994). Teaching is performance: Reconceptualizing a problematic metaphor. *American Educational Research Journal*, *31*(1), 3–25. https://www.jstor.org/stable/1163264

Spry, T. (2001). Performing autoethnography: An embodied methodological praxis. *Qualitative Inquiry*, *7*(6), 706–732. https://doi.org/10.1177%2F107780040100700605

Spry, T. (2011). *Body, paper, stage: Writing and performing autoethnography*. Walnut Creek, CA: Left Coast Press.

Turner, V. (1969). *The ritual process: Structure and anti-structure*. Chicago, IL: Aldine Publishing.

Turner, V. (1974). *Dramas, fields, and metaphors: Symbolic action in human society*. Ithaca, NY: Cornell University Press.

Turner, V. (1982). *From ritual to theater: The human seriousness of play*. New York: PAJ Publications.

Turner, V. (1988). *The anthropology of performance*. New York: PAJ Publications.

Turner, V., & Bruner, E. M. (Eds). (1986). *The Anthropology of Experience*. Chicago, IL: University of Illinois Press.

Part II

Narrative, Art, Dance, and Music

Chapter Six

"Hip-Hop Just Saved Me"

Rap Music Engagement as a Music-Based Intervention for Substance-Addicted Youth

Alice Marianne Fritz and Kamran Afary

"Into my heart an air that kills" wrote A. E. Housman (1896), thereby summarizing into seven syllables the almost ineffable ache that accompanies a realization of things lost, never again to be regained. Like the fictional "Shropshire Lad" who narrates this poem, many youth today, including those with little or no formal education in language use and composition, use simple, everyday, and often even slang vocabulary to articulate profound frustration, suffering, and perseverance. Rap music has made accidental poets of hip-hop identified young men and women, who find in the rap genre a channel through which to express their stifled voices.

A constellation of factors in the postindustrial urban landscape of the South Bronx in the mid-1970s gave birth to the now global cultural force known as hip-hop, and its most prominent feature, rap music (Rose, 1994). Since its inception, this musical genre has allowed disenfranchised individuals on the socioeconomic fringe to tell the stories of their struggles. Tricia Rose's (1994) *Black Noise: Rap Music and Black Culture in Contemporary America* describes rap expressivity as an outlet to reflect on issues that concern inner-city youth, including "poverty, fear of adulthood, the desire for absent fathers, frustrations about black male sexism, female sexual desires, daily rituals of life as an unemployed teen hustler, safe sex, raw anger, violence, and childhood memories" (p. 18). Today, rap music has been embraced by youth (and by adults) everywhere, across cultural and ethnic divisions, who continue to associate it with the chronicling of disadvantaged socioeconomic conditions, dysfunctional familial relationships, and the often vast discrepancy between desire and lack. This use of rap music as a narrative vehicle for the problems facing youth living in high-risk environments has often led to the composition of lyrics with negative messages and implications, as when rappers glorify "thug life" as a way for deprived youths to cope under harsh conditions. *Gangsta rap*, a subgenre of rap music, has been a particular target of those who malign rap for reinforcing antisocial attitudes and behaviors. But just as the complexity of rap allows it to articulate both antisocial and prosocial messages, rap music is interpreted and used by its adherents in both destructive and constructive ways. Instances in which rap music acted as a conduit for positive change among at-risk youth have been documented in the literature, and researchers have advocated for the integration of rap into therapy (for example, Elligan, 2000), school counseling (for example, Gonzalez & Hayes, 2009), and social work (for example, Travis & Deepak, 2011). This chapter considers the potential that rap music offers for the promotion of prosocial attitudes and behavior in youth, specifically within the context of substance abuse intervention. As will be made apparent in the literature review that follows, the bulk of research done with regard to substance use and rap music engagement has been from a psychological perspective. The current chapter is an attempt to engage with this phenomenon from a communication studies perspective, using a narrative approach. To illustrate the therapeutic potential of rap music for individuals presenting with substance use disorder (SUD), we offer the case example of an adolescent male who credits rap expressivity as a significant factor that inspired the positive change in his own life. The impetus for the present essay arose when one of the authors encountered this adolescent, and thereby discovered the natural support group that this youth had spontaneously formed with a few substance-using friends. The exemplary case highlighted in this chapter did not occur in a psychotherapeutic context; rather, it demonstrates the positive effects of rap music engagement in non-clinical, everyday settings. Nevertheless, it is expected that the insights gleaned therein may be of interest for professionals working with at-risk adolescents who may wish to incorporate rap music into their youth work strategies.

LITERATURE REVIEW

We begin this section with a brief, and necessarily reductionistic, overview of substance use among teens and common psychotherapeutic approaches to this problem, before progressing to a discussion of how rap music engagement may complement such traditional interventions.

Substance Use Disorder among Youth

According to the fifth edition of the *Diagnostic and Statistical Manual of Mental Disorders* (*DSM-5*), substance use disorder (SUD) is diagnosed when an individual presents with at least two to three pathological symptoms associated with the disorder, including intense craving for a substance, withdrawal effects that accompany cessation attempts, and compulsive use of a substance even when such use impedes an individual's functioning in the areas of school, work, or other obligations (APA, 2013). In a 2014 survey conducted by the Substance Abuse and Mental Health Services Administration (SAMHSA, 2015), approximately 2.3 million adolescents (9.4%) in the United States aged 12–17 admitted to using illicit drugs of some kind. These included the use of marijuana (7.4%), but also more harmful substances such as cocaine (0.2%) and heroine (0.1%) (p. 3). Adolescents living in low-income households reported more illegal drug use than those living in households whose income exceeds the Federal Poverty Level (FPL). A discrepancy based upon household income likewise exists among individuals who abuse or are dependent upon an illicit drug, with a higher percentage of drug abuse or dependence reported by those living in households without health insurance or whose income is below the FPL. Substance abuse among adolescent populations can lead to social, legal, and physical complications, and may be particularly troubling since brain trauma stemming from drug or alcohol abuse during this critical developmental stage may lead to lasting neurocognitive deficits (Squeglia, Jacobus, & Tapert, 2009). Furthermore, drug dependence syndromes (for example, drug tolerance, withdrawal symptoms, emotional and physical problems, etc.) have been shown to manifest more quickly with adolescent-onset drug use (Chen, Storr, & Anthony, 2009).

Psychotherapeutic Approaches to Treatment of Substance Use Disorder

Currently, there are multiple treatment strategies in the field of substance abuse counseling, reflecting a variety of psychotherapeutic paradigms. In addition, there are self-help groups for individuals with SUD, of which the best known are Alcoholics Anonymous (AA) and Narcotics Anonymous (NA). Those programs are not guided by trained helping professionals, but rather rely upon members to support and encourage each other to discontinue addictive behaviors. At a typical AA speaker meeting, group members relate personal stories relating to their addiction, the negative consequences of the addiction, and their efforts toward recovery, an act of storytelling that facilitates "bonding to the group, and to the fellowship of AA, by establishing a sense of shared experience" (Nowinski, 2003, p. 60). This can be said to parallel the sense of community generated when rappers "spit" about their personal struggles, including drug addiction. In fact, rap music engagement may hold considerable promise in helping individuals with SUD in their change efforts.

During traditional talk therapy sessions, the focus is often on the problematic behaviors that prompted the intervention, rather than on the abilities, strengths, and skills the clients possess which could be harnessed to substitute well-being promoting behaviors for health-inhibiting ones. One treatment approach that has been employed by SUD service providers is that of solution-focused counseling (SFC). In contrast to problem-focused approaches, the solution-focused counselor emphasizes "those things in the client's life that have gone well and continue to go well" (Osborn, 2012, p. 151), and exhibits confidence that the client's own abilities and strengths will inevitably lead to positive change. Themes in rap music often convey empowering messages (Travis, 2013; Travis & Deepak, 2011), and the selection of self-affirming rap songs by the service provider may support strength-based treatment approaches. Another established therapy that has demonstrated effectiveness for chemical dependency intervention is the cognitive-behavioral approach. Rap music may be incorporated into therapy sessions in a way that aligns with essential features of cognitive-behavioral interventions, as when clients are encouraged to compose lyrics they could repeat to themselves whenever they encounter emotional or cognitive triggers that induce craving to use. This strategy parallels the "self-talk" clients in cognitive-behavioral therapy are taught to engage in as a coping skill (Osborn, 2012).

Certain basic assumptions of both solution-focused counseling and cognitive-behavioral therapy are shared by counselors who employ narrative therapy. All three treatment strategies refrain from equating the patient with the disease, and instead emphasize the extrinsic nature of the client's presenting issues. The practitioner working from a narrative therapy approach recognizes that it is the clients who are "experts" on their own needs, motivations, and psychological impediments (Payne, 2006). The therapeutic process starts with the therapist inviting the client to talk about something in the client's life that is causing distress (Payne, 2006). The result is often a *problem-saturated description* characteristic of the dominant way in which the client frames their experiences at that point in time (Payne, 2006, p. 11). In *Narrative Theory: An Introduction for Counsellors*, Martin Payne (2006) explains why these first-person narratives are the important underlying roots of the client's dysfunction, and are the targets of the change effort from a narrative therapy perspective:

> The stories do not just comprise a neutral linguistic representation of memory; they are also *influential*. These stories, or narratives, come to form the matrix

> of concepts and beliefs by which we understand our lives, and the world in which our lives take place; and there is a continuing interaction between the stories we tell ourselves about our lives, the ways we live our lives, and the further stories we then tell. (Payne, 2006, p. 20; emphasis in the original)

In conversation with the therapist, this self-story is gradually deconstructed as the client volunteers additional self-disclosures, some of which may contradict the original story (Payne, 2006). Ultimately, the revision of their problem-saturated dominant story allows clients to adjust the lens through which they perceive themselves and their reality. It is easy to see the influence of narrative therapy on hip-hop-integrated therapy, which similarly advocates encouraging clients to write about specific concerns in the form of song lyrics, which are then discussed and interpreted with the therapist (Gonzalez & Hayes, 2009).

The treatment strategy employed depends in large part upon how one conceptualizes addiction itself. On a micro level, it may influence what methods a particular practitioner uses; on a macro level, it may impact which public policies are adopted to deal with this problem. Viewing addiction as a disease that is inseparable from the diseased organism may result in the pathologizing of the client presenting with addiction issues. Relatedly, seeing addicted individuals as those who have persistently made bad choices, when smarter options were available, contributes to spiking incarceration rates and harsher penalties for illicit drug users. The issue is further bemuddled by uncertainty surrounding the phenomenon of addiction itself, with one extreme faction claiming it to be a myth (for example, Davies, 1997). These kinds of perspectives do not appear to have produced optimal outcomes, and helping professionals working from both the solution-focused and cognitive-behavioral approaches prefer to isolate the presenting issue (that is, the substance addiction) from the individual.

VALUE OF RAP MUSIC ENGAGEMENT IN DEVELOPMENTAL INTERVENTIONS AND EVERYDAY SETTINGS

Raphael Travis Jr. (2013) includes the various change efforts directed at youth under the umbrella term "developmental interventions," which is defined as "the health promotion and prevention aspects of education, therapy, and youth work" (p. 141). Counselors, social workers, researchers, and other helping professionals have documented the value of developmental interventions that integrate a rap music engagement component (for example, DeCarlo & Hockman, 2003; Elligan, 2004; Gonzalez & Hayes, 2009; Kobin & Tyson, 2006; Travis & Deepak, 2011). For example, Beats Rhymes and Life (BRL) is a mental health service provider based in Oakland, California, that focuses on hip-hop therapy as a culturally sensitive therapeutic modality for helping marginalized youth (BRL, Inc., n.d.). According to their website, the organization's hip-hop therapy model produces the desirable outcomes of improved client mood and self-esteem, decreased risk behaviors, and more favorable attitude toward mental health services. In addition to such successful examples of rap music deployment in schools or by mental health service providers, youth have been found to use rap music therapeutically outside of professional contexts, within their everyday lives (Travis, 2013). Without prompting from mental health professionals, these individuals actively seek engagement with rap music as a tool for coping with and overcoming negative life events and psychological distress. Such informal music interventions, lacking the presence of professional music therapists to guide the sessions, have been referred to as *music-based interventions* rather than music therapy (Hohmann et al., 2017). Often, adolescents who are going through stressful situations are reluctant to seek out helping professionals or to articulate their anxieties in clinical environments. Deterrents to seeking counseling or therapy include cynicism toward the therapeutic process or mistrust of mental health professionals (Tillie-Allen, 2005). Moreover, the reticence of adolescent males may be amplified in African American and Latino youth due to cultural expectations (Alvarez, 2012).

In an episode of the hip-hop themed TV show *Empire*, the protagonist, Lucious Lyon, is grilled on the violent messages that so often permeate rap songs. Coming to rap music's defense, Lucious points out that "there's hope in the fact that these kids are expressing their anger with music and poetry and not with a 12-gauge shotgun" (Daniels, Strong, & Chaiken, 2015). Although the analogy Lucious uses may be an extreme one, rap music has been reported to promote healthier attitudes and behavior in adolescents living in hazardous environments (DeCarlo & Hockman, 2003), where the choice of whether to pick up a mic or a gun may be a real dilemma. However, the potential benefits of rap music engagement go beyond being a substitute for antisocial activities. Don Elligan, who in 2000 coined the term *rap therapy* and was one of the first clinicians to integrate the then as yet untested modality of rap music into psychotherapy, outlines a therapeutic process that includes encouraging clients to compose their own rap lyrics "to help work through the presenting issue" (Elligan, 2012, p. 36). Listening to or creating rap songs can potentially pacify angry emotions, and expressing oneself through the art form of rap can be used for "cathartic release"; rapping can be a safe way to vent negative emotions (Elligan, 2012, p. 27; Travis & Deepak, 2011). V. Thandi Sulé (2016), studying a sample of college students, found that performing rap songs allowed the students to release tension by expressing, in an innocuous way, their discontent (for example, toward the socioeconomic status quo), which, left unsaid, would have caused stress. Using rap expressivity as an outlet for stressful thoughts and emotions may be particularly beneficial for some populations, including African American and Latino adolescent males, as they belong to a culture wherein members are taught from a young age to "be tough, conceal pain, hide emotion, and deal with problems on their own" (Alvarez, 2012, p. 121). The stress-reducing potential of rap music engagement holds important implications for substance abuse interventions, as stress and anxiety are major factors leading to relapse, driving individuals to revert to drug-taking behavior after a period of abstinence (Nobre & Castilho, 2009).

A distinguishing aspect of rap music that sets it apart from other musical genres is its emphasis on the spoken word; rap aficionados often pay more attention to the lyrics and rhymes than to the melodies of rap songs (Kobin & Tyson, 2006). Another salient characteristic of rap music is its personal narrative aspect. Rap music facilitates the expression not only of emotions, but also of the experiences that gave rise to those emotions. George Yancy and Susan Hadley (2012), in their introduction to *Therapeutic Uses of Rap and Hip-Hop*, call modern-day rap artists the inheritors of the important responsibility of the West African *griots* of yore: that of "telling and retelling collective and individual stories" (p. xxxi). When a narrator tells their own story or the story of their community to an audience, the lived experiences that are narrated assume a new importance; they are validated through the implicit recognition that those lived experiences were valuable narrative fodder.

Adolescents may be more vulnerable to certain kinds of problems, including depression symptoms (Susman & Rogol, 2004), than individuals in other age groups (Arnett, 1999). The emotional vulnerability of inner city adolescents is often compounded by environmental threats indigenous to urban settings, such as "lower parental education, exposure to violent crime, single parenthood," and other by-products of economic privation (DeCarlo & Hockman, 2003, p. 47). A combination of normal adolescent stress and environmental hazards could result in intense negative emotions such as anger, depression, or despondency. The literature provides ample evidence of the therapeutic value of music engagement in general, in part due to the important function of music listening as a mood regulator (Bogt et al., 2016; Groarke & Hogan, 2016). Individuals often listen to music to modulate a negative affect and promote a more positive one (Shäfer et al., 2013).

Thematic aspects of rap music can potentially enhance its therapeutic value, as when songs express themes, motifs, or ideas that are empowering to the listener or performer (Travis, 2013). Empowerment has been defined as "any attempt to gain power over decision making, opportunities, or the meaning ascribed to one's life" (Travis & Deepak, 2011, p. 207). Many at-risk youth live in oppressive social and economic conditions that are inimical to a sense of personal agency; to those adolescents, the empowering messages found in some rap songs may inspire faith in one's own ability to survive a traumatic past, transcend an adverse present, and build a better future (Travis, 2013). Closely connected to the construct of empowerment are those of self-esteem and resilience; both are important target areas in psychotherapy involving youth (Ierardi & Jenkins, 2012). Travis (2013) notes that within rap music, empowerment, self-esteem, and resilience themes are common, and messages in rap songs are often about "esteem enhancing strategies," or "strategies for overcoming life obstacles" (pp. 147–148).

On the one hand, rap expressivity allows youth to vent their angers, frustrations, fears, and other negative emotions, while on the other hand, it allows them to create messages of personal empowerment, resilience, and coping. An emphasis on these types of empowering messages in rap songs may allow at-risk youth to perceive themselves as capable of overcoming problems and effecting positive outcomes in their own lives. Previous researchers have conducted analyses of major themes emerging from commercial hip-hop songs (Kobin & Tyson, 2006; Tillie-Allen, 2005; Tyson et al., 2012). Edgar Tyson, Konstantin Detchkov, Erin Eastwood, Aussa Carver, and Amanda Sehr (2012) concluded that popular rap songs were dominated by four general themes that could be broken down into twenty-one subthemes. The broad thematic categories were social criticism, social empowerment, humanistic values, and negative behavior criticism (Tyson et al., 2012). The subcategories encompassed under the major category of social empowerment included "personal empowerment," "praise of family values," "praise of work and achievement," "praise of education," and "praise of women" (Tyson et al., 2012, pp. 107–109). Beyond an examination of the lyrics of commercial rap songs, which may be shaped somewhat by the demands of the market or the predilections of record label executives, it is also important to look at the kinds of themes that emerge when young people are prompted to write their own lyrics. Aaron Lightstone (2012) conducted a thematic analysis of the rap lyrics in songs written by residents at a youth shelter to assess the therapeutic potential of the songs' contents. Lightstone's (2012) analysis yielded the following nine general themes: (1) authenticity and emotional expression; (2) rapper as critical theorist; (3) boasting; (4) rap battles/insults; (5) drugs; (6) evidence of group process; (7) spirituality; (8) violence; and (9) musical wordplay.

Although some of the messages in rap music may have negative implications when they glorify violence, romanticize the gangsta lifestyle, or objectify women, even such "high-risk themes" (Travis, 2013, p. 150) may offer something uplifting for individuals who focus upon the self-empowerment aspect and affirmation of their self-image such lyrics arouse (Travis & Deepak, 2011). Raphael Travis Jr. and Anne Deepak (2011) observe that lyrics narrating the attainment of material success in the face of structural obstacles may be perceived as empowering regardless of the means through which such success is depicted as being achieved. Similarly, messages describing the subjugation of others through aggression or sexual domination may be experienced by the listener as empowering even as they promote risky attitudes and behaviors (Travis & Deepak, 2011). Furthermore, although a thorough discussion of the issue of sexism and misogyny in hip-hop is beyond the scope of this chapter, it is worth noting in passing that some scholars and cultural observers take issue with the characterization of rap music as monolithically sexist (Azikwe, 2011). Those scholars point to successful female artists who rap about women navigating sexual politics, surviving domestic violence, and struggling against economic lack; or female rappers who "create a progressive, feminist space within hip-hop's hyper-masculine universe" (Azikwe, 2011, p. 137). In the process, not only do these female rappers exhibit a lyrical virtuosity equal to that of their male counterparts, but they also present images of powerful women that their fans could use as blueprints by which to model their own personas. Female rappers like Queen Latifah, for instance, assume a respected maternal posture from which to speak to audiences about political-economic issues affecting the Black community, while the "sistas with attitude" persona is exemplified by rappers such as Lil' Kim and Foxy Brown, who present themselves as powerful women in full charge of their sexuality (Keyes, 2012). Ultimately, the "conflicting, inconsistent grey areas of hip-hop" (Azikwe, 2011, p. 137) is a complex cultural terrain that conveys messages which audiences can interpret as either, or even both, empowering or oppressive.

The potential benefits of rap music engagement have motivated therapists working with adolescent clients to include a hip-hop component as part of their developmental interventions, in both individual and group work settings. Alonzo DeCarlo and Elaine Hockman (2003) compared client reactions to standard group therapy sessions and sessions using rap music engagement, which were similar to the traditional therapy sessions but related discussions of key issues (morality, anger management, etc.) to lyrics of rap songs. Three groups of African American male adolescents, including a group of violent offenders, another group of status offenders, and a third group comprised of young males with no criminal record, were asked to rate their impressions of the usefulness of the group therapy sessions they attended. All three groups indicated preference for the rap therapy sessions for helping them build prosocial skills. In terms of affect, 100% of DeCarlo and Hockman's (2003) participants reported enjoyment of the rap therapy sessions, and 81% reported feeling excited about upcoming meetings.

A strong connection with social ties is a crucial factor for optimal functioning in youth (Travis, 2013). In group therapy contexts, the inclusion of a rap music component may facilitate bonding between group members. Scott MacDonald and Michael Viega (2012), who led a rap song-writing program for children living in a high-risk neighborhood, assert that the process of cocreating rap songs helped the children "feel connected to other group members" (p. 169). Similarly, Lightstone (2012) lists the collective creative experience of making rap music as a potential advantage of synergizing conventional therapy with rap music engagement. During rap music therapy sessions with youth living at a shelter, the author noted instances in which members would encourage one another to rap or sing, or reference the lyrics of another member in their own rap, thereby signaling attention to and validation of the fellow group member's work. More importantly, members would use their rap lyrics to demonstrate they understood and have felt the pain experienced by other members, and to also encourage others in the group to maintain a positive outlook and take positive actions, such as staying in school (Lightstone, 2012).

As Travis (2013) points out, music engagement is used by both youth and adults as a coping strategy: "They already use music as a strategy for help without any professional help" (p. 143). Researchers have suggested that rap music engagement can facilitate provider-client communication in substance abuse interventions, as when therapists and clients collaboratively explore themes in rap songs that relate to addiction (for example, Baker, Dingle, & Gleadhill, 2012; Kobin & Tyson, 2006). Incorporating rap music into substance abuse interventions can enhance the effectiveness of treatment by reducing client resistance to therapy and by increasing motivation to attend sessions (Kobin & Tyson, 2006).

The above discussion illustrates how the idea of rap-integrated developmental interventions have gained acceptance among practitioners. There is by now no lack of research exploring the utility of rap music in clinical contexts. However, studies documenting how rap music engagement is being used by youth themselves, independent of helping professionals, as a music-based intervention (Hohmann et al., 2017) are rare. As the following case example demonstrates, even in the absence of attendance mandates, such as court-ordered therapy sessions, rap music engagement can motivate hip-hop identified youth with substance abuse problems to attend regular meetings to rap about the issues pertinent to their lives. We present this case example to support the idea that rap music engagement is an appropriate and effective therapeutic component for certain populations. Furthermore, an analysis of two rap songs written by the subject is presented to supplement previous research into the themes that are prominent in both commercial rap music and songs written by amateur rappers. The lyrics were written by the subject of the current case study, and show the kinds of themes that are relevant to youth with SUD. These themes will be compared with the themes previously identified by Tyson et al. (2012) and by Lightstone (2012).

The following research questions constitute the primary foci of the present study: (1) How does a self-formed counterpublic support group come into being, and what is the nature of such a group? (2) How is rap music and storytelling integrated by the group's members? (3) What themes can be identified in a close reading of the rap songs composed by a member of this group? and (4) How does rap expressivity allow individuals to reframe their problem-saturated stories into a more empowering narrative?

METHODOLOGY

As narrative is a main focus of the present paper, both in terms of its relevance in the therapeutic context for substance-addicted individuals, and as a key feature of rap expressivity itself, we will provide a narrative analysis of two rap songs composed by our subject, Diego (pseudonym). Narrative analysis has acquired popularity among researchers working within various fields, and the specific strategies used in the analysis can differ accordingly, with the most common being the psychological, biographical, and discourse analysis approaches (Merriam, 2002). The term "narrative" can be applied to a wide range of rhetorical texts, from "literary works to diaries and written autobiographies, conversations, or oral life stories obtained in interviews" (Lieblich, Tuval-Mashiach, & Zilber, 1998, p. 3). That Diego's rap songs revolve around unified subjects, contain descriptions of events which follow a temporal sequence, and establish causal links between the events (Foss, 2009) justify assigning them the label of narrative texts. Following the strategy outlined by Sonja Foss (2009) in her *Rhetorical Criticism: Exploration and Practice*, the objective(s) of each song was identified, and the specific features of the songs were then dissected to reveal how they contributed to attaining the objective(s). A characteristic of narrative criticism is its use of subjective reading, and the current study makes no claim to providing definitive interpretations of the polysemantic narratives presented below. Notwithstanding its element of subjectivity, narrative analysis can be a valuable tool for the social science researcher, and its methods "can be considered 'real-world measures' that are appropriate when 'real-life problems' are investigated" (Lieblich, Tuval-Mashiach, and Zilber, 1998, p. 5). Moreover, triangulation can help overcome limitations associated with qualitative research (Lindlof & Taylor, 2011). In the present research, triangulation involved the use of two investigators and two sources of data (the song lyrics and interview transcripts). To minimize any potential bias that may seep into subjective interpretations, the authors first independently enumerated themes each discerned in the song lyrics. Subsequently, the lists of themes were compared and discussed, until agreement was reached as to which themes were best supported by the data.

In the pages that follow, we consider narrativized accounts of personal experience from a communication perspective that focuses on how narrative devices are used in the creation of those stories, and attempts to discover the storyteller's objectives through analysis.

A CASE EXAMPLE OF RAP MUSIC ENGAGEMENT AS A MUSIC-BASED INTERVENTION

One of the authors met Diego when he enrolled in her public speaking class at a public university in the western United States. For their first major speech, students were asked to tell the class about a group or community they were a part of, and to elaborate on why membership in this community was important to them. With a candor that surprised the author, Diego shared in his speech that when he was 12 years old, he became addicted to crack cocaine. Now 18, he had been drug-free for the past three years and was, obviously, in school working toward a college degree. What was less obvious, but what the author came to realize after observing him over the course of the semester, was that Diego was not merely going through the motions like so many other students, but was intent upon working hard in his classes, earning good grades, and carving out a future for himself. During his speech, Diego revealed that he was part of a small group of friends who all had experience with substance abuse, and who were all also deeply into rap music. They would meet once a week to "spit," bringing lyrics composed over the previous week to share with the group. By regularly meeting and indirectly discussing their problems and feelings through the vehicle of rap, Diego's small group of former substance users approximates an informal self-help group. Diego attributed his success in thus far remaining sober partly to these rap sessions with friends who had or were going through experiences similar to his own. When the semester ended, the author approached Diego and asked him if she could interview him and document his experiences. He readily granted his consent, and in the course of two semi-structured interviews (the first lasting two hours, the second one hour), which were subsequently transcribed, Diego described his experiences with addiction, the constant struggle to stay clean, and how creating rap music helped him in that struggle. The two songs analyzed in the pages that follow were voluntarily shared by Diego during the interviews, without prompting by the researchers (although transcripts for both pieces were requested after the interviews to ensure that interpretation was based on accurate versions of the artist's lyrics).

When asked about the rap artists he listens to, Diego named old-school rappers like A Tribe Called Quest, Wu-Tang Clan, and Tupac as a few of his favorite rap artists. Diego is deeply immersed in the hip-hop culture, as evidenced not only by his attempts to create his own rap music, but also by a phase he went through during which he would paint graffiti, perhaps the most publicly vilified aspect of hip-hop culture, on public walls. When grafitti-writing first appeared on subway cars and stations in New York City in the late 1960s, both city officials and the local newspapers declared war on the activity (Castleman, 2012). Before long, a graffiti bill was passed that made it illegal for anyone to write or draw on any public property, or even to carry an open aerosol paint can in a public place (Castleman, 2012). Graffiti-writing remains an arrestable offense, and Diego acknowledges his own recklessness, especially as he recalls the times when he would attempt to spray paint billboards in broad daylight.

Diego was 12 years old when he smoked crack for the first time. At that impressionable young age, the absence of a role model who could have had a positive influence on Diego was unfortunate. During the interview, he spoke wistfully of wanting an older male figure in his life to guide him, but his father appears to have been too busy running the family business to spend much time with Diego.

> Nobody really played the role of like, an older brother to check me or anything, so anytime I saw an older male I would look up to him no matter what it was they were doing, and unfortunately, all of them happened to be doing bad stuff. So, like, my first time that I was looking up to someone, it was something negative that I looked up to. My sister's friends, for example . . . well, we live in a gang neighborhood, it's not so active anymore, but she went out with a gang member of that gang, and he introduced me to knowing about that gang life. I ended up wanting to join a gang. (personal interview, June, 2016)

Besides introducing him to gang life, his older sister's boyfriend, Diego's surrogate brother figure, also introduced him to crack cocaine. But it was during a trip to Mexico when Diego was 14 years old that his substance abuse truly spiraled out of control. Aware that his cousin in Mexico knew all the places to score drugs, Diego convinced his mother to leave him with the cousin for a month, while she herself stayed with Diego's grandmother, a three-hour drive away. It was easy to convince the cousin to take him to a drug dealer. Diego described his first trip to the dealer's, comparing entering the "drug lord's office" to walking into "a candy store." For the duration of this vacation in Mexico, Diego smoked crack every day, and by his own admission, that was when "everything went downhill." Upon his return home, Diego realized that it was harder to procure drugs in the United States than in Mexico. He began to engage in lying and stealing behavior, "crack-head stuff," to feed his crack habit.

> I would just find myself outside of grocery stores and coming up with some bullshit story that I needed a dollar to get on a bus, and I would just do that every day, just take money from people, just to go buy drugs or get drunk or something. I started stealing a lot, like from people, from stores and everything, y'know? Running from cops, hiding from helicopters, running from police dogs and everything . . . just, it was all, like, that's what I believe was rock bottom. I just didn't care . . . yeah. (personal interview, June, 2016)

Diego was expelled from the high school he was attending at the time, and he ran away from home. Ultimately, Diego broke into his own home to steal from his parents. The incident forced Diego's parents to take action to curb his out-of-control behavior, and they placed him into a rehab facility, where he remained for ten months. A staff member at this facility introduced Diego to journaling, and Diego began regularly writing down his thoughts and feelings. While Diego and his group of friends had already been rapping even before his compulsory stay at the rehab center, his new-found interest in journaling informed the rap lyrics he created after he left the facility and reconnected with the group. Diego acknowledges that initially, his lyrics tended to be dark and full of anger. He would write about violence, even about killing someone. But putting his anger and aggression into his lyrics seemed to have allowed him to sublimate those turbulent emotions in a way that eschewed repercussions:

> It actually helped because I knew that if I weren't to write about this, I'd probably express this anger in a different way . . . it's better that I wrote that, instead of just burning this bridge with this person, just because I didn't like him. It's better that I wrote that instead of telling someone to their face. (personal interview, June, 2016)

Seeing his friends again upon his return from the rehab center, Diego suggested the idea of rapping sessions to them, and an informal "rap group" was formed as their meetings became more regular. Despite each member's issues with substance use, professional counseling was not a resource Diego and his friends sought out, at least not voluntarily. As mentioned earlier, for some youths, there are attitudinal and cultural reasons to shun professional therapy. Such apprehensions may have motivated Diego and his friends to create a space for themselves where they could exchange personal narratives through the act of rapping. Nancy Fraser (1990) describes groups that allow members who feel marginalized by the dominant society to "invent and circulate counterdiscourses to formulate oppositional interpretations of their identities, interests, and needs" (p. 67). The group that grew organically out of Diego and his friends' life struggles, including those with substance abuse, their shared interest in rap music, and their need for a support system, bears the hallmarks of the subaltern counterpublics described by Fraser (1990). That the group chose to compose their own rap lyrics, rather than consume the lyrics produced by commercial rap artists, may also be interpreted as a countercultural act insofar as it demonstrates resistance against industry-produced hip-hop. The tension between a desire to create authentic lyrics documenting their lived experiences and the need to capitulate to industry dictates in order to sell albums is one that commercial rap artists constantly contend with. Record producers, advertising agents, and marketing strategists leave their imprint on every commercially produced album; in some cases, the effect of commodification is manifested in the way it "domesticates and defuses rap of some of its subversive energy" (Watkins, 2012, p. 703), resulting in a finished product presumably more palatable to a mainstream (and predominantly white) audience. It has also been argued that the proliferation of gangsta rap owes more to deliberate design by record label executives than to the MCs' autonomous artistic expression. The appropriation and commodification of rap music by major record labels influence the thematic content of rap songs, with MCs pressured to rap about the gangsta or thug that has become the primary signified associated with the urban African American male (Wright, 2012). Diego's partiality toward old-school rappers may indicate an affinity for a more authentic, prelapsarian use of the rap medium, before rap music's thematic proclivities were refocused by dominant institutions.

Although Diego professes an interest in writing, his preferred style of rap is freestyling, which he believes to be the most direct path to authenticity. Still, he explains that his chief goal in introducing his friends to rapping was to motivate them to write. The way he recounts his "founding" of the rap group shows that he takes pride in having initiated his friends to the art of rapping. Earlier during the interview, Diego revealed that while he was using, he would goad peers into trying crack too. In getting his friends to share his interest in composing rap lyrics, Diego was propelling them toward a constructive activity rather than the detrimental behavior he had previously instigated:

> I started doing it, spitting. And I kinda introduced some friends to it . . . and they tried it, and it was fun and they liked it. It feels good, like I really sparkled this up for these people, they like it, y'know? So this is like, our way of bonding. And it just keeps us busy, I know that there's worse things we could be doing. Sometimes we communicate to one another through that. (personal interview, June, 2016)

For Diego, the effort to stay clean is a never-ending battle, and temptation arises from sources both expected and unexpected. Working alongside his father on a drywall installation job can turn into a major test of his will to resist relapse, as the drywall's white, powdery detritus reminds Diego of another white, powdery substance on which he once relied to feel good. A few friends, whom he had met in junior high, were already into the graffiti scene when Diego "brought the rapping thing in." Prior to his stay in the detox facility, spending time with those friends inevitably meant consuming alcohol, if not other mind-altering substances. Upon his return home, against warnings from the rehab counselors about associating with former friends and re-immersing himself into an environment rife with behavior he was now trying to avoid, the desire to keep writing and rapping impelled Diego to rejoin the group. They were people who were into the same music as Diego and they were the only group of people he knew who were "down to rap" with him. When the group of friends first began to "spit," alcohol abated self-consciousness and boosted self-confidence ("Everybody knew they sucked at that time, but after a few drinks they're not gonna care"), facilitating everyone's amateur performances. Upon his re-entry into this group, Diego initially allowed himself to accept the beer and cigarettes that were offered, although he refused anything else. Eventually, he convinced the others to forego the alcohol and drugs as well, and just to focus on the "spitting." The budding rappers soon realized the increased gratification that comes from creating rhymes while sober. Ultimately, the focus of their meetings became the display of their growth as rappers and their burgeoning mastery over rhyming. Equally important was the opportunity afforded by those meetings to share symbolic representations of whatever events or thoughts were currently occupying the minds of those present. Their get-togethers, once an occasion for these young men to get high, became a reason for them to stay sober. As Diego himself put it, their meetings were "my little escape, to not be messing around."

Having goals, both short-term (for example, getting good grades for the current school term) and long-term (becoming a teacher someday), helps Diego stay focused, as does forming friendships with new acquaintances and deepening his relationships with his family. The desire for interpersonal connection comes across as a profound need that Diego mentioned several times during the interviews. Not surprisingly, this need often surfaces as a prominent theme in the songs that Diego writes. Among the songs Diego has composed, there are two which appear to hold particular significance for him. He volunteered to perform both songs for one of the authors and provided copies of the lyrics, which are reproduced below (with the composer's consent). In the analysis of those lyrics that follows, major objectives of the rhymed narratives will be discussed, as well as their main themes. Interpretation of the lyrics was based upon close readings of the two texts, and was informed as well by known biographical information about our subject obtained through the interviews.

NARRATIVE ANALYSIS

The first text is a song Diego wrote for his sister:

"Mi Luz (My Light)"

I feel like I'm gettin' fat
-tuated I'm glad
you made it

to this point in your life
in which you open up your ears
and open up your mind.
Opened up your eyes.
Now to your peripherals
Is the fact that I feel where you placed what was real; ya sister role.
I kinda missed you tho.

Now that I grasped you
it's time that I ask you
Don't feel like I'm tryna attack you.
I'm glad to
Fix all the bad news
But did you have to
Make shit such a hassle?
– Nevermind that.
That's a burden broken
Let's leave it behind.
I'm hopin' our vibes back.
I feel like I got my life back

'Cuz you're everything to me
Sometimes blood could fuck it up
But now when something's up I showed you how we're settling things.
The bettering things
They barely think
We're telling the things
To one another
N that's because we love each other

It's the things that love do.
My heart and my mind
Made it right, now when I hug you
It's all I want in my life, I'm feeling right that's what's up, Luz. (Diego, 2016)

In the interviews with Diego, references to relationships are brought up repeatedly: his relationship with his parents, his closeness to his godfather, his yearning for a friend in an unfriendly high school environment. This rap song expresses a longing for a closer relationship with a sibling. There are clues here that past events have driven a chasm between brother and sister—the narrator misses her, suggesting a period of estrangement, either due to physical distance or less obvious etiologies. At one point, the speaker seems about to berate Luz over something she did, however, "Did you have to make shit such a hassle" is as close as the narrator comes to describing her actions; exactly how Luz made a "hassle" of things is not elaborated upon. Amia Lieblich, Rivka Tuval-Mashiach, and Tamar Zilber (1998), in their *Narrative Research: Reading, Analysis, and Interpretation*, point out that researchers interpreting a life story should pay attention to instances in which significant elements are left out of the narrative, as their importance may be suggested by just such marked omission. Conflict is the spark that fuels every narrative, yet, in this story, the crucial incident that constitutes the conflict of the narrative is *left out.* This very exclusion highlights the importance of the mysterious incident, and, more importantly, how the incident is being handled. According to Walter Fisher (1984), for whom the narrative impulse is a basic and universal feature of human nature, individuals glean *good reasons* from the stories they encounter, which suggest proper courses of action and can be used to guide decision-making and behavior. With regard to the unspecified incident that happened, although the listener is given no particulars, the lyrics reveal that Luz acted in a manner at some point which led the narrator to question whether she had deprioritized her role as a sister. This situation places the two at a crossroads. Three possible courses of action are available to the actors in this drama: they could terminate their relationship, or at least avoid future interactions with each other; one party could exact revenge upon the other; or the incident could be overlooked and the relationship preserved. The speaker's conspicuous avoidance of any detailed elaboration of the discord between him and his sister implies a conscious decision to overlook the incident in question. The narrator realizes that the best course is to leave whatever unpleasantness happened between the two in the past, rather than let the incident contaminate their present relationship. With the decision to move past the conflict, the story of how "blood could fuck it up" is no longer the dominant narrative—the revised story is one that focuses on how messes could be cleaned up, injured feelings could be mended, and estranged relationships could be reinvigorated. Whatever it was that drove a wedge in between the siblings, there are references throughout the song to Luz's status as a member of the narrator's family, and the love the narrator feels for her: "Your sister role," "You're everything to me, " "we love each other," "when I hug you, it's all I want in my life." The narrator is reminded that his sister is capable of being a good listener, if she would only open up her ears and open up her mind. The implication is that by listening carefully, she will be able to hear his side, and by clearing her mind of preconceptions, she will be able to understand issues from his perspective. This communication is both important and inevitable, because the two love each other. The main narrative objectives revealed by this close reading are that of conflict resolution, the restoration of order, and the renewal of a relationship after a period of estrangement.

Themes in "Mi Luz (My Light)"

A primary theme of this song is *relationship dynamics*, which Katrina McFerran (2012) found was a key theme that emerged from her examination of songs written by her teenage clients. Relationship dynamics is also a frequent focus of therapeutic interventions (McFerran, 2012). References to *vision/perception* abound in this song. "Luz" is used both as a name for the addressee and as the Spanish word for "light." Luz is a sibling with a flaw: imperfect perception. Failing to perceive her own role in the relationship clearly, she has downgraded her responsibilities as a sister to subordinate importance. The narrator rejoices that Luz has finally opened up her eyes; her vision has now acquired a clearer focus, presumably because she has matured (she has made it to a point in her life, a psychological milestone, when the puerility of one's childhood is cast aside). Connected with this theme is the tension between *emotion and reason*, between the "heart and mind," another theme that can be identified in this song. Events viewed in a clear light (that is, with a clear head) are more likely to yield rational conclusions, while, in the heated moment of an ongoing argument, words and behavior are highly susceptible to misinterpretation. Blood, with its dark hue and its infamous ability to stain, is used here as a metaphor for family, but also as a reference to things that can muddle or confuse, leading to imperfect perception or interpretation of a situation. The text suggests that it is precisely because Luz is "blood" (family) that the potential for conflict is increased; an observer sees with impaired vision that which is too close.

A close reading of this text also reveals the theme of *restoration of broken things*. The narrator is "glad to fix all the bad news," which can be interpreted as mending the previously damaged relationship between him and his sister. Significantly, the narrator also acknowledges that some damages are beyond repair and can only be left behind. The proximity of this line to the line "I feel like I got my life back" may be a deliberate attempt to link the idea of a thing wrecked beyond repair and a person's life wrecked past a salvageable point. In recounting his past as a substance addict, Diego acknowledges there were periods when he was using such a large quantity of crack cocaine that he must have come close, on multiple occasions, to dying from an overdose. Although this song is not specifically about drug use, those intense experiences from his days as a user can be expected to interject themselves into much of Diego's artistic output. The inclusion of these lines, then, may represent messages to himself, reminding Diego of the potentially fatal consequences of substance abuse.

Finally, this is a song that emphasizes the theme of *love*. Communication is portrayed as a precursor to love, while positive outcomes are represented as its products. Love is allowed to flourish when siblings open up their ears, eyes, and minds to each other, and "tell things" to one another. The result of such open communication are "settling things" and "bettering things," terms that connote a return to order and equilibrium (that is, problems are settled) and hope (that is, things will get better). Although the "hard stuff" Diego wrote when he first started composing rap lyrics may have served some cathartic purpose, positive lyrics such as those in this song, about the importance of resolving sibling conflict and maintaining close ties with one's family, may serve as more inspirational reminders of why he needs to remain sober.

The next song contains a more overt and emphatic antidrug message:

"Letting a Plant Rot"

Your momma said don't be chillin' with kids on your block
'Cuz she noticed a change by the way you talk
So young and free who would put your good life to waste?
You forgot all of the good things taught when you were raised
Only 12 years old—but that was just a number—to you
But who knew the cruel things that you'd do?
Now somebody reckless and the hectic streets had taught
That it was cool to get into that street talk.
They were your friends and what the hell did she know?
Nothing, just how to buy you out of that street clothes
Black jeans long white socks, Nikes, hat on top
Baggy jeans to look hot, and that lean in your walk.
Your taste had changed
And you started to hate the cops
After your first time experiencing buying some rock
The dealer said that they were simply a bust
And you had your chance to give back all of the stuff—
But you didn't
And showed it off like a hypocrite with religion
Claiming their goodness after a mission.
Years passed and this act became a habit
Too many conflicts with your life
And the results were tragic.
But it was nothing
You ignored it with your vision distorted
You made a new friend, a new problem with Captain Morgan
A junkie, a wino, your parents called you "marijuano"
And sometimes it hurt, but you didn't cry though . . .
And when they said,
"Ayo, your brain's dead,"
You answered, "The drug is my treasure, the friend I found like James read."
Something ironic: It was Sirach
Then you moved up 'cuz bud was the gateway
14 years old now & bigger mistakes made
You started digging that yay
And life was about money made
You liked that acidic like it was Minutemaid
And I ain't talking about lemonade
Stayed the highest like an ace of spades
You even got kicked out of where your people stayed,

Broke in, and what's there left to say—you were a shame

No athlete but you played a sport
Competitive crack fiend
Winning 8–balls to snort
You thought it was something magical like "HOKUS POKE"
Thought you were strong but I guess you're not
Fool
You overdosed. (Diego, 2014)

Focalization, or the "lens through which we see characters and events in the narrative" (Abbott, 2008, p. 73), provides important clues toward deciphering a narrative text. One intriguing aspect of the above song is its focalization: the story is told from the point of view of a heterodiegetic narrator (Genette, 1983), who is addressing a substance-addicted young person, tracing the young man's life from his initial experience "buying some rock" to his ultimate overdose. And yet, this is clearly an autobiographical narrative; the addressee is obviously Diego himself. Details of this story correspond to what Diego revealed about his life during the interviews: the addressee was 12 years old when he "forgot all of the good things taught when [he was] raised" and started associating with the wrong friends and using illicit substances; the addressee was abusing "yay" (crack cocaine), and he broke into his own house, the home his exasperated parents had previously kicked him out of. However, although Diego mentioned during one of the interview sessions that there were "multiple times where, I believe I should've gone to the hospital because maybe I might've been like, overdosing," he is, of course, still alive. Sam Larsson, John Lilja, Therese von Braun, and Yvonne Sjöblom (2013) observed that personal narratives serve a dual function of revealing one's life experiences to others as well as of contributing to the teller's identity formation. The psyche is comprised of different sub-identities (Larsson et al., 2013), and this song demonstrates that the ascendant voice currently dominating Diego's psyche (represented by the heterodiegetic narrator) has "killed" his self-destructive part-identity. The heterodiegetic narrator is far from a neutral observer: rather, he takes a clearly evaluative position vis-à-vis the protagonist—in fact, this unnamed main character emerges as the villain of the story through the critical and contemptuous language used to describe him. By thus vilifying the substance-addicted Diego, the narrator legitimizes his present governance over Diego's psyche—this autobiographical rap song tells not only the story of Diego as he used to be, but also introduces us to this new master self, the Diego as he is today. This, then, is a major objective that can be identified from this life story: the construction of a new identity—a clean, sober Diego arising out of the ashes of his former reprobate self—and the legitimization of this identity's "killing" of that drug-abusing sub-identity and assumption of primacy.

For young men abiding by implicit cultural sanctions against the sharing of revelations concerning personal troubles, innermost thoughts, and feelings, rap offers a safe way to communicate such intimate content. Their spontaneously formed counterpublic forum allows Diego and his friends to share personal stories with each other away from the scrutiny of oppressive entities in the shape of their parents, law enforcement, and other authority figures in their lives. The creation of their own lyrics also hints at a rejection of commercially produced rap music. These aspects of the group reflect its members' counterpublic tendencies, and within the safe confines of their private "spitting" sessions, Diego and his friends exercise control over their own cultural production, made for their own consumption. However, rap music is not, ultimately, an art form intended for private enjoyment; unlike journaling, or even the writing of poetry, rap music has, since the days of its inception when the early DJs would convert parks and streets into impromptu block parties (Rose, 1994), been a public phenomenon. A rapper is motivated to create a rap song by something within themself that demands translation into tangible form, and the end product is then addressed outward to a hip-hop savvy public. Rap music is meant to be performed for an audience. Diego's song, created within the context of the counterpublic group he is a part of, reflects the somewhat paradoxical nature of counterpublic spheres as it assumes at once an inward *and* outward orientation (Asen & Brouwer, 2001). As discussed above, the song's inherent message is, on one level, addressed to Diego's own part-identity. At the same time, however, its message is also meant to be disseminated *outward* to a wider public. Speculating on who the target audience for this song might be yields a second objective of this text. A rap song can best be appreciated by those with an affinity for hip-hop, of course, but the specific language employed in this piece also requires listeners to understand the slang references to drugs and drug use in order to decipher its meaning. To the uninitiated, the jargon of substance abuse may prove unintelligible: "bud" (marijuana), "yay" (crack cocaine), "acidic" (a play on "acid" for LSD), "8–balls" (3.5 grams of cocaine, a commonly purchased quantity). Therefore, the intended audience is not only hip-hop identified youth in general, but in particular, those who are familiar with drug-related slang, perhaps because they too are users of illicit substances. Interpreted in this light, the lyrics become a cautionary tale warning other young people who may be engaging in the same deleterious behaviors that Diego himself was involved in not to go down the same self-destructive path he has traveled.

Themes in "Letting a Plant Rot"

The predominant theme of this song is *drug use*. Drug-related themes are so pervasive in commercial rap music that songs containing such themes have achieved the status of a distinct subgenre: "cocaine rap" (Frere-Jones, 2006). Popular rappers like Jay-Z, Gucci Mane, Kanye West, Eminem, Pusha T, and Travis Scott, to name but a few, either describe drug use or recount the adventures of drug dealers resourcefully evading the law, often in ways that portray the use or sale of illicit substances as glamorous or at least as being without severe consequences. Unlike the depiction of drug use in those songs produced by a commercialized rap industry, Diego's lyrics convey an oppositional representation of drug use and its effects. Drug use was also a major theme identified by Lightstone (2012) in his analysis of rap lyrics written by youth undergoing hip-hop-infused therapy. Lightstone (2012) attributed the frequent mention of drug use to its prominent role in the lives of his participants.

Imperfect vision emerges as another important theme of this song. The protagonist's own vision is distorted, both physically as a result of his drinking and drug use, and metaphorically—he is blind to the "tragic" consequences of his drug habit. Flawed vision afflicts the character of the mother as well. Diego revealed during an interview session that at the height of his drug use, he was smoking crack on a daily basis, "for like a month. It's like I started losing my color, turning yellowish and whitish, and it was just like—I just looked terrible." And yet, the mother failed to see the signs of his addiction ("what the hell did she know?/Nothing"). She only noticed a change in Diego when she heard him talk (aggressively? Did she first note the transformation during an argument?), his speech peppered with street argot.

Another overlap between the themes uncovered by the present analysis and those identified by Lightstone (2012) is that of *authenticity*. Within the hip-hop tradition, "keepin' it real" is a valorized motto, while "posers," those who pretend to be something they are not, are especially despised. With the clarity of vision that his present sobriety confers, Diego seems to be mocking his younger self for affecting all the clichéd postures and props of counterfeit coolness: the street talk, the baggy jeans, the unnatural lean in his walk. This aversion toward inauthenticity is again manifested a few lines later, echoed in the allusion to falsely pious hypocrites "claiming their goodness after a mission," who don religious habits like costumes, the same way Diego wore the attire of a street thug to play that stock character. Although here too, as in the song Diego wrote for his sister, relational dynamics appear as an integral theme, the figure of the mother is not portrayed with any discernable affection in this song. Besides her inability to recognize the drug addict her son had become, the lyrics expose another symptom of her ineffective parenting: her attempt to use money to manage his behavior. Rather than communicating with her son using the authentic currency of open discussion and loving concern, she commodifies their relationship by endeavoring to "buy [him] out of that [*sic*] street clothes." But merely changing someone's clothes is, of course, a superficial fix, and such artificial measures cannot but fail to solve any real problems.

Interpersonal relationships is another theme that can be detected in this song. References to the mother or parents ("momma," "she," "parents," and "your people") occur five times; the word "friend" is repeated three times. As in the song discussed earlier, here too Diego's need for interpersonal connections is revealed through the lyrics. SUD takes its toll not only on users' physical, mental, and psychological health (all of which may be encompassed by the reference to pain: "sometimes it hurt"), but on their relationships as well. The addict addressed in this song arguably reaches a point of no return when he chooses the deceptive comfort of drugs over his family and social ties: "The drug is my treasure, the friend I found."

Diego's creation and use of this life story as an aid toward personal healing and sobriety are, coincidentally, consistent with narrative therapeutic techniques that direct clients to externalize their presenting issues. From a narrative therapeutic standpoint, doing so disrupts thinking patterns that equate the individual with the presenting problems, and, in collaboration with the therapist, clients may come to perceive how they can change the unhealthy relationships they have formed with their problems (Clark, 2014). In the above song, Diego's refusal to be defined by the self-destructive behaviors in which he once took part is evident. He distances himself from the problem-saturated story of his past life by attributing all those negative behaviors to a sub-identity and disassociating his present self from that former self. The "killing" of the "bad Diego" at the end of the song represents a symbolic termination of the relationship between Diego and his substance use problem. What is exceptional is that Diego's use of this strategy occurred spontaneously, without the guidance of a helping professional in the context of a narrative-focused intervention. This may offer support for the attractiveness of narrative therapy as a treatment option, by itself or as part of a hip-hop-based intervention, insofar as the current case study demonstrates that an individual would choose to employ narrative therapeutic strategies of his own volition.

CONCLUSION

This chapter explored rap music engagement as a treatment modality for substance-addicted youth, and highlighted the example of one organically formed group of substance-using adolescents who used rap expressivity to articulate their experiences. While much research has previously been done on hip-hop-infused therapeutic interventions, the extant literature predominantly reflects a psychological approach. The present study examined the phenomenon from a communication perspective, and this perspective informed the narrative analysis presented above.

The current case study lends support to the view that rap music-based substance-use interventions can be a clinically efficacious therapeutic approach. Although we focused on a case example of a youth presenting with SUD, insights gleaned from this case illustration and the analysis of song lyrics can prove pertinent for practitioners, educators, and researchers working with youth exhibiting other deleterious conditions, such as aggression, depression, high-risk sexual attitudes or behaviors, etc. That Diego and his friends autonomously chose to hold regular jam sessions, during which they would discuss, using their rap lyrics as a starting point, issues surrounding their addiction and recovery process, demonstrates their inherent interest in this musical genre as an expressive vehicle. As Nakeyshaey Tillie-Allen (2005) observed, an important aspect of rap music that makes it attractive as a treatment modality is its mass appeal to youth, which helps to diminish their resistance to receiving therapy. Adolescents with SUD, who may otherwise shun professional help due to mistrust of practitioners or a negative perception of the therapeutic process in general, may be more willing to attend sessions that incorporate an activity they find meaningful and enjoyable, such as listening to and/or creating rap songs. Additionally, hip-hop infused therapy has been postulated to enhance the client-provider relationship, as it heightens perception of the therapist's empathy and relatability (Kobin & Tyson, 2006). It is those same service providers who play a key role in the diffusion of innovative practices (Herbeck, Hser, & Teruya, 2008; Osborn, 2012). As more and more practitioners recognize the therapeutic promise of rap music engagement and incorporate it into their treatment strategies, certain types of individuals may be better served as a result, particularly hip-hop identified adolescents.

Rappers often use rap music to rewrite the story of their lives, replacing the socially marginalized victims they used to be with a more empowered entity, the central agent in their own dramas. Through their rhymed narratives, told to the accompaniment of a hip-hop beat, Diego and his friends constructed new identities for themselves, and replaced problem-saturated stories with ones that affirmed positive values (of love, family, reconciliation, etc.), promoted personal growth and responsibility, and discouraged destructive behavior. Rap music itself was once a fringe art form associated with marginal peoples, cultures, and locales, before its indomitable forward shift led to its current centralized position among the most popular musical genres worldwide. At least part of the appeal of hip-hop is its ability to bring its practitioners and artists out of obscure, marginal positions, and rap artists have used their music to draw attention to themselves, their posses, and their neighborhoods. Although the limited accessibility of the record industry may mean that the fruits of their labor may never reach a wider audience, their rapping nevertheless holds tremendous inherent value for Diego and his group as they engage in the constant struggle to resist relapse.

REFERENCES

Abbott, H. P. (2008). *The Cambridge introduction to narrative* (2nd ed.). Cambridge, UK: Cambridge University Press.

Alvarez, T. T., III. (2012). Beats, rhymes, and life: Rap therapy in an urban setting. In S. Hadley & G. Yancy (Eds.), *Therapeutic uses of rap and hip-hop* (pp. 117–128). New York, NY: Routledge.

American Psychiatric Association (APA). (2013). *Diagnostic and statistical manual of mental disorders* (*DSM-5*) (5th ed.). Arlington, VA: American Psychiatric Association.

Arnett, J. J. (1999). Adolescent storm and stress, reconsidered. *American Psychologist, 54*(5), 317–326. https://doi.org/10.1037//0003–066x.54.5.317

Asen, R., & Brouwer, D. C. (2001). Introduction: Reconfigurations of the public sphere. In R. Asen & D. C. Brouwer (Eds.), *Counterpublics and the state* (pp. 1–32). Albany, NY: State University of New York Press.

Azikwe, M. D. (2011). More than baby mamas: Black mothers and hip-hop feminism. In G. Dines, & J. M. Humez (Eds.), *Gender, race, and class in media: A critical reader* (3rd ed., pp. 137–144). Thousand Oaks, CA: Sage Publications.

Baker, F. A., Dingle, G. A., & Gleadhill, L. M. (2012). "Must be the ganja": Using rap music in music therapy for substance use disorders. In S. Hadley & G. Yancy (Eds.), *Therapeutic uses of rap and hip-hop* (pp. 321–336). New York, NY: Routledge.

Bogt, T. F., Vieno, A., Doornwaard, S. M., Pastore, M., & van den Eijnden, R. J. (2016). "You're not alone": Music as a source of consolation among adolescents and young adults. *Psychology of Music*, 1–17. https://doi.org/10.1177/0305735616650029

BRL, Inc. (n.d.). Hip hop theraphy. *Beats Rhymes and Life*. Retrieved from http://brl-inc.org/

Castleman, C. (2012). The politics of graffiti. In M. Forman & M. A. Neal (Eds.), *That's the joint: The hip-hop studies reader* (2nd ed., pp. 14–22). New York, NY: Routledge.

Chen, C.-Y., Storr, C. L., & Anthony, J. C. (2009). Early-onset drug use and risk for drug dependence problems. *Addictive Behaviors*, *34*(3), 319–322. https://doi.org/10.1016/j.addbeh.2008.10.021

Clark, A. A. (2014). Narrative therapy integration within substance abuse groups. *Journal of Creativity in Mental Health*, *9*(4), 511–522. https://doi.org/10.1080/15401383.2014.914457

Daniels, L., Strong, D., & Chaiken, I. (Writers), & Daniels, L. (Director). (2015, January 14). The outspoken king [Television series episode]. In W. Calhoun & D. Strong (Producers), *Empire*. Chicago, IL: Fox/Imagine Television.

Davies, J. B. (1997). *The myth of addiction* (2nd ed.). New York, NY: Routledge.

DeCarlo, A., & Hockman, E. (2003). Rap therapy: A group work intervention method for urban adolescents. *Social Work with Groups*, *26*(3), 45–59. https://doi.org/10.1300/J009v26n03_06

Diego [pseud.]. (2014). "Letting a Plant Rot." With permission of the author.

Diego [pseud.]. (2016). "Mi Luz (My Light)." With permission of the author.

Elligan, D. (2000). Rap therapy: A culturally sensitive approach to psychotherapy with young African American men. *Journal of African American Men, 5*(3), 27–36. https://www.jstor.org/stable/41819404

Elligan, D. (2004). *Rap therapy: A practical guide for communicating with youth and young adults through rap music.* New York, NY: Kensington.

Elligan, D. (2012). Contextualizing rap music as a means of incorporating into psychotherapy. In S. Hadley & G. Yancy (Eds.), *Therapeutic uses of rap and hip-hop* (pp. 27–38). New York, NY: Routledge.

Fisher, W. R. (1984). Narration as a human communication paradigm: The case of public moral argument. *Communication Monographs*, *51*(1), 1–22. https://doi.org/10.1080/03637758409390180

Foss, S. K. (2009). *Rhetorical criticism: Exploration and practice* (4th ed.). Long Grove, IL: Waveland Press.
Fraser, N. (1990). Rethinking the public sphere: A contribution to the critique of actually existing democracy. *Social Text, 25/26*, 56–80. https://www.jstor.org/stable/466240
Frere-Jones, S. (2006, December 17). Coke is it: Rap's drug obsession. *The New Yorker*. Retrieved from http://www.newyorker.com/magazine/2006/12/25/coke-is-it
Genette, G. (1983). *The narrative discourse: An essay in method.* (J. E. Lewin, Trans.) Ithaca, NY: Cornell University Press.
Gonzalez, T., & Hayes, B. G. (2009). Rap music in school counseling based on Don Elligan's rap therapy. *Journal of Creativity in Mental Health, 4*(2), 161–172. https://doi.org/10.1080/15401380902945293
Groarke, J. M., & Hogan, M. J. (2016). Enhancing wellbeing: An emerging model of the adaptive functions of music listening. *Psychology of Music, 44*(4), 769–791. https://doi.org/10.1177/0305735615591844
Herbeck, D. M., Hser, Y. I., & Teruya, C. (2008). Empirically supported substance abuse treatment approaches: A survey of treatment providers' perspectives and practices. *Addictive Behaviors, 33*(5), 699–712. https://doi.org/10.1016/j.addbeh.2007.12.003
Hohmann, L., Bradt, J., Stegemann, T., & Koelsch, S. (2017). Effects of music therapy and music-based interventions in the treatment of substance use disorders: A systematic review. *PLoS One, 12*(11), 1–36. https://doi.org/10.1371/journal.pone.0187363
Housman, A. E. (1896). "Into my heart an air that kills." *A Shropshire Lad*. London: K. Paul, Trench, Treubner, & Co.
Ierardi, F., & Jenkins, N. (2012). Rap composition and improvisation in a short-term juvenile detention facility. In S. Hadley & G. Yancy (Eds.), *Therapeutic uses of rap and hip-hop* (pp. 253–273). New York, NY: Routledge.
Keyes, C. L. (2012). Empowering self, making choices, creating spaces: Black female identity via rap music performance. In M. Forman & M. A. Neal (Eds.), *That's the joint: The hip-hop studies reader* (2nd ed., pp. 400–412). New York, NY: Routledge.
Kobin, C., & Tyson, E. (2006). Thematic analysis of hip-hop music: Can hip-hop in therapy facilitate empathic connections when working with clients in urban settings? *Arts in Psychotherapy, 33*(4), 343–356. https://doi.org/10.1016/j.aip.2006.05.001
Larsson, S., Lilja, J., Von Braun, T., & Sjöblom, Y. (2013). General theoretical perspectives of narrative analysis of substance use-related dependency. *Substance Use & Misuse, 48*(13), 1294–1305. https://doi.org/10.3109/10826084.2013.815537
Lieblich, A., Tuval-Mashiach, R., & Zilber, T. (1998). *Narrative research: Reading, analysis, and interpretation.* Thousand Oaks, CA: Sage Publications.
Lightstone, A. J. (2012). Yo, can ya flow! Research findings on hip-hop aesthetics and rap therapy in an urban youth shelter. In S. Hadley & G. Yancy (Eds.), *Therapeutic uses of rap and hip-hop* (pp. 211–251). New York, NY: Routledge.
Lindlof, T. R., & Taylor, B. C. (2011). *Qualitative communication research methods* (3rd ed.). Thousand Oaks, CA: Sage Publications.
MacDonald, S., & Viega, M. (2012). Hear Our Voices: A music therapy songwriting program and the message of the Little Saints through the medium of rap. In S. Hadley & G. Yancy (Eds.), *Therapeutic uses of rap and hip-hop* (pp. 153–171). New York, NY: Routledge.
McFerran, K. (2012). "Just so you know, I miss you so bad": The expression of life and loss in the raps of two adolescents in music therapy. In S. Hadley & G. Yancy (Eds.), *Therapeutic uses of rap and hip-hop* (pp. 173–189). New York, NY: Routledge.
Merriam, S. B. (2002). Introduction to qualitative research. In S. B. Merriam & Associates (Eds.), *Qualitative research in practice: Examples for discussion and analysis* (pp. 3–17). San Francisco, CA: Jossey-Bass.
Nobre, M. J., & Castilho, V. M. (2009). Drug abuse. In E. J. Kerr & O. E. Gibson (Eds.), *Substance abuse: New research* (pp. 83–108). New York, NY: Nova Science Publishers.
Nowinski, J. (2003). Self-help groups. In J. L. Sorensen, R. A. Rawson, J. Guydish, & J. E. Sweben (Eds.), *Drug abuse treatment through collaboration: Practice and research partnerships that work* (pp. 55–70). Washington, DC: American Psychological Association.

Osborn, C. J. (2012). Psychotherapeutic approaches. In D. Capuzzi & M. D. Stauffer (Eds.), *Foundations of addictions counseling* (2nd ed., pp. 142–164). Boston, MA: Pearson.

Payne, M. (2006). *Narrative theory: An introduction for counsellors* (2nd ed.). London: Sage Publications.

Rose, T. (1994). *Black noise: Rap music and Black culture in contemporary America.* Middletown, CT: Wesleyan University Press.

Shäfer, T., Sedlmeier, P., Städtler, C., & Huron, D. (2013, August 13). The psychological functions of music listening. *Frontiers in Psychology, 4,* 1–33. https://doi.org/10.3389/fpsyg.2013.00511

Squeglia, L. M., Jacobus, J., & Tapert, S. F. (2009). The influence of substance use on adolescent brain development. *Clinical EEG and Neuroscience, 40*(1), 31–38. https://doi.org/10.1177/155005940904000110

Sulé, V. T. (2016). Hip-hop is the healer: Sense of belonging and diversity among hip-hop collegians. *Journal of College Student Development, 57*(2), 181–196. https://doi.org/10.1353/csd.2016.0014

Substance Abuse and Mental Health Services Administration (SAMHSA). (2015). *Behavioral Health Barometer: United States, 2015.* HHS Publication No. SMA–16–Baro–2015. Rockville, MD: Substance Abuse and Mental Health Services Administration, 2015. Retrieved from http://www.samhsa.gov/data/sites/default/files/2015_National_Barometer.pdf

Susman, E. J., & Rogol, A. (2004). Puberty and psyhcological development. In R. M. Lerner & L. Steinberg (Eds.), *Handbook of adolescent psychology* (2nd ed., pp. 15–44). Hoboken, NJ: John Wiley & Sons.

Tillie-Allen, N. M. (2005). Exploring hip-hop therapy with at-risk youth. *Praxis, 5,* 30–36.

Travis, R., Jr. (2013). Rap music and the empowerment of today's youth: Evidence in everyday music listening, music therapy, and commercial rap music. *Child and Adolescent Social Work Journal, 30*(2), 139–167. https://doi.org/10.1007/s10560–012–0285–x

Travis, R., Jr., & Deepak, A. (2011). Empowerment in context: Lessons from hip-hop culture for social work practice. *Journal of Ethnic & Cultural Diversity in Social Work, 20*(3), 203–222. https://doi.org/10.1080/15313204.2011.594993

Tyson, E. H., Detchkov, K., Eastwood, E., Carver, A., & Sehr, A. (2012). Therapeutically and socially relevant themes in hip-hop music: A comprehensive analysis of a selected sample of songs. In S. Hadley & G. Yancy (Eds.), *Therapeutic uses of rap and hip-hop* (pp. 99–114). New York, NY: Routledge.

Watkins, S. C. (2012). Black youth and the ironies of capitalism. In M. Forman & M. A. Neal (Eds.), *That's the joint: The hip-hop studies reader* (2nd ed., pp. 691–713). New York, NY: Routledge.

Wright, K. (2012). Rise up hip hop nation: From deconstructing racial politics to building positive solutions. In M. Forman & M. A. Neal (Eds.), *That's the joint: The hip-hop studies reader* (2nd ed., pp. 519–526). New York, NY: Routledge.

Yancy, G., & Hadley, S. (2012). Introduction: Give 'em just one mic: The therapeutic agency of rap and hip-hop. In S. Hadley & G. Yancy (Eds.), *Therapeutic uses of rap and hip-hop* (pp. xxiii–xlii). New York, NY: Routledge.

Chapter Seven

Preferred Cultural Mediums of Healing

Rapping into Identity

Travis Heath and Jacobo Mesa Ramirez

The phrase carried with it a certain jolt to the system: witness protection. I, Travis Heath, had heard the phrase before, but it was usually in the context of movies or television shows. These mediums tried to convince me that people with this label forced upon them were violent and unpredictable. I glance over at the clock and see that it is just a few ticks from when our work is scheduled to commence. I shake my body in hopes that it will help shake my mind, and perhaps more importantly, my soul, of any preconceived notions. I breathe deeply a couple of times and head to the waiting room.

As I round the corner, I see Jay (a pseudonym), a twenty-one-year-old man, sitting on the couch with his right leg nervously bouncing. He makes eye contact with me as I approach. He gives me a quick nod as one would do to a person one is acknowledging in passing. When I stop a few feet in front of him, he seems confused and a bit on edge.

"What's up?" I say kindly. "I'm Travis." I hope Jay will receive my words as an initial, albeit probably unexpected, gesture of camaraderie. Over seventeen years working with young people entangled with the criminal injustice system in Los Angeles, California, and Denver, Colorado, has taught me that first impressions matter. I have also learned, somewhat paradoxically, that people who come in with the most difficult reputations are actually the easiest to work with, provided that I do something outside of the classical therapeutic *script*. This history is a calming companion.

Jay's eyes shout a message of surprise and befuddlement. As a relatively young therapist with brown skin, long dreadlocks, and tattoos, this was not the first time eyes dispatched such correspondence.

"Should we head up?" I inquire matter-of-factly. Jay nods affirmatively.

As we pass through the office door, Jay slowly pulls down the hood of his black sweatshirt and arranges it to rest on his shoulders. In doing so, it reveals more clearly the tattoo on the left side of his face. I quickly recognize it as a symbol of a local street gang. He sits on the couch but does not allow his body to be fully consumed by its cushions.

Sitting, rather tentatively, Jay more fully takes in the room. He pays close attention to some of the windows, almost as though he is canvassing the security of this new environment. As this looks to be of some importance to him, I make sure not to interrupt his process.

After twenty more seconds or so, Jay sits back a little bit deeper into the couch. I begin my first query in a measured tone.

"Do you mind if I ask if you've ever done anything like this before, Jay?"

"Yeah, I have," he replies.

"Do you mind if I ask if you found it to be helpful or not so helpful?"

Jay looks me in the eyes in a way that almost feels like he is trying to determine whether or not I am someone who can be entrusted with his truth. I act on this intuition and say, "And whether it was great or not helpful at all, please know that all that matters to me is how you experienced it, okay?"

After taking some time to let my follow-up comment permeate his being, Jay proceeds with caution. "It was pretty much a joke. Those fools don't understand me. They are like these white women all dressed up talking nonsense, just talking noise. Like my problems can be fixed by taking some deep breaths and counting to ten or some shit."

Jay chuckles aloud, demonstrating just how preposterous the suggestions still seem to him.

"Jay, did those past therapists, by chance, take any time to figure out what you thought might be helpful or did they just tell you what they thought would be helpful?"

Jay snickers before saying sarcastically, "I'm a delinquent. What would I know?"

"Do you suppose you may have seen and heard things in your life that they haven't?"

"For sure."

"And do you suppose that those things you've seen and heard might lead to knowledge about the world they just don't have?"

Jay cocks his head just a little bit to the right. It starts to feel as though there might be a slight opening to invite Jay onboard to a new kind of therapy, the likes of which he probably has not experienced before. I feel a touch of excitement and the spirit of possibility starting to build inside of me.

Perhaps this could be the first opening into knowledge that Jay has that often is not valued, the building blocks of what a narrative therapist might call a counter story that can be constructed to challenge more dominant societal stories that are often told about people in the criminal justice system.

"Do you think you might have answers in there," I ask leaning in closer and pointing to his chest, "that only you have the key for?"

"Yeah, but I wish I knew where the fucking key was." Jay's tone is a mixture of intrigue and resignation.

"Do you think that might be the work we should do in here together? Would that be more helpful than the kind of work you've done in therapy before?"

Jay nods.

"When was the last time you remember having the key in your possession?"

"I notice it mostly when I do poetry and art."

"Poetry and art, huh?" I say with a burgeoning smile. "How many people are aware of these talents that are opened with this key, Jay?"

"My mom knew about my drawing. I won this contest in like fifth grade. I drew this picture of The Joker. You know, from Batman?" He pauses to check in. I nod as a larger smile pulls on the corners of my mouth. "It got put on display in this mall by my house for like a whole month."

"You must have been quite the artist, even back in fifth grade, huh? Do you mind if I ask you about the poetry talent you mentioned, Jay?" He nods his assent. "How does poetry make its appearance in your life?"

"Mostly making rhymes, making raps." The pace of his speech begins to quicken. "I've rapped since I was a kid, maybe like seven years old. Most of my raps have been about living the G-Life. These are the ones my homies hear."

"Jay," I say in an inquisitive tone, "I'm wondering if there are other rhymes that perhaps your homies don't hear?"

"Yeah, I also make some rhymes about my family and stuff. Recently I became a father, so I've also been making rhymes about my little man."

"Wow, you just became a father? Congratulations! Jay, is it okay if I ask you some more about the diversity of your rhyming ability?"

"That's cool."

"Would it be fair to say your rhyming ability is versatile? Like, can you rap about a lot of different parts of life?"

"I can pretty much rap about anything," he replies without hesitation.

"Can we call upon that ability to rap about anything in our work together in here, Jay? Could this, by chance, be a way we locate that key we were talking about earlier?"

"I'm down to give it a shot."

"Do you mind if I ask what kind of rap you prefer? Do you prefer to write your rhymes or freestyle?"

"Both," he says emphatically.

"Would it be alright if I asked you if any rhymes are brewing about what we've talked about in here so far today? Can you locate any inspiration, or should we keep on moving along in our conversation like we have been?"

Jay pauses, trepidation emanating from his being. "Are . . . like . . . can we do that?"

"Rap?" I reply.

"Yeah." Jay proceeds with care. "Will it still count?"

"What do you mean by count?"

"Will my PO [probation officer] count it as the classes I have to take?"

"Yes, it will," I reassure him. "Probation has given me the freedom to do what works for people rather than forcing them to do something that doesn't. Does this sound like an okay plan for us to pursue?"

Jay nods affirmatively, his body seeming to release some of the trepidation that had been following him.

"Do you have any paper I can use?" Jay asks. I walk over to my desk, remove a fresh pad of paper from the top drawer, and hand him a pen.

"Thanks. Actually, do you have a pencil? Sometimes I have to erase, you know what I mean?"

I reach into the right pocket of my jeans, remove a pencil, and hand it to him. Jay graciously accepts.

"This might take a few minutes." He speaks in a tone that is almost asking for permission.

"Jay, please take as long as you need. I'm not in any kind of rush."

Jay now looks settled into the couch in a new way. I can almost see the wheels turning as he scribbles quickly on the pad, taking time to erase when he needs to. After about five minutes he looks up. "Alright, I got something."

"Would it be helpful to let the rhyme out in here or would it be best for the lyrics to stay on the paper?"

Jay smiles briefly and says, "Let's do this thing." He begins rapping . . .

Note: Due to sensitivity and identifying features in some of Jay's original lyrics, Jacobo Mesa Ramirez, a writer and rapper, coauthored this chapter by creating new lyrics that maintain the spirit of the original story but also adequately maintain Jay's confidentiality.

Who is this? My therapist? Brown skin, tattoos, and dreadlocks. I don't get this.
I was asked, have I ever done anything like this in the past? Was it helpful or not and how the experience advanced?
Then the question I think is can I even trust this man?
My past experience is just people all talking nonsense. Tell me take a deep breath count to ten. I really doubt it. Don't you think I've tried to relax? Dawg I'm anxious.
We're born with a target on our backs gotta stay dangerous.

Peace seems preposterous when you're labeled a delinquent.
I guess that's what happens when you live the life I'm living.
I've heard some things that others should not have to be hearing. I have seen some things that the eyes should not be sight-seeing and I'm broken.
Slowly trying to pick up the pieces make them whole again. There is a hole in my heart bet you can feel the depth.
The hole is shaped like a key and it sits right on my chest, but lately I'm coughing up phlegm. This world sometimes it makes me sick.
The key is one I have to craft just like when making art and rap.
Gotta keep up my persona when talking with homies so they only hear my raps about thugging, that's about it.
I also rap about life and how it's too intricate complicated to say the least.
Plus, I got a kid want to see him do better than me. Years of trauma haunting we could break the cycle free.
Want to live for my kids, at one point that kid was me. (lyrics by Jacobo Mesa Ramirez)

I notice myself bobbing my head in unison with Jay as the rhyme progresses. As he finds his way to the end of the first performance, I let out a "whoot!" and clap. I notice Jay sits up just a touch straighter than he has been.

"Did any of these ideas make their way into your past conversations in therapy?" I ask.

"Are you kidding?" Jay's lips assume the shape of a smirk.

"Instead of doing therapy the way it's been done to you before can we make this experience about looking for the key to your knowledge? What might the knowledge you just dropped teach us about where you want to go?"

"It's all about my son, man." His voice is now booming with conviction. "You know, my father was never around growing up. When I found out I was going to have a son, my whole life changed. That's when the DA offered me the deal. I was going to do twenty-five to life. I would never be around for my son. That was unacceptable to me, man. So, I snitched. I'm a fucking snitch. There's no coming back from that shit. The G-Life is all I've ever known. My uncle would send me out with drugs to deliver when I was like seven. I didn't even know what I was doing. He would just be like, 'Yo, go take this shit over there.' I started selling rocks when I was like thirteen."

"What does it say that you would give up the only life you ever knew to be a father?" I speak in a voice I hope Jay will recognize as compassionate.

A tear begins to flow down Jay's cheek and his top lip quivers a bit. "He means everything to me, man. From the moment I found out my girl was pregnant I knew what I had to do."

I swallow deeply, feeling we may be touching on something that could become core to the work we might do together, before asking, "Where did this knowing come from?"

"I don't know." Jay sits in contemplation for a few seconds. "But I feel bad because I snitched on my homies, you know? I let them down. Where was my loyalty?"

"This might sound like a weird question," I say cautiously, "but have you noticed that there are different kinds of loyalties?"

"What do you mean?" Confusion hangs from Jay's brow.

"Like, is the kind of loyalty you showed your homies different from other kinds of loyalties you've seen or experienced in your life?"

"For sure! Loyalty in the G-Life is like this crazy kind of loyalty. My parents never said I love you, but my homies did. Like I'll bust a cap for you. There's crazy loyalty in what I did for my hood. But really, when you needed someone and you were at your lowest, they weren't really there. It's like loyalty on the surface, but it doesn't really always run deep down sometimes. It's hard to explain."

Wanting to continue to ensure that loyalty doesn't get storied as a unitary construct that traps Jay in the position of being disloyal should he choose anything other than his previous life as a gang member, I inquire, "Is there a different kind of loyalty you practice with your son or is it the same as the G-Life?"

Jay's eyes once again well up with tears. "I used to have this tough gangster front. It's whatever. I figured out, like damn, I do want my family. I know I'm a good dad. I'll do anything for my son. I change his diapers. I changed his first diaper. I want to do shit with my son that my parents never did with me."

"Can I ask you how old your son is, Jay?"

"He's 5 months old."

"Now, I know he can't speak yet, but if he could and I asked him about what he loved most about his dad, what do you think he would tell me?"

Jay starts fidgeting with the thumb and index finger of his right hand. "He would say I have a big heart. I've always taken care of everybody in my hood. If I had five bucks and you had none, we both got five bucks."

I look at the clock and realize that time is running away from us. In an attempt to try and bring our first meeting to a close, I ask, "Does this feel like an okay direction we've been going together today?"

"Yeah, it's good. You're not a goofy like those other therapists."

"What do you think about continuing to invite rap music into our conversations? Do you think rap might have the potential to take us places that just talking couldn't?"

"Yo, I've known it could do that for a long time," Jay asserts.

"Do you think this might be part of that knowledge that exists in the locked vault inside you like we were talking about earlier?" I ask this question in hopes that he might remember this as I did. "Maybe rap music is a key to get in there?"

Jay leans back on the couch and lets out a small sigh. “When I was in prison, I used to write rhymes almost every day. Without them I don’t know how I would have made it through.”

“Jay, now that you are out of prison and no longer a part of the G-Life would you say that you are creating a new identity?”

“Yeah, and it’s so fucking hard. Some days I just feel totally lost. Being a regular civilian is not a life I’m used to.”

“Jay, would you be up for doing a little writing between now and the next time we meet?”

Jay nods affirmatively.

“What do you think about writing a rhyme about how you imagine your identity recreating itself as a father and a civilian and bringing it with you for next time?” I notice myself trying to be precise in my use of language knowing that the words we choose now could over time become representative of the identity he might prefer to live into.

“That’s cool,” he replies.

As the meeting comes a close, I walk Jay down to the main office door. His ride has not yet arrived. I notice this stirs up some anxiety. Jay positions his body to the right side of the door to the minimize the chances he might be seen. I offer to grab him a chair so that he might sit down, but he declines. The anxiety only seems to intensify.

“I have to drive through my old neighborhood to get here,” Jay says in a disconcerted tone. “They have a hit out on me. All it takes is one person seeing me, and BANG! It’s over.”

Jay mimics the firing of a gun with his right hand. This action in combination with the way Jay says the word bang with such emphasis viscerally rattles my being. I am uncertain how to respond. With my mouth still trying to catch up to my brain and heart, Jay peers around the corner once more. “Oh, there’s my ride. Peace.”

“Okay, I’ll see you next week, brother,” I reply.

“For sure.”

I watch as Jay walks at a hurried pace to the car, his head on a swivel. I notice my stomach churning with discomfiture. As I head back up to my office to grab my belongings, I experience the feeling of my stomach doing somersaults.

I get in my own car and start the ignition. Music begins emanating from the car’s speakers. I quickly turn it down, not wanting it to get in the way of my contemplation. Questions begin cycling through my head. Isn’t coming to have a conversation with me supposed to provide at least some kind of relief? Well, perhaps he did feel some of that while we were in conversation? But what good is that if he fears for his life commuting to and from our meetings?

My mind flashes back to recent conversations I have had with probation officers. “Why don’t they show up to therapy?” they would ask. When confronted with all it took just for Jay to make it to and from our first conversation, I wondered if they were asking the wrong question. Perhaps the better question is why people in Jay's set of circumstances *would show up at all* given the existential threats they were carrying with them on a daily basis.

I awake the next morning with more clarity in what I must do. I call and speak to Jay and ask if it might make things easier if I were to come to him rather than him having to worry about coming to me. Jay politely declines and tells me it would be no problem. I push a little harder letting him know that I do not want him to put his life at risk on behalf of our conversations. Jay begrudgingly accepts my offer, but he lets me know this arrangement could get complicated as he somewhat frequently changes his place of residence as an added safety measure. He tells me he will be staying with his mom next week when we are due to meet, and we agree to meet at her house.

Six days later I pull up to the projects where Jay's mother lives. I navigate up the stairs to the fourth floor where the apartment is located to the sounds of children playing and honking horns on the crowded adjacent street. As I take a deep breath and steel myself for the conversation to come, Jay opens the door before I have a chance to knock. He ushers me in quickly and shuts the door behind me.

"What's up, brother?" he asks in a friendly tone. I feel a sense of near instant comfort in him adopting the same language I have been using to greet him.

"It's great to be here, brother. Please tell your mother thank you for lending us this space."

As I look around, I take a few moments to metabolize the tight surroundings of the one-bedroom apartment. A pair of Air Jordan sneakers have been kicked off to the right side of the door. Five Virgin Mary candles rest on the mantle with the smell of freshly burned incense saturating the air. A half-eaten bowl of cereal sits on the kitchen table with the flakes slowly bobbing in the milk. Jay clears some of the belongings off the couch for us as we sit down. "Sorry, that's where I've been sleeping."

The fickle nature of Jay's life reveals itself in a way that only being in this space could truly do justice.

"Thanks for coming over here," Jay continues.

"It's the least I could do. I don't want you having to worry about making it to and from my office."

While Jay does not verbally respond to my words, his body seems to indicate a sense of increasing solidarity. I wonder if he thought I would not show up. Should I ask him about this? I mull the possibilities as the silence between us grows.

"Most therapists don't like leaving their little offices," quips Jay.

"That's a true story! Are you surprised that this therapist left his?" I follow my comment with a friendly, iconoclastic smile.

"Nah, I knew if you showed up that you're a real one."

While Jay's words fill me up a little, it feels weird to be getting any kind of extra credit for something that seems like it must be done for the good of our work. I quickly pivot.

"Jay, I wonder if we might revisit what we were talking about at the end of our last conversation? Would that be alright with you?"

"I've been writing." Jay flashes a toothy grin.

"Is this writing that would feel comfortable to share in here, or is it something you would rather keep in your pocket?"

"I wrote just for this meeting, homie, so we might as well do it."

Jay takes some time to connect his phone to the television in the living room. He tests the speakers. As he begins playing a beat through his phone onto the TV, I realize fairly quickly he had prerecorded this track. The beat begins to capture my mind moments before the lyrics exit the speakers.

Note: Again, the coauthor of this chapter, Jacobo Mesa Ramirez, a writer and rapper, created new lyrics that maintain the spirit of the original story but also adequately maintain Jay's confidentiality.

My father was never there when I was growing up, and the only love my family showed was in the form of tough love.
When I was young my uncle would send me out with drugs. I didn't even know at the time what was going on.
He would tell me "take that shit over there" started selling rocks before I knew what a drug was, and that's a shame, but who is the kid to blame?
When we're young we're mostly just products of the environment. The places which we're placed in influence thoughts and behaviors.
Imagine this, a kid figuring out what life is, delivering an unknown substance to his neighbor. The streets are filled with violence a bloody trail of paper. And I want a life that's better for my kids forever.
I used to have this tough gangster front, it's whatever.
Always had a big heart, share what I have with my neighbors. Figured out my family comes first that's what's most important.
The hood say that they love me, but it's only on the surface. Gotta think about the future. What are my priorities?
I knew when I saw my son there that he meant more to me than the G-life. I swear sometimes it feels like it got a hold on me.
There's different kinds of loyalties. Transitioning from doubt to self-belief. The only life I've ever known, how could I just up and leave it often defeated by self-doubt?
At least I'm alive and breathing. I fear I won't know what to do, in quote to quote what's normal . . . the past it sticks around, and it doesn't work to avoid it. I get paranoid when my way of doing things isn't working.
But isn't that what life's about: living, loving, learning. Although it can be scary it's time to find my own purpose.
A way of doing things is different sometimes makes me nervous, but I know I have more to offer than just what's on the surface. So, let's take a look behind the curtains, inner purpose of the person, with money can't be purchased, for something we're all searching.
(lyrics by Jacobo Mesa Ramirez)

After taking some to metabolize Jay's lyrical offering, I move our conversation forward with a phrase he turned near the end of the rhyme. "Jay, would I be right in saying this rhyme is giving us a little peak behind the curtain of your life?"

He nods affirmatively.

"What have you been seeing behind there?

Jay sighs deeply. "I'm scared to die because of my son. I've never felt fear before. I didn't used to be scared of dying. We know we're banging death. I came out of prison, and I was really sensitive. It was different. But I'm still a fucking snitch."

"Jay, is choosing to value fatherhood the same thing as being a snitch?"

Jay's face twists with discomfort at my question. Angst seems to almost drip off him the way it drips off one's body on a particularly hot and humid day. I wonder if he is having trouble finding words. Then, his head drops quickly toward the ground as if aided by an anchor.

"I got jumped by old buddies at the store this week. I have to learn how to walk away from shit like that. They were a rival gang. They spit on me, and that's where I lost it. I'm still trying to find who I am. I have to let the past go and not keep holding on. There's no reason to keep glorifying it and reminiscing. I feel like the gang unit used me, too. As soon as the trial was over, they don't do shit for me except try and get info about what's going on in the streets. My mom's afraid if I get a job, they are going to find me and kill me. But probation is on my ass about getting a job all the time, and if I don't, they say they'll revoke my shit. What the fuck am I supposed to do?"

It feels as though despair has Jay by the collar. I consider how much longer I should explore this particular topic with him.

"Would it be fair to say the G-Life and snitching are complicated stories that run pretty deep, maybe even so deep that probation and other people in your new life can't quite understand?

"Yeah, it's always there. My cousin said I could rob or sell drugs? I said, 'Nah, I can't do it. I'll get addicted to it again.' I miss the loyalty and respect I had. My cousins bring it up all the time."

"Do you think sometimes people, especially people who have never lived it, look at the G-Life as all bad?"

"Oh, hell yeah!"

"Are there elements of that life that you would like to carry with you, or do you feel it best to let it go entirely?"

Jay lets out an audible snicker. "That's true, but no civilian has ever asked me that before. They just always tell me to get out. Even my girl was always saying that."

"As a civilian, Jay, I only know of the G-Life through story. To be honest, I don't feel positioned to tell you what to do one way or the other. Can I invite us to use your knowledge on this topic since it's the kind of knowledge

I couldn't possibly have? Maybe there are elements of the G-Life that will serve you well as you move towards this new identity?"

"I know we talked about how loyalty gets fucked up in the G-Life, but my homies were like my family. My dad wasn't there. My mom had her own shit going on. But family is real. We all need family."

I see an opening to perhaps invite Jay into reconsidering how family might look in his life now as compared to how it looked even just a few short months ago. "Are you carrying that sense of family with you now with your son and your girl, Jay?"

"That's for sure. It's an even better sense of family if you ask me."

"Are there other elements of the G-Life you'd like to carry forward?"

Jay takes a prolonged pause and seems to drift somewhere else. I wonder if the place he's traveling is one of importance, and I take care not to interrupt his journey. A tear slowly cascades down his cheek. Other tears follow as if in a race to reach the bottom of his cheek first. "I've done shit I can't even talk about, horrible shit. I'm a bad person. This is the part I don't think I can ever get over. I have violent dreams sometimes. I wake up freaking out. When I'm awake tires scratching do that, too. Also, people running. Cars pulling up fast on me. When people walk with hoodies on it makes me nervous."

I worry that shame may be trying to take over our conversation and wonder if this might be creating blemishes on his new identity canvas. This stirs a sense of urgency in me. A question flies out of my mouth that I have never asked of anyone previously. "Jay, do you think systems that behave badly sometimes invite good people to do bad things?"

Jay's face takes the shape of a person experiencing utter confusion. I chuckle to myself as I realize that my question was one deeply rooted in the jargon and theory of a practice that is likely quite foreign to him. I quickly appreciate that for the question to do the work I hope for it to do, I must make it more relatable.

"Sorry, Jay. I know that question was a little weird. Can I give it another shot?"

Jay graciously obliges with a quick nod of his head.

"Thank you. Do you think if you grew up down the road in the rich area of town you would have found yourself engaging in the same activities you did living the G-Life here in the projects?"

A wry smile finds its way onto Jay's face. "Nah. I would have been playing tennis and polo and shit."

We both share a quick laugh together.

"The day you came out of the womb, Jay, you weren't destined to be labeled a criminal?"

"I guess not." Jay's body leans into the conversation ever so slightly.

"Might I ask how it is that you found yourself tangled up with the law?"

Jay replies without hesitation. "I had no choice. My dad and my uncle were part of the G-Life. I was basically in it since birth. It's like the family business. You do what you gotta do to make ends meet, you know what I mean?"

"Would it be fair to say that you were just doing what kids who live the G-Life do rather than being a bad person?"

Jay's face slowly assumes a look equal parts gradual surprise and possibility. It is as if a small portal of hope is starting to open ever so slightly. "Damn, I'm going to have to think about that right there."

"Would it in any way be helpful to write a rhyme about this or would it be best to just continue talking about it next time we meet?"

"I've just got to try and wrap my head around it."

I glance at the clock on the microwave about twenty feet away, and it says 4:57 p.m. I feel a slight jolt as I come back to the realization that I'm not in my office as I am so enthralled by our conversation that I have forgotten. As I prepare to get up and leave, I once again thank Jay for his hospitality and ask him to pass this sentiment along to his mom. We agree to meet again next week at the same time. Jay and I exchange dap, and he opens the front door for me.

In the days that follow, I carry with me a sense of hope and invigoration with regard to where our future conversations might take us. The day before I am to meet with Jay again, I get a call from him. His voice projects a sense of distress. "We can't meet this week. It's too dangerous, man. I'm at my cousin's house. They found out I was at my mom's."

I reassure Jay that I would feel just fine coming to meet him at his cousin's house, but he is adamant that I not come. Not wanting to push the issue, I ask if we might reschedule. He says, "I'll holler at you, brother."

This interaction leaves me unsettled. Questions do jumping jacks in my mind. Is Jay okay? Should I do more to try and ensure his safety? A couple of minutes later, some other questions, that have more to do with me than him, follow in hot pursuit. Is this his way of opting out of our meetings? Are our conversations perhaps not proving to be of much value to him?

I feel flummoxed. I let out a deep sigh. As I sit down on the park bench where I fielded his call, I take a moment to breathe in the surroundings. I watch three young boys playing soccer. I study the pigeons as they study me. I listen to the wind blowing through the leaves of the trees. Perhaps nature will reveal some kind of direction?

I feel my phone buzz. Reluctantly, I pull it from my pocket and look at the slew of incoming email. I notice one of them is from Jay with the subject line, "Check this rhyme!" I open the email and inside is an audio file as well as a document with lyrics. I feel a sense of hope restored to my body. I scramble for my headphones in my other pocket, connect them to the jack, and begin listening to the song as I read the lyrics.

Note: As mentioned earlier, the following lyrics are by Jacobo Mesa Ramirez, a writer and rapper, who created new lyrics to maintain Jay's confidentiality.

I'm scared to die, but I'm scared to live. And with the life I lived before, I knew this was what came with it.
We know we're banging death. When I came out of prison, I was really sensitive I'm scared to die cause of my kid.
Before I never feared death when there was not much to live for.
I have to let the past go still trying to find who I am. You can't possibly understand half of what I've been through.
Call me a snitch, in my situation what would you do?
This runs deeper than a wound and takes some time to heal, too.
If you've never lived it from the outside it looks different. Born into this shit. You could call it the family business.
Still getting temptations to go back. It's an addiction. It's like once you get that hit you just go back for more, you fiending.
Found a family in the streets. My real one wasn't there for me. I guess it's a full circle.
Coming out the womb I was not labeled a criminal. I did what any kid would have done if they had to.
What I did before still haunts me sometimes, makes me miserable. Waking up in cold sweats, violent dreams get physical.
Born in a system that oppresses expressed by aggression. Can I even move forward, and what will be the end of this?
This is what they want me to tell myself but forget it. My kids will not feel the baggage of this weight that I've been carrying . . . for generations.
I must walk down this road even if it may be wearying. Bury my regrets and move forward very progressive.
I know it won't be easy, but shit, it's never really been in the first place. (lyrics by Jacobo Mesa Ramirez)

A large smile overtakes my face. An astonished chuckle flies from my mouth. The rhyme has momentarily transported me to another world. The curious look of a passerby reminds me that I am in a public place. I collect myself and begin the journey back to my office. After a brisk fifteen-minute walk, I sit down at my computer and compose a quick reply to Jay's email. I let him know that I am very much looking forward to meeting with again when the opportunity presents itself.

Three days later, I receive a text from Jay in the morning saying that he wants to meet. He is staying with a friend and gives me the address. I have a full day of conversations with people lined up, but I do not want to let this opportunity pass. I ask if I might come over after my day is over around 8:30 p.m. Jay agrees.

As I walk out of my office after a long day of teaching and therapeutic conversations, I notice myself feeling a little weary. I wonder if I have made a mistake by agreeing to see Jay so late. As I put the address he gave me into the GPS on my phone, I start to feel a bit of a second wind kick in.

I pull up to the small house of his friend, and I see Jay peering out the window. He quickly hops to attention and opens the front door for me. We exchange dap. Jay's face reveals a paradoxical sense of restlessness and relief. We each sit down on a folding chair at a small kitchen table.

Our conversation begins with an interaction he had in a local department store earlier that day.

"Everyone thinks I'm a gang member until they talk to me," he says with a curious smile. "Probably because of my tattoos they think I'm a mean ass tough guy, but I'm actually gentle and not intimidating."

"You know, Jay, I'm struck by something. Is it okay if I share it with you?"

He nods his head for me to continue.

"I'm wondering if there is a deep care that travels with you in your life for people?"

Jay takes a few seconds to ponder my question. "Yeah, I think that is part of the new person I'm trying to be, you know what I mean?"

I give his words time to settle. "Here's the thing, I have no doubt what you're saying is true, Jay. But I just can't help but wonder, do you think this care has always traveled with you in some way, even when you were a gangster?"

Jay is quick to dismiss my query. "Nah, to be a gangster you have to be cold-blooded."

Undeterred, I continue. "Wait, wait. You mean to tell me that if I knew you during your days as a gangster, I wouldn't have experienced any of this care that I have felt in all of our conversations since I first met you?"

My question seems to push Jay into a deeper state of contemplation. After sitting in silence for about thirty seconds, Jay's eyes begin to indicate that something might be stirring.

"I just thought of this, but even when I was a gangster, I was never mean to civilians. I started this thing with my gang that we never rob civilians, never hurt them."

"Was this a new thing that started under your leadership, Jay?"

"Yeah, before we would rob people just to act hard. It was stupid."

My voice gets a little more measured and quieter as I ask, "Maybe that care has been there all along?"

"I guess so." Jay's body settles into the hard confines of the chair as though something was pushing on him. The silence seems to be doing some kind of important work. Jay's being perks up.

"You know, I would warn people in my hood with kids when shit was about to go down so they could go inside and get in the basement. I had them on a group text. They didn't choose this life. They would call me because they knew I would take care of the neighborhood. During Thanksgiving I would buy all the moms like twenty turkeys and twenty pumpkin pies. I would deliver these to every family in my hood."

I can feel myself being moved by Jay's stories. A lump forms in my throat. As I start my next question my voice cracks ever so slightly. "Do you think that the legal system and other civilians typically know about this deep care that helps drive your living?"

"No, they just think I'm some Mexican, gangster piece of shit. This is why I can't be this new person here in this city. I need a fresh start."

A mist of hopelessness begins to settle over us. Before I can formulate my next question, Jay's phone dings. A message pops up on the screen. He takes a quick glance at the message. Then he picks up the phone, drawing it closer to his face, and an alarm sounds in his eyes.

"You've got to go," he says hurriedly. With uncertainty about what the contents of the text message were, I am in a state of confusion. A longer glance at Jay's face lets me know the magnitude of the urgency he is feeling.

"It's not safe. You gotta get the hell out of here." Jay carefully looks out the window, making sure to not move the curtain. "C'mon," he says lightly guiding me to the door. He escorts me to my car and tells me to leave as quickly as I can. I feel my heart pumping a little faster than I am accustomed to. My mind is fuzzy as I drive away.

I talk to Jay the next afternoon on the phone. He explains to me that one of his old homeboys tipped him off that his former gang knew where he was, and that they were coming for him. The conversation leaves me feeling as though he has a deep desire to ensure my safety, which only increases the bond I share with him. Jay ends the call by telling me he will let me know when we can have another conversation.

After this, it becomes clear to me that I have to redefine what *therapy* is. If we have fifteen minutes on Tuesday and twenty more on Friday, I'll take it. I start asking myself quite a number of questions about my field. How is it that we have decided therapy sessions must last one hour? How have we decided that these meetings must take place in the often haughty office of a professional? How have we decided that they must include conversation to the near exclusion of other potential models of healing?

These questions inspire me to call Jay with a proposal for a new kind of *therapy*, one where he lets me know when he has a bit of free time and feels like he is in a safe space. Then, I will let him know if I can come meet him, or even speak on the phone.

Over the next month, Jay and I have a series of mini-meetings. With each one I notice a continuing frustration and urgency in Jay's being. On a random Thursday I meet Jay at a friend's apartment where he is staying.

"I finally got a job for a couple days, but there were Bloods there," he says with a look of uneasiness. "I left because of safety concerns. I used to have a gun, but now I don't. I don't want to hurt nobody. If I'm meant to die,

I can't stop it. I've thought about slangin' again. I have no other resources to get legit money, but I have a bunch of other resources from the streets. If I was caught and with a gun, that's thirty-two years. That's my son's whole life. I have more to lose than to gain."

I feel the heaviness of Jay's dilemma. "What does it say about you, Jay, that you are trying to stay legit despite all of these forces working against that?"

Jay's shoulders straighten up ever so slightly. "I know I'm not who I was back in the day. I found my old journal from prison with all my old raps. I can see the difference. My good friends say I bring leadership. I know I'm a better person than I was. When I'm with my son, I feel joy. But if you keep knocking at the Devil's door, he's gonna answer."

"Hey Jay, do you remember this line from one of your rhymes a few meetings ago? For some reason it just came to my mind." I search my phone nearby for the specific lyrics. "Okay, here it is."

> I must walk down this road even if it may be wearying. Bury my regrets and move forward very progressive. (lyrics by Jacobo Mesa Ramirez)

"If you were to bury your regrets and move forward, can you imagine how that might look?"

Jay's face becomes sullen. "That's the thing, I don't know how I can do that here. My best friend wore a wire on me for two years. It's hard to understand what's real and not real. Every day I live my life with regret. When I was everybody's ATM, everybody loved me. I don't show my emotions because I'm afraid they'll take advantage of me. I don't do Lean or Percocet because of my son. Without him I'd probably be in jail. You know, it was easier in jail. There was a schedule. I started so much shit as a gang member and it follows me now. Can't take the bus. These dudes started shit with me on the bus. It's easy for my PO and them to say at least I'm free because they don't have to deal with the anxiety."

Jay's face drops toward the floor. Tears begin streaming down his face. I move my body just a bit closer to his in hopes it might provide a sense of solidarity. He looks up and we embrace as the tears come faster.

Within a flurry of teardrops, Jay admits, "I stole diapers and wipes for my son. I didn't want to look like a loser, but I don't know how else to get money. I don't want my son growing up angry because they killed his dad. My cousins told me people are getting consequenced because I'm still alive. I think about all my friends that passed away, and then all the bad stuff I did because of it. I'm free, I guess, but I'm not really free. I'm not free like an ordinary citizen. I would work at McDonald's, I'd work anywhere, but I can't because I could get killed. I have to get out of this city, but I'm trapped."

Jay takes some time to collect himself. I opt not to say anything, feeling that words might take up unnecessary space. Jay takes a deep breath. "I feel better when I come here. I'd release my feelings in anger in the past. Now I also think about my decisions more. If I go to jail, I would live up to what everyone thinks of me."

"Would you be living up to what others think of you or down to what they think of you?" I inquire gently.

"Down," he replies forthrightly.

"If you were to live up to what we think of you, what might that look like?"

Tears well up again in Jay's eyes.

"May I give you that question to carry with you until we meet again, Jay? Would you be up for writing a rhyme about it?"

Jay nods affirmatively. On my way out he forgoes the typical male hug that mandates an arm-bar between our torsos and hugs me tightly with two hands. I do the same. Moments after leaving the apartment, I start to wonder if that hug knew something that perhaps I didn't.

Two weeks pass without as much as a text from Jay. While I don't wish to be a bother, I start to wonder if everything is okay. I try to text and call him. The number is disconnected. I have no luck trying to contact him by email, either. I start to worry. I reach out to Jay at least once every week for the next month. Still no response.

Over a month later, I find an email in my inbox from an email address I don't recognize with "It's me" in the subject line. Sufficiently intrigued, I open the email. It's from Jay, sent from a new email address. It reads as follows: "Hey brother. I had to leave the state. I can't be the person I want to be there. I don't want to die. . . . I'm with my son and my girl. We are going to make a new life. I already have a job out here, and I don't have to watch my back all the time. Listen to the rhyme in here. It will explain it better than I can. Peace, Jay."

I click to open the audio file and begin listening to the song that he attached to the email.

Note: As mentioned earlier, Jacobo Mesa Ramirez, a writer and rapper, created new lyrics for this chapter that maintain the spirit of the original story but also adequately maintain Jay's confidentiality.

Looks can be deceiving. You know the old saying don't judge a book before you read it. Assumptions on the surface can be misleading.

People see tattoos on my face and they probably think I'm like a demon. When they never read a single chapter of my story or bothered to flip the pages to find out what my true strength is.

I've always cared for others but who has really cared for me? Witness protection don't even guarantee safety. I'm faced with two options either death or a long time in prison.

The person who I was before could not keep on living. The path I traveled ultimately led to destruction.
Witness protection was only trying to get info. They did not make me feel safe, so I keep my guard up. It's simple.
Took some things with me that helped me to build up my character, but who I was before cannot continue going down that road.
Deep care for the people, I don't want to see them cry alone. Working against all opposing forces tryna stay legit. I'm not who I was in the past I can see the difference.
My good friends, they telling me that I bring leadership. knock . . . knock . . . That's the devil tryna get in. If we keep knocking on his door he will answer, best believe it.
My best friend wore a wire on me . . . for two whole years. It's hard to understand what's real and what's not with what we feel.
Every day I live . . . my life with regret. . . . Everybody loves you when you are an ATM. . . . Withdrawing cash from you and not heard from . . . ever since.
The spiritual bank deposit is one I must put in, and I can't give that to nobody else. That's only for my kin.
Build myself over the years so my kid can be free, and that's exactly the purpose and reason why I had to leave.
Will I live down or up to what everyone thinks of me? I can't be the person that I know I want to be, in this fucked up city that I grew up in. I don't wanna die but don't want to be scared of living. (lyrics by Jacobo Mesa Ramirez)

My throat begins to feel tight. The tightness makes its way up my face and squeezes a tear from my left eye. I know what this rhyme means. Jay is *really* gone. He has decided to leave the state, maybe even the country. Perhaps his journey to a new location helped life feel just a little more possible.

Jay still sends me rhymes every so often. I listen, metabolize, and reply, often with the same kinds of questions I would ask if we were sitting together. His rhymes bare his soul, and one could argue this is much more important for the work we were doing than his physical presence. While I miss our embodied meetings, I am thankful for the technology that allows us to stay connected through song and the written word.

I do not know if most folks would classify what Jay and I are doing now as psychotherapy. This realization pestered me only for a short time. I discovered that whether or not others would call it psychotherapy is secondary to whether or not Jay is finding some measure of healing in it. Just as Jay rapped, "I could not heal in the environment I was trapped in," perhaps he also could not heal using often unwittingly colonizing forms of psychotherapy from Eurocentric traditions?

Recently in some of our written correspondence, I ask Jay what he would call the work we engage in. He replies, "Freedom Fighting where the gun is the rhyme."

I type in response, "Is using rhymes to take up the fight of freedom the key we were looking for all along?"

Jay replies, "Yeah. I can actually live life now."

And perhaps that is the most we can ask from any attempt at healing.

Narrative therapy is a way of working originally pioneered by David Epston and Michael White in the 1980s. Rather than being influenced by psychiatry and psychology, Epston and White spent a great deal of time reading about anthropology, Foucauldian French philosophy, and feminism, among other topics. This helped inspire narrative therapy and community work to look at people and problems as separate. That is, problems are socially constructed and not housed solely inside the physical bodies of people. Moreover, narrative therapists view people as being multi-storied and their identity as fluid and shaped by systems that espouse ideas about who people are supposed to be. In this way, narrative therapy has always tried to pay close attention to power and to the ways in which power structures can impact how people have come to view themselves or others as problematic (White & Epston, 1990).

Narrative therapists are thus focused on helping people through coauthoring counter-stories, which are stories that exist alongside the more dominant stories that are being told about their life. For example, in Jay's case, he is looked at as a gang member and a criminal. This account has become the dominant story of his existence and is being upheld by societal systems with a great deal of power (that is, the criminal injustice system), making them feel as though they are absolute truth. My job as a therapist, through the use of narrative therapy questions, is to begin the process of unearthing stories about Jay that are not being told by these more dominant systems. As was revealed, Jay is a loving father and someone who cared a great deal about those in his community. These are counter-stories that offer new possibilities for how Jay's life might be storied.

Epston and White also advocated that narrative practices value voices and ideas that come from local cultures and communities, often referred to as local knowledges, rather than from more global, expert knowledges. Thus, narrative therapists ask many questions without the presupposition of knowledge. These questions are designed to invite and to privilege the knowledge of the client rather than more professionalized ideas or assessments. Such questions are at the heart of narrative practice, and as such, it is important that those questions and the dialogue that results from them be represented in sufficient detail in Jay's story. In addition, rather than mandating a canonical approach, narrative therapy encouraged the work to assume a stance of adventure (White & Epston, 1990). The aforementioned factors, along with narrative therapy's commitment to justice-doing, have helped make the approach fertile ground for new and radical ways of working (Reynolds, 2010).

In the last decade, narrative thinkers have, with increasing momentum, started exploring anti-colonial approaches to therapy as alternatives to the now nearly ubiquitous multicultural approach (Akinyela, 2014; Heath, 2018; Polanco, 2016). Anti-colonial approaches tend to assume a stance of cultural democracy, which allows people to have a say in their own healing through use of their own cultural ideas and traditions as opposed to inviting people to heal within more dominant, Eurocentric paradigms (Akinyela, 2002). These ideas and traditions could take many forms. This chapter specifically looked at the use of rap music by Jay as a preferred medium of healing (Heath, 2018).

Jay's story was presented in the form of an autoethnography. The method for this particular story can probably best be described as evocative autoethnography (Bochner & Ellis, 2016). This approach seeks to help the reader feel as though they are a part of the story through present-tense, first-person storytelling. It writes the *researcher* into the story and acknowledges that researchers are part of the same world as the participants. The hope is that the reader will feel like they are sitting in the room with the therapist and their conversational partner. Evocative autoethnography typically tries to avoid making intellectual or academic interpretations about what is happening in the story, and instead, endeavors to leave the reader with a felt sense of the encounter, content with the fact that some therapeutic mysteries will remain mysterious.

Often students report a disconnect between understanding a theory of psychotherapy and actually being able to put that theory into practice. Autoethnography is being explored as a bridge to praxis and as a pedagogy for teaching narrative therapy in a way that is less technical, more soulful, and explores the use of preferred mediums of healing (Epston et al., 2016; Heath & Arroyo, 2014, 2015, 2016; Polanco, 2011). Early returns have shown autoethnography to be an intriguing way to help people take what has traditionally been a bit of esoteric practice and start to *feel* the practice and embody it in their own work (Vogel Mitchell, Heath, & Epston, 2017; Carlson et al., 2017). This approach steers teachers and writers away from telling people about theory as an introduction to narrative therapy and instead invites them into feeling the work through first-person stories. It is a sort of reverse engineering of the traditional process of teaching and learning psychotherapy.

REFERENCES

Akinyela, M. (2002). De-colonizing our lives: Divining a post-colonial therapy. *International Journal of Narrative Therapy and Community Work*, *1*(2), 32–43. http://www.narrativetherapylibrary.com/media/downloadable/files/links/0/2/022Akinyela_2.pdf

Akinyela, M. (2014). Narrative therapy and cultural democracy: A Testimony view. *Australian and New Zealand Journal of Family Therapy*, *35*(1), 46–49. https://doi.org/10.1002/anzf.1041

Bochner, A., & Ellis, C. (2016). *Evocative autoethnography: Writing lives and telling stories.* New York, NY: Routledge.

Carlson, T., Espton, D., Haire, A., Cortuillo, E. M., Huerta Lopez, A., Vedvei, S., & McAllum Pilkington, S. (2017). Learning narrative therapy backwards: Exemplary tales as an alternative pedagogy for learning practice. *Journal of Systemic Therapies*, *36*(1), 94–107. https://doi.org/10.1521/jsyt.2017.36.1.94

Epston, D., Heath, T., Ingamells, K., & McCallum Pilkington, S. (2016). Exemplary tales: Virtual apprenticeships. *Journal of Systemic Therapies*, *35*(2), 56–70. https://doi.org/10.1521/jsyt.2016.35.2.56

Heath, T. (2018). Moving beyond multicultural counselling: Narrative therapy, anti-colonialism, cultural democracy and hip-hop. *International Journal of Narrative Therapy and Community Work*, *3*, 42–47.

Heath, T., & Arroyo, P. (2014). "I gracefully grab a pen and embrace it": Hip-hop lyrics as a means for re-authoring and therapeutic change. *International Journal of Narrative Therapy and Community Work*, *3*, 31–38.

Heath, T., & Arroyo, P. (2015). Spitting truth from my soul: A case story of rapping, probation, and the narrative practices. Part I. *Journal of Systemic Therapies*, *34*(3), 77–90. https://doi.org/10.1521/jsyt.2015.34.3.77

Heath, T., & Arroyo, P. (2016). Spitting truth from my soul: A case story of rapping, probation, and the narrative practices. Part II. *Journal of Systemic Therapies*, *34*(4), 80–93. https://doi.org/10.1521/jsyt.2015.34.4.80

Polanco, M. (2011). Autoethnographic means to the end of a decolonizing translation. *Journal of Systemic Therapies*, *30*(3), 42–56. https://doi.org/10.1521/jsyt.2011.30.3.42

Polanco, M. (2016). Knowledge fair trade. In L. L. Charlés & G. Samarasinghe (Eds.), *Family therapy in global and humanitarian contexts: Voices and Issues from the field* (pp. 13–25). New York, NY: Springer.

Reynolds, V. (2010). *Doing Justice as a Path to Sustainability in Community Work*. PhD diss., Tilburg University. Retrieved from https://www.taosinstitute.net/Websites/taos/Images/PhDProgramsCompletedDissertations/ReynoldsPhDDissertationFeb2210.pdf

White, M., & Epston, D. (1990). *Narrative means to therapeutic ends.* New York, NY: Norton.

Vogel, M. G., Heath, T., & Epston, D. (2017). A tale of an exemplary tale in the classroom: An accidental inquiry of the restoration of beauty. *Journal of Systemic Therapies*, *36*(1), 78–92.

Chapter Eight

Music Therapy

An Ethnographic Approach to Understanding How Music Therapists and Adolescent Patients Communicate and Perform Community

Melanie Frontz Kramer and Kurt Lindemann

Music affects every person differently, depending on the context, the type of music, and the emotional, physical, and spiritual state of the person. Many of us are not aware of the fact that the soundtrack keeps playing. Music lingers in the background of our busy lives, existing in the shadows. This is the power of music.

In 2013, for her master's thesis, the first author, Melaine Kramer, immersed herself in the Music Therapy (MT) culture at the California School of Music Therapy (CSMT) (a pseudonym). The CSMT works with children and adults of all ages who suffer from a variety of physical and neurological limitations. Through this research, we explored the concepts of music, communication, and community construction. The following is a condensed version of the study written with the assisstance of coauthor Kurt Lindemann.

LITERATURE REVIEW

Below you will find a brief overview of how and why music is being used therapeutically as a complementary and alternative medicine with many populations, including adolescents with neurological limitations, developmental disabilities, and behavioral challenges.

Musical Communication

Music is a common form of complementary and alternative medicine (CAM) partially due to music's communicative properties. Music and communication are interconnected and apparent in human interaction. Consuming music is part of people's daily lives (Larsen, Lawson, & Todd, 2010), as is communication. Throughout daily interactions, many times we are communicating with, through, and about music.

Listening to, performing, and composing music are ways of sending messages to ourselves intrapersonally, and to others interpersonally. The fascinating nature of music, when purely instrumental, is that it can be a form of nonverbal communication, conveying messages and expressing emotions that may not be expressed by words (Crowe, 2004).

Communication is one of the main purposes of music (Crowe, 2004). Studies have shown that it is likely that music was actually one of the, if not the first, types of human communication (Crowe, 2004). Some researchers argue that all human communication is musical (Trevarthen, 2002). Charles Inskip, Andrew MacFarlane, and Pauline Rafferty (2008) suggest that music is itself a language, and those who enjoy it do so through musical experiences. David Hargreaves, Raymond MacDonald, and Dorothy Miell (2005) in their edited book *Musical Communication* propose a closer look at real-life situations in which individuals are engaging in musical activities while interacting with others to expand on this model of musical communication. This review of literature will do just that, starting with a definition of MT.

Music Therapy

Many organizations have developed definitions for MT, its goals, and its components. One working definition that encompasses multiple definitions reviewed for this study is presented by Kenneth Bruscia (1998) in his *Defining Music Therapy*: "Music therapy is a systematic process of intervention wherein the therapist helps the client to promote health, using music experiences and the relationships that develop through them as dynamic forces of change" (p. 20). Depending on the needs of a patient, MTs employ specific interventions keeping in mind the main goal: health, with an emphasis on music *experiences* (Bruscia, 1998). Simply involving music in a therapeutic session is not the strategy of a music therapist; it is engaging in music experiences.

MT is being used in a variety of settings and has had positive results with patients. The following populations have experienced positive transformation through MT: individuals with developmental disorders such as cerebral palsy, autism spectrum disorder, Down's syndrome, and attention-deficit hyperactive disorder (Brown & Patel, 2005); individuals with post-traumatic stress disorder (PTSD) (Bensimon, Amir, & Wolf, 2008); individuals with depression (Maratos et al., 2008); those who suffer from addictive behaviors including substance abuse (Dingle, Gleadhill, & Baker, 2008) and eating disorders (Dokter, 1994); palliative care patients (Gallagher et al., 2006); dementia patients (Koger, Chapin, & Brotons, 1999); and stroke patients who have acquired speech aphasia and apraxia (Hurkmans et al., 2012). MT is used in many settings to help with a variety of symptoms, many of which are communicative in nature. Colwyn Trevarthen (2002) argues that because all communication is inherently musical, communicative limitations may also be mended through the use of music. Because of the connection between music, communication, and the brain, MT strategically helps a variety of populations.

Music and the Body/Brain

Music has a significant effect on humans' cognitive and motor skills. The brain reacts in intense ways to musical phenomena. When humans listen to music, many different parts of our brain are stimulated. Heinz Gregor Wieser (2003) explains that rhythm stimulates the cerebellum, musical melodies and harmonies activate the temporal lobe, consonant music stimulates the right frontal lobe and orbitofrontal cortex, dissonant sounds activite the gyrus parahippocampalis, and discriminating pitch causes us to use our planum temporale. Early and higher cognitive skills can be developed through MT such as sensation, perception, discrimination, concept development, thinking, reasoning, behavior, motivation, learning, memory, intelligence, creativity, imagery, language, speech, and consciousness (Crowe, 2004). Performing music also draws on complex processes (Crowe, 2004). Those making music must be aware of their body position and posture to physically be able to produce sound (Crowe, 2004). They must employ proper kinesics to cause their body to move, including their muscles, joints, and bones. Music affects other parts of the body as well, such as blood pressure and heart rate (Crowe, 2004). The effects music has on the brain and body are very important to the use of music as a CAM therapy and practice.

Music with Adolescents

One group of individuals that has guided more recent literature on MT is adolescents, particularly those with disabilities, mental illnesses, emotional/behavioral challenges, and those at risk (McFerran, 2010). Whether neurotypical or not, all adolescents seem to have a deep bond with music (McFerran, 2010). Additionally, they are in a phase of their lives in which they are beginning to question the world around them and form their own opinions about life that will shape the people they become (McFerran, 2010).

Both individuals with developmental disabilities and adolescents with emotional/behavioral challenges are stigmatized in our society. We might expect MT interventions for those with developmental disabilities to look different from those used with other adolescent populations, but the therapeutic goals for both are similar. Although some disabilities manifest themselves physically and neurologically, there are other inevitable symptoms on a social/psychological level (Butler & Zeman, 2005) that should not be overlooked. Many of these psychological/social effects are experienced across the adolescent population. Thus, C. Butler and A. Z. J. Zeman (2005) argue for a "'bio-psycho-social' approach to illness" (p. i31), which identifies not only the symptoms patients suffer biologically but also the psychological and social effects that are caused by a disease that on the surface seems purely biological. Although some disorders remain incurable, there are CAMs that can alleviate symptoms suffered by patients even if simply at the quality-of-life level.

Community Construction

The previous paragraphs have provided an overview of how music affects the brain and the body, which affects our communication, both verbally and nonverbally. The implications of these interconnections go beyond the individual self and affect the society at large. When MT began emerging as an official profession, therapists were more concerned with one-on-one treatment than they were with outside cultural and social forces, which are the very forces that plague their patients every day (Ruud, 2004). More recently, the MT field is expanding its horizons as MTs are acknowledging that illness often goes beyond medical disabilities and disorders (Ruud, 2004). Illness may begin as a simple diagnosis with medical treatments, but disempowerment can not only enhance an illness (Ruud, 2004), but perpetuate it. MTs understand that music is an important tool that can give power to the powerless and make visible the invisible (Ruud, 2004). Some researchers who have made this shift are now focusing on MT as a communicative process of creating community within a community. They have begun a movement called Community Music Therapy (CoMT), a term coined by Gary Ansdell and Rachel Verney in 2000 (Pavlicevic & Ansdell, 2004).

Community is more of a process than a place (Ansdell, 2004), and it occurs through communication. So how do we define and conceptualize community in the context of CoMT? The following paragraphs will illuminate the overarching dimensions of community that previous literature has highlighted which lustrates which aspects of community this research will focus on.

Each dimension of community discussed below is a tension/balance because the process of community building is complex. The first dimension of community is autonomy versus togetherness, also referred to as individualism vs. belonging (Ansdell, 2010; Delanty, 2003). This is a continual tension that is negotiated in community formation. Ansdell (2010) illustrates that the construction of "communication communities involve(s) the active search for belonging, understanding and communication in often unpromising circumstances" (p. 45). Individuals within a community must feel not only that they belong to the group, but also that they are able to be independent when outside of the group.

A second dimension of community within literature is the balance between being private and public. Music should not be contained in the private sector, but it should permeate throughout society causing a "ripple effect," as Mercédès Pavlicevic and Gary Ansdell (2004) discuss in their introduction to *Community Music Therapy*. MT may start in one, small context, but expand to further saturate a larger context.

The third dimension of community is the performance of identity. Communities must be performed through communication (Ansdell, 2010; Delanty, 2003). By "perform," Gerard Delanty (2003), *Community*, and Ansdell (2010) are not referring to typical concert-performances with a physical stage and audience. "Performance" in this context is referring to Goffman's (1959) idea of identity performance. Erving Goffman's (1959) *The Presentation of Self in Everyday Life* compares life to a stage in arguing that "life itself is a dramatically enacted thing" (p. 72). We are the performers in our everyday interactions with others and we choose to enhance certain aspects of ourselves while omitting others. Through these communicative performances, others come to view us in a certain way, and we in turn view ourselves in a certain way.

The fourth dimension of community is the creation of a healing environment. This dimension is the most difficult to achieve. A combination of the first three dimensions, and whether all of the tensions are successfully negotiated, determines whether or not a healing environment is created, and to what extent. This healing environment is often where transformation may occur.

Adolescents who suffer from neurological or psychological limitations are especially in need of a community in which to belong. Many of them have communication limitations that perpetuate their alienation from society. Organizations can and are using music as a medium to accomplish goals with adolescents with neurological limitations, developmental disabilities, and behavioral challenges.

Research Question

The concepts of music, communication, and community are deeply intertwined on many levels. These concepts unite to foster certain goals while dealing with tensions. In order for MTs to be successful in constructing community with their patients through the use of musical communication, they must embody many roles. Meanwhile, patients perform their limitations as individual expressions while attempting to belong. This is a beautiful and complex process that should be expanded on in future research on MT, performance studies, and communication. This research is designed to begin this exploration by answering the following research question.

> RQ: How does the communication within the context of MT encourage community building for adolescents?

METHODS

In this study, qualitative ethnographic methods are employed from a pluralistic interpretive perspective (Tracy, 2013). Kramer attended MT sessions as a "play participant" (Tracy, 2013) conducting observations while also taking part in activities. She also spent time with MTs including before and after MT sessions. Additionally, twelve interviews were conducted of eight certified MTs and one guitar instructor.

Analysis/Results

Guided by therapeutic narrative analysis (Aldridge & Aldridge, 2002), we analyzed all forms of data and identified five overarching patterns that answered my research question: autonomy, connections, motivation/encouragement, togetherness, and individuality. The following excerpts are from the Kramer's fieldnotes and interviews.

6:00 p.m. Mentors and music therapists arrive and set up instruments and songbooks around the room. It is 6 p.m. and I am one of the first of fifteen volunteer mentors to show up at the day school for this week's jam session.

The room is filled with musical instruments. There is a piano by the door, drums of all sizes spread throughout, three microphone stands, and a guitar. As I begin to drag chairs into the room, Jill states that fifteen students will be in attendance. I start to wonder how thiry chairs are going to fit in this small room.

Other volunteers help me place songbooks around the room, one for every two chairs for each mentor/mentee pair. Jill welcomes the new volunteers as they arrive, thanking them for coming. She asks that they put their names on nametags, then enter the room to help with the setup. I brand myself as "MEL" for the evening. Fitting every letter of my name on this nametag would be like trying to squeeze thirty chairs into this circle. Chair legs are overlapping, and microphone cords are beginning to tangle. Looks like we will be getting close tonight!

Once the room is set up, volunteers gather and take a seat. The MTs pull out a big white binder and begin to tell each of us who our mentees will be for the evening. Mentees and mentors are paired up based on the mentor's skills, experience, and personality. They go around the circle telling each mentor a few important facts about their unique mentee. First: name. Second: age. Third: instrument of choice. Fourth: musical experience. Fifth: diagnosis. I start to wonder what it would be like if the larger society saw these students like this, as actual people with hobbies and interests. Instead, much of society sees one thing first: diagnosis. Today, I am paired with a lovely girl. Name: Sofia. Age: 17. Instrument of choice: Voice. Musical experience: Student of one-on-one music lessons and performer of various recitals. Diagnosis: Cerebral Palsy. This would be far too much information to put on Sofia's nametag, so we will ignore all the labels and brand her as "Sofia," and "Sofia" only.

The following sections will help illuminate the findings of this study as they pertain to the research question. Community is made up of four dimensions: the tension of autonomy versus togetherness, the balance between the private and the public, the performance of identity, and the creation of healing environment. All of the patterns give us insight into how these dimensions are communicatively constructed. The four patterns found in the data are expanded upon separately in this chapter, but they are all interrelated.

Connecting the Notes: Communicating Connections

Through the initiation of relationships between mentors and mentees, MTs are able to facilitate a unique connection that students may not have the opportunity to experience in any other situation. Most of the students who attend jam sessions are either almost out, or are out of the school system, making it challenging to form relationships with people outside of family. A major goal of MT with adolescents is fostering rewarding and positive social relationships. The following excerpt is a portion of the grant application that the therapists wrote to pitch their idea of the jam sessions to potential funders:

> Pairing youth with special needs with mentors (high school and college students) will facilitate positive relationships and peer friendships through modeling social skills. These connections with mentors will provide safe, consistent, and trusting settings for our students with special needs to further understand and develop non-verbal and verbal social cues, communication styles, conversational mannerisms, and one-on-one and group dynamics. The need for our target population to strengthen these essential life skills is a key component for successful inclusion in schools and integration in the community.

The creation of connections between youth with special needs and other high school/college students has a variety of benefits for both types of students.

By connecting with mentors of a similar age, students are able to observe the socially acceptable communicative behaviors so that they can then enact those behaviors in the larger community. The following paragraphs and interview excerpts will further describe this pattern and how it relates to MT, communication, and community.

Emma, a certified music therapist, explained that connections in general are what separate MT from music education. When referring to her sessions with at-risk youth, Emma described:

> Music therapy, instead of something you do to someone, it's something you do with someone. So it's very much about the process, how they're interacting with you, how they're interacting with each other, so I guess that would be the main difference is music education is very didactic. Whereas MT is more process-oriented and it's not so much about how much the kids learn. It doesn't matter if they learn to play the drum in eight different rhythms. It's more about what happened before during and after that little bit of drumming. Did people make eye contact? Or actually share a smile—the people that were just beating each other up at lunch? They're making more connections; it's more about the connection than just learning how to do something. (Emma, personal interview, February 4, 2013)

By thinking about music in this way, we can discover the important role of communication in the context of MT. Music therapists understand that although they may not be able to cure their patients of whatever they are suffering from, they can facilitate communication (Ansdell & Pavlicevic, 2005). They create a place where the students are able to openly communicate and interact with one another while mending communicative limitations. Through experiences, patients are able to more intimately communicate and connect with their mentors, their therapists, and each other.

In addition to connections between volunteers/mentors and students/mentees, MTs who work with teens with special needs sometimes create very close personal connections with their patients and the patients' families. When responding to a question about a time when closeness was experienced with a patient, Zoe, a music therapist who works primarily with youth that suffer from neurological limitations, told the following story:

> I . . . got really close to the family. The boy had autism and Down syndrome. When I first started seeing him he didn't really like many people . . . but he could be very strong, and he could run off and throw things and hit people, but we developed such a relationship over that time that his parents were wanting me to do more than just the music. . . . And so I became his personal care assistant. So I would bring him out into the community. I'd take care of him. . . . So that shows tons of trust because nobody else really understood

> him, I suppose . . . the mom once said, you know, if her and her husband were to pass away, I'm the only person that they would want to take care of him. (Zoe, personal interview, March 12, 2012)

From this story, and many others, we were able to begin to understand the importance of connections between therapists and families, particularly with youth and adolescents who suffer from neurological limitations. MTs are able to encourage more use of the therapeutic strategies in a home setting. They can encourage parents to engage in certain therapeutic activities with their children. When parents continue therapeutic strategies within the home setting, community building grows outside of the session itself and helps youth with their social development so that community integration on a larger scale is more feasible.

Although the creation of connections with patients was consistent across various populations of adolescents, the creation of connections with parents/families was not. For example, when dealing with at-risk youth who have grown up in difficult situations such as foster homes, or youth who are in rehabilitation for substance abuse issues, a *close* relationship with the patient may not always be the goal. Also, a relationship with the parents may not even be an option, as many of these students do not even have relationships with their own families. Fay, a music therapist whose main passion is working with at-risk youth, told Kramer that "developing a close relationship is not one of my goals. I would say developing a trusting relationship is very important. They need to trust me" (Fay, personal interview, January 30, 2013). This trusting relationship is still a type of connection, though it may be in a different form. Fay is given a short amount of time to help her patients as much as possible. Developing a close relationship is not needed to reach the objectives at hand. Instead, making patients feel safe and respected so that they can begin their own processes of personal growth is more important. The amount of time a group of individuals will spend in the particular group has an influence on the way community is constructed and the way connections play a role in that process.

In addition to human connections, connections students feel with their instruments of choice facilitate a unique bond between students and their teachers, mentors, and therapists. Not every student enjoys playing the drums, or the guitar, or the keyboard. Likewise, not every student feels comfortable singing in front of others. Students in the jam sessions are matched with mentors that have experience with the same chosen instrument to create common ground. The fact that students and patients feel that they are able to connect with a certain type of music or instrument keeps them interested in MT and returning week after week.

The facilitation of this connection was apparent in Zoe's description of the initial assessment of a patient. She mentioned that this first assessment is very important in terms of affecting whether or not that student returns for future MT sessions. She said:

> It's mostly nonverbal assessment. It's reading their eye contact, reading where they're looking, what their body language is saying. It's just a ton of assessment, throwing different instruments at them and seeing what they gravitate towards, whether it's the piano, or they like to strum the guitar, they like to play drums . . . and so then after that it's creating that bond and relationship with the child in like ten, fifteen minutes, and then . . . kind of talking about okay here's what I saw. I start off with, is there that natural music ability? Is it how the music created a soothing, you know a soothing feeling. It calmed them down. It helped put down that barrier in wanting to connect with me and communicate with me more. (Zoe, personal interview, March 9, 2012)

By engaging in nonverbal assessment, therapists can determine which instruments the students are drawn to. Telling students to find their favorite instruments and play them during an assessment session can motivate the patients to form this connection with the instruments of their choice. Once therapists find out a student is drawn to a certain instrument, they provide positive feedback to the patient when the patient plays that certain instrument. After facilitating this connection, they are able to further unite with their patients and open the doors for enhanced communication. Allowing the patients to make this connection point with the songs and instruments allows MTs to have a better understanding of what motivates the patients. With this knowledge, MTs can better plan patient-specific interventions that aid in community construction.

Voices in Unison: Communicating Togetherness

7:00 p.m. Welcome/opening/introduction song. At 7 p.m., once all the students arrive at the jam session and they are with their mentors, it is now time for the introduction. Lexi gets the students excited about the night by yelling, "Who's ready to jaaaaaammm?" The students are ecstatic. At this point Lexi says, "Okay let's start out by saying hello!" This is when the hello song begins and everyone sings along.

> When you see someone for the first time
> We smile at them and say hello
> When you see someone for the first time
> We smile at them and say hi
> We can wave
> Look at their eyes
> Shake hands
> Give a high five

These verses repeat, and the students are encouraged to look at their neighbor and do what the song says. Then they walk around the room and repeat the actions.

Following the "hello song," Lexi sings another song so that everyone begins giving compliments to one another. In the middle of the room, Jill has a white board where she writes down all of the nice compliments the students give to one another. If a student says a somewhat simple compliment like "nice hair," the therapist will sometimes offer critique and tell the student some other examples of compliments like "you're very beautiful," or "great job playing your instrument." By encouraging the students to interact with one another, the MTs are helping to facilitate important connections. While connections between mentors/mentees, students/instruments, therapists/families, and therapists/patients were discussed separately in the previous section, all of these bonds combined create for an environment in which patients are able to feel comfort, safety, and enjoyment as a whole group. Thus, in these environments they can learn various social development skills with each other that can later be transferred into the community at large.

By making adolescents feel like they belong to this group, therapists can begin to teach important social skills and can encourage their students to integrate into the community. This section will explain how the communication of togetherness offers insight into the research question for this paper.

What separates the first pattern (the creation of connections) from the second (communication of togetherness) is at what point the two occur in the process of community construction. Connections must be formed early on in order to catapult the remaining patterns. A connection could be a one-time occurrence, and once it repeats, togetherness can be fostered. A one-time connection can make a difference in community building, while togetherness must be an ongoing characteristic of a group in order for the strength of community to be sustained.

In addition to encouraging community integration, the communication of togetherness can begin to facilitate meaningful experiences for students. Humans desire and need a sense of belonging (Baumeister & Leary, 1995). Some researchers have found that individuals with social connections are more likely to survive than those without (Holt-Lunstad, Smith, & Layton, 2010). Positive interactions with others are an important aspect of every human's health, including the health of adolescents. A sense of belonging becomes particularly important during the process of individuation-separation (Lapsley & Edgerton, 2002). Adolescents are beginning to develop new relationships outside of the family that affect what kind of people they become (McFerran, 2010). Whatever group they feel belongingness with will influence their identities (McFerran, 2010). Therefore, the communication of togetherness in the MT context can give adolescents a positive place to belong.

One of the most common interventions therapists use in group settings that help promote togetherness are drum circles. Within drum circles, all members are given a percussion instrument and they work together as a group by listening to one another and playing a cohesive rhythm. When a music therapist leads a drum circle, they are motivating the students to play the same rhythm as a group. This is a unique setting in which the therapist is able to foster enhanced nonverbal communication between the members of the group. Fay, who works at a rehabilitation center for teens, explained:

> You get a groove going and there's this energy that starts to flow, and a connectedness that many of us have never experienced before, in fact even adults quite often have not experienced that feeling until they've been in a really good drum circle or something. So for them, it's this new way of relating and something inside of them opens up where they start to feel kind of their soul and they start to feel something different. And yet it's connected. So, once they get a taste of that feeling it makes them less likely to go back (and use drugs). Even the most superficial of people that come in are changed by that experience, because for the first time in their life they get close to this deeper way of relating to their peers. (Fay, personal interview, January 30, 2013)

Finding this alternative way to relate to peers is an important experience for at-risk youth. They feel so much pressure to fit into a social group. Providing a group where they can belong that has positive goals is a good alternative to the groups in which they are used to belonging. As the group continues, students are able to encounter a feeling of togetherness that encourages personal growth. Fay further elaborated on this:

> They're among their own age group so they're more natural in their interactions with each other. They know what each other is going through and for them to build their own trust in their own peer group, they begin to trust and be more honest with them and to be learning to learn how to cope and to be learning to learn how to say "no," to be learning how to relax in their own peer group. And they need to also expand their worldview and they can do that by hearing other people's stories. Then they know that they're not alone and they're not some kind of weirdo. They know that they're not weird at all. (Fay, personal interview, January 30, 2013)

Once students feel that they belong to this group, they can begin engaging in self-disclosure and reciprocation, as opposed to holding everything in.

As part of the observations conducted for this interview, Kramer became a member of a band which also included two adolescents and the therapist.

Both adolescents in this band are on the Autism Spectrum. One boy played the drums, the other played the piano, the therapist played guitar, and Kramer became the singer. They had weekly sessions, and they practiced and recorded songs. This band environment gives these students a feeling of belonging. They come together, practice songs, listen to one another, make decisions, develop a common interest, and create common goals. This type of social belonging is difficult for them to engage in daily.

Zoe, the therapist who runs this band, explained in two separate interviews the importance of being a band and learning group cohesion for these boys:

> They think their goal is to make music, and to get through the songs, and to hopefully be able to perform and have fun. Whereas my goals for them are the social interaction, the communication, being able to listen to each other. . . . In some case I'll bring in how important it is as a band to be listening to each other, to be able to stop and finish together. (Zoe, personal interview, March 9, 2012)

By practicing listening to one another, the band members are learning social skills that can improve their communication in their everyday lives. Another strategy Zoe used to encourage togetherness was to give the band a name. They spent a whole session on choosing a band name. Having an official name made them feel like they were part of something important.

Adolescents, through MT sessions, are able to engage in open communication and self-disclosure, which helps them experience a unique form of companionship. The communication of togetherness encourages further developed social skills, which can eventually transfer into the larger community outside of MT sessions.

The Power of the Percussionist: Communicating Autonomy

7:05 p.m. Drum circle/rhythm warm up, take turns leading solos. Volunteers pass out different types of drums and percussion instruments: djembes, little drums, larger drums, congas, bongos, tambourines, and mallets. One therapist stands in the middle of the drum circle and begins to play her drum. Soon the entire group is following. The therapist models ways to lead a drum circle, guiding the group to follow her rhythm. She raises her drum up and the group starts hitting their drums harder. She lowers her drum and we quiet down. She signals a rumble, and everyone hits their drums as loud and fast as they can. Then she puts her two hands up, and signals us to stop. We do so in one cohesive bang. This start to the drum circle gets all of the students excited, ready for another round. The therapist then invites students to come up and lead the drum circle. Some students are eager to lead. Others feel more timid and sink down in their chairs, avoiding eye contact. She asks students who would like to lead the next drum circle to choose students who are ready for the limelight, while also motivating those who do not feel ready to lead the group yet.

Doing this allows them to build community within their group therapy sessions, and to also understand different roles they can play out in the larger community, particularly the role of an autonomous individual.

The role of communicating autonomy is present in the formation of many communities, and the balance between communicating togetherness and communicating autonomy can be a complicated one (Ansdell, 2004). As Delanty (2003) and Ansdell (2010) describe, one of the most obvious tensions in community formation is the balance between encouraging autonomy and togetherness, simultaneously. The following paragraphs describe what this looks like and how MT is a unique environment in which this balance is achieved.

One MT, Lexi, ensures within her sessions that students are able to develop a sense of ownership once they begin to improve as a band, which is very empowering. During an interview, Lexi expressed what it is like to see such progress in her students, "It has been cool to see them . . . really developing that sense of ownership over the group where they are excited about taking the music out and performing it" (Lexi, personal interview, December 17, 2012). Being in a band with other peers of similar ages and similar diagnoses, these students have a safe place where they can learn more complex communication skills, such as negotiation and conflict management. A sense of pride can begin to develop which leads to improved self-esteem. In *Music and Soulmaking: Toward a New Theory of Music Therapy,* Barbara Crowe (2004) demonstrates that as MT patients begin to realize that they are developing a skill that people deem worthy across cultures, their confidence increases.

Similarly, at-risk youth have a need for autonomy and control and a need to feel a sense of ownership over their lives. MT Autumn has done work all over the state, as well as abroad in countries like Kenya. She said the following about the group of adolescents she currently works with in one of the roughest neighborhoods in Los Angeles:

> Well first of all I think that one of the main reasons (making them leaders) works so much is because . . . they're having such a hard time is that they're never in a power position. Their teachers, their parents, the police, and the society. Everyone's sort of telling them what to do and who to be. . . . So when you make them a leader, it's a really positive thing with those roles. Otherwise gangs will give you that feeling, right? So hopefully this is another alternative to that is to empower them to be leaders within the group. . . . And it absolutely would impact everything. . . . So I think if they're getting power in a positive

> way they don't seek it outside of the group in negative ways. (Autumn, personal interview, February 2, 2013)

MTs are able to communicate autonomy to their students and by doing this they give power back to students. Instead of taking their power away to be sure they do not make the wrong decisions, giving them a little bit of power can help them realize they need to take control over their lives by making the right decisions. Adolescents, on the verge of becoming young adults, experience individuation-separation, a time in which they are gaining autonomy from their family and making new connections with peers around them (Lapsley & Edgerton, 2002). Giving them a dose of what it is like to make negotiations and choices can help them begin to prepare for adulthood which helps facilitate autonomy.

Adolescents in these small groups are all experiencing the need for autonomy and can understand one anothers' situations. MTs are able to give students the opportunity to lead their group of peers, which can empower each student separately, and therefore unite them. If no one student is empowered, it would be more difficult to foster a sense of community because patients would have an *us* (patients) and *them* (therapists) experience. Having the students lead each other fosters a sense of ownership among patients where they can have pride in what they are doing collectively. Not only do these students need a space where they are able to take control, they also need a place where they can feel safe to express their own identities, which will be further illustrated in the following section.

Performance of Self: Communicating Identity/Expression

7:40 p.m. Improvisation jam/youth select songs from songbooks. For the past twenty minutes, the students have been able to interact with the guest musician. Now is the time they have been waiting for. Instead of following the guest musician's creativity, they get to express their own. Instead of being told to play the song choices of the guest musician, they get to choose what songs they would like the group to play. They get to play shakers, or drums, or keys, or sing into the microphone. Or, they can just get in the middle of the circle and dance. This is their chance to express their individuality.

The fourth and final pattern represented in the data collected for this research is MTs' communication of identity and expression. MTs are able to encourage adolescents in their construction of community on both a micro and macro level through communication.

Many youths with special needs have come to live with this stigma that they are different from the rest of their peers. They are taught certain ways to live within the molds of a *normal* teenager. With this constant pressure, it is a relief to find a safe place where their individuality can be expressed. Creative expression is an emotional *release*. Adolescents, in order to be encouraged to build community with one another, must feel that their collective group is a safe space to be able to *release* whatever emotions they may be bottling up inside.

The process of releasing is essential to the pattern of communicating identity/expression. Many times, adolescents do not have the best use of their words to express a feeling. They may not even know that they have a feeling. Communication, in this sense, is not always intentional. What makes this interesting in the context of MT is that when individuals play and perform music, different parts of the brain are activated that are not activated during regular speech (Taylor, 2010). This helps individuals access something that they would normally not be able to access: a memory, a thought, a feeling. And, as they are *musicing*, they are processing that and communicating that; it is getting released. One reason music is helpful in this process, as Emma shared, is because one can self-express without words:

> I think because of the fact that you don't have to say what you're feeling. Because I think teens also sometimes don't know how to express how they are feeling. They themselves can't say, "I feel this" to themselves. They maybe are just feeling it. (Emma, personal interview, February 4, 2013)

The nonverbal properties of music can help students self-express.

One way in which MTs encourage students to self-express during a session is through drum *conversations*, which are purely instrumental and nonverbal. One student will bang on a drum, and another student will respond on their drum. The students have freedom to express emotions to one another through drum conversations. They can bang on a drum to release built-up anger, or they can play a steady rhythm if they are in need of a more calming conversation. Autumn talked about how she was able to foster self-expression with one of her students in a program she leads with at-risk teens:

> I definitely think they can express themselves and their uniqueness. Music lends itself to that. I think being flexible is really important because a lot of that stuff doesn't just pop up unless you make space for it. Like I have one kid who . . . doesn't read very well, and he doesn't write in my class, but he is a freaking amazing drummer. And he loves to do beats with pencils on desks. What would most teachers say? "Stop; stop drumming on your desk!" Right? So for me I'm like, well, I brought drums, but let's play with pencils on a desk. It's still music. (Autumn, personal interview, February 2, 2013)

Students who feel that their self-expression is a positive thing feel more motivated to engage in creative activities. They are less afraid to express their individuality, so they feel safer opening up to their peers.

One of the goals of therapists who work with at-risk youth, adolescents with special needs, and adolescents with substance abuse addictions is to let the pain emerge and be released. In sessions with adolescents who suffer from eating disorders, the emotional nature of music is essential. Erin, a therapist who specializes in working with teens who suffer from eating disorders, enlightened me on the way music can serve as a vehicle for healing for these adolescents.

> Music can be very non-threatening, so it can open up the discussion and open up the process of all the things that are involved in that recovery or treatment. . . . We use music to stimulate that. We might analyze song lyrics. We might create a song; we do a lot of song writing. We also do a lot of self-expression . . . a lot of the women I've worked with, it's hard for the to express themselves in an organic kind of way. . . . So just to be able to be more open in that way is a lot easier with music almost as a transitional object. "Well we're going to do this, but hey do you see what you're doing while we do this? You're being you; you're expressing yourself how you want to express yourself today." (Erin, personal interview, January 13, 2013)

These women feel that they are not good enough for society's idea of *perfection*. Thus, they resort to this place where they are stuck and unable to move forward. An ability to self-express could contribute to progress for these individuals, and even a breakthrough.

Through *musicing*, adolescents are able to discover more about themselves. As one therapist shared, "They get into this zone, and they discover this really exciting part of being alive is being in the creative process. When they discover that, they discover their uniqueness, they discover who they are in the process" (unnamed, personal interview, February 4, 2013). Music can help our next generation with having a sense of self (Crowe, 2004; McFerran, 2010). According to Erik Erikson (1963) in *Childhood and Society*, when young people are in their adolescent years, they will either experience the construction of self-identity, or they can become confused about their role and lack a sense of self. Music is a medium through which adolescents are able to self-express through this process of negotiation aiding in a successful identity formation. Without self-expression, some youth are not able to understand their own value. By giving them a voice, we can begin to validate them and to show them that their thoughts and experiences are important to those within the larger community.

CONCLUSION

The previous sections have answered the research question, "How does the communication within the context of MT encourage community building for adolescents?" The findings illustrate that, in the context of MT with adolescents, MTs promote community construction by illuminating connections, communicating togetherness, encouraging autonomy, and facilitating a safe place for the creative expression of individuality. Through communicative strategies, adolescents are able to begin building a sense of community within their small groups. This helps them learn how to more successfully integrate into the community.

As therapist Zoe expressed, "as you move forward, showing how what we do in the MT session is going to transfer outside. That's the ultimate goal" (Zoe, personal interview, March 9, 2012). Lexi mentioned a similar goal: "so moving forward because he is turning 18, so vocationally, how can he integrate into the community, how can he have a skill or a leisure activity that he can do basically for the rest of his life" (Lexi, personal interview, March 9, 2012). And finally, Jill described, "for the older kids we really shift in our goals to what can be functional for them in the community" (Jill, personal interview, December 13, 2012). This shift in objectives is consistent across the board. As children become teenagers, MTs are mostly concerned with micro and macro community building rather than other goals. They shift their objectives because the teens are moving toward adulthood in a society that does not provide sufficient resources for this population:

> There is a huge breakdown once students leave the school setting. There isn't a lot of services or things for them to be doing out of the community and so there is really . . . a huge drop off . . . for instance, the California Department of Education in 2000 there were approximately 650,000 youth with special needs between 0–22 in California and a lot of these individuals have like brain injury, multiple disabilities, speech and language impairment, autism. Then they have deficits in social skills, emotional expression and communication, and then in 2010 this number had increased to 670,000. So despite these increasing numbers state funding for services has decreased. (Jill, personal interview, December 17, 2012)

The need is growing more quickly than the means to fulfill it. Lexi demonstrated how MT can be a bridge to community:

> Music therapy for, especially I see it, as kids start to get older music therapy can be a bridge to community, can be an entrance point especially as they are getting older and maybe there isn't necessarily a place for them in the society or in the community. I think music could be something that brings people together. (Lexi, personal interview, December 17, 2012)

MT has the potential in adolescent populations to form the "ripple effect." Music in the private sector never has as much influence on communities as does music that permeates throughout our society (Pavlicevic & Ansdell, 2004). So, maybe this idea of taking the private into the public and giving music back to the people has the potential to transform our community, one mini-community at a time.

> You have a community within every single session. That's your little mini community. But the idea is that as we grow as a profession and as these kids go out into the world, they're spreading it and it's getting bigger and bigger. . . . What I always say is that "I want to give music back to the people." Like it's not just about entertainment; it's not about something you have to spend a ton of money for or just not participate in if you're not amazing. It's for everybody, which is how it's been for thousands and thousands of years . . . music *is* how you rise up from the trenches. (Autumn, personal interview, February 2, 2013)

REFERENCES

Aldridge, D., & Aldridge, G. (2002) Therapeutic narrative analysis: A methodological proposal for the interpretation of music therapy traces. *Music Therapy Today* (online), 1–23. Retrieved from http://pdf.aminer.org/000/329/031/structure_and_interpretation_of_music_concepts_music_from_a_computational.pdf

Ansdell, G. (2004). Rethinking music and community: Theoretical perspectives in support of community music therapy. In M. Pavlicevic & G. Ansdell (Eds.), *Community music therapy* (pp. 65–90). Philadelphia, PA: Jessica Kingsley Publishers.

Ansdell, G. (2010). Reflection: Belonging through musicing: Explorations of musical community. In B. Stige, G. Ansdell, C. Elefant, & M. Pavlicevic (Eds.), *Where music helps: Community music therapy in action and reflection* (pp. 41–62). Burlington, VT: Ashgate Publishing Company.

Ansdell, G., & Pavlicevic, M. (2005). Musical companionship, musical community: Music therapy and the process and values of musical communication. In K. Miell, R. MacDonald, & D. J. Hargreaves (Eds.), *Musical communication* (pp. 193–213). New York, NY: Oxford University Press.

Baumeister, R. F., & Leary, M. R. (1995). The need to belong: Desire for interpersonal attachments as a fundamental human motivation. *Psychological Bulletin, 117*(3), 497–529. http://doi.org/10.1037/0033–2909.117.3.497

Bensimon, M., Amir, D., & Wolf, Y. (2008). Drumming through trauma: Music therapy with post-traumatic soldiers. *Arts in Psychotherapy, 35*(1), 34–48. https://doi.org/10.1016/j.aip.2007.09.002

Brown, K. A., & Patel, D. R. (2005). Complementary and alternative medicine in developmental disabilities. *Indian Journal of Pediatrics, 72*(11), 949–952. https://doi.org/10.1007/BF02731671

Bruscia, K. E. (1998). *Defining music therapy* (2nd ed.). Gilsum, NH: Barcelona Publishers.

Butler, C., & Zeman, A. Z. J. (2005). Neurological syndromes which can be mistaken for psychiatric conditions. *Journal of Neurology, Neurosurgery and Psychiatry, 76*(suppl. 1), i31–i38. https://doi.org/10.1136/jnnp.2004.060459

Crowe, B. J. (2004). *Music and soulmaking: Toward a new theory of music therapy.* Lanham, MD: Scarecrow Press.

Delanty, G. (2003). *Community.* London, UK: Routledge.

Dingle, G. A., Gleadhill, L., & Baker, F. A. (2008). Can music therapy engage patients in group cognitive behaviour therapy for substance abuse treatment? *Drug and Alcohol Review, 27*(2), 190–196. https://doi.org/10.1080/09595230701829371

Dokter, D. (1994). *Arts therapies and clients with eating disorders: Fragile board.* Philadelphia, PA: Jessica Kingsley Publishers.

Erikson, E. H. (1963). *Childhood and society.* New York, NY: W. W. Norton.

Gallagher, L. M., Lagman, R., Walsh, D., Davis, M. P., & LeGrand, S. B. (2006). The clinical effects of music therapy in palliative medicine. *Support Care Cancer, 14*(8), 859–866. https://doi.org/10.1007/s00520–005–0013–6

Goffman, E. (1959). *The presentation of self in everyday life.* New York, NY: Bantam Doubleday Dell Publishing.

Hargreaves, D. J., MacDonald, R., & Miell, D. (2005). How do people communicate using music? In K. Miell, R. MacDonald, & D. J. Hargreaves (Eds.), *Musical communication* (pp. 1–25). New York, NY: Oxford University Press.

Holt-Lunstad, J., Smith, T. B., & Layton, J. B. (2010). Social relationships and mortality risk: A meta-analytic review. *PLoS Medicine*, *7*(7), e1000316. https://doi.org/10.1371/journal.pmed.1000316

Hurkmans, J., de Bruijn, M., Boonstra, A. M., Jonkers, R., Bastiaanse, R., Arendzen, H., & Reinders-Messelink, H. A. (2012). Music in the treatment of neurological language and speech disorders: A systematic review. *Aphasiology*, *26*(1), 1–19. https://doi.org/10.1080/02687038.2011.602514

Inskip, C., MacFarlane, A., & Rafferty, P. (2008). Meaning, communication, music: Towards a revised communication model. *Journal of Documentation*, *64*(5), 687–706. https://doi.org/10.1108/00220410810899718

Koger, S. M., Chapin, K., & Brotons, M. (1999). Is music therapy an effective intervention for dementia? A meta-analytic review of literature. *Journal of Music Therapy*, *36*(1), 2–15. https://doi.org/10.1093/jmt/36.1.2

Lapsley, D. K., & Edgerton, J. (2002). Separation-Individuation, adult attachment style, and college adjustment. *Journal of Counseling & Development*, *80*(4), 484–492. https://doi.org/10.1002/j.1556–6678.2002.tb00215.x

Larsen, G., Lawson, R., & Todd, S. (2010). The symbolic consumption of music. *Journal of Marketing Management*, *26*(7–8), 671–685. https://doi.org/10.1080/0267257X.2010.481865

Maratos, A., Gold, C., Wang, X., & Crawford, M. (2008). Music therapy for depression. *Cochrane Database of Systematic Reviews*, *1*, CD004517. https://doi.org/10.1002/14651858.CD004517.pub2

McFerran, K. (2010). *Adolescents, music, and music therapy: Methods and clinicians, educators and students.* Philadelphia, PA: Jessica Kingsley Publishers.

Pavlicevic, M., & Ansdell, G. (2004). Introduction: "The ripple effect." In M. Pavlicevic & G. Ansdell (Eds.), *Community music therapy* (pp. 15–31). Philadelphia, PA: Jessica Kingsley Publishers.

Ruud, E. (2004). Foreward: Reclaiming music. In M. Pavlicevic & G. Ansdell (Eds.), *Community music therapy* (pp. 11–14). Philadelphia, PA: Jessica Kingsley Publishers.

Taylor, D. B. (2010). *Biomedical foundations of music as therapy* (2nd ed.). Brandon, SD: Barton Publications.

Tracy, S. J. (2013). *Qualitative research methods: Collecting evidence, crafting analysis, communicating impact.* Malden, MA: Wiley-Blackwell.

Trevarthen, C. (2002). Origins of musical identity: Evidence from infancy for musical social awareness. In R. A. R. Macdonald, D. J. Hargreaves, & D. Miell (Eds.), *Musical identities* (pp. 21–38). New York, NY: Oxford University Press.

Wieser, H. G. (2003). Music and the brain: Lessons from brain diseases and some reflections on the "emotional" brain. *Annals New York Academy of Sciences, 999*, 76–94. https://doi.org/10.1196/annals.1284.007

Chapter Nine

Comfort and Catharsis

Critical Reflections on Therapeutic Dance Practice

Gregory J. Langner

In the final, wildly excruciating throes of graduate school—a point in my life marked by a litany of stressful circumstances—I danced. *Cicadas*, a performance I premiered in the spring of 2019 with a small ensemble alongside other dance projects at the avant-garde Art Klub stage in New Orleans, Louisiana, not only coincided with all of my educational and professional demands at the time, but also in many ways helped me to meet those demands. As a discipline largely characterized by the commingling of artistic expression and physical exertion, dance has usually helped me to cope with the different tensions and anxieties that I collect in my day-to-day life; but *Cicadas*, specifically, drew inspiration from those tensions. I found the piercing hum of the cicada bug deeply comforting after first moving across the country to complete a doctorate in a region and climate almost entirely unfamiliar to me. The piece was an approximately twelve-minute, three-person contemporary performance physicalizing the back and forth between anxious discomfort and fleeting moments of relief that many experience when abruptly immersing themselves in a new culture with new surroundings. *Cicadas* allowed me to pay homage to that solace, but also in a way allowed me to replicate it. That is, as an ensemble, our bodies in the performance would shift from near-violent convulsions accompanied by tightly-controlled wanderings across the stage, to gentle and more loosely- or extemporaneously-controlled full-body gestures that instead *alleviated* our tensions. These were moments during which we could simply be, and breathe; moments I found lacking at the time in much of my life beyond dance.

The sequential process of devising, rehearsing, and performing *Cicadas* indeed helped me to recapture a much needed sense of comfort and catharsis (emotional release) by way of my body's expressive impulses and my conscious desire to connect with other dancers through synchronous meditative choreography. I aim in this chapter to unveil the capacity for the dance production process to facilitate such comfort and catharsis for all dance practitioners (hereafter also *practitioners*), regardless of dance discipline or degree of experience. Following the chapter's introduction, I explore the therapeutic capacity of dance production through the vibrant network of stimuli that collectively define the process as more complex and substantive than dance performance alone. I then more deeply assess how culturally conditioned bodies can better achieve catharsis by using dance deliberately to discover entirely unfamiliar possibilities for self-expression. Finally, I reflect critically on the potential that dance communities possess to foster, intentionally or otherwise, supportive environments in which all practitioners can grow, reflect, and simply more comfortably *be* in a cultural environment that otherwise functions to inhibit comfort with oneself.

Therapeutic, healing experiences certainly occur outside the clinical setting all the time. Framing the dance production process (hereafter also *dance process* or *dance production*) as an aggregate avenue for finding comfort and reaching catharsis helps me to characterize the phenomenon of catharsis- or alleviation-through-dance as dance practitioners already know it to exist. As a Performance Studies researcher and practitioner, I can also note here that my discipline—sometimes recognized as a sub-discipline of both the performing arts and of Communication Studies, in that performance can be understood as a form of "aesthetic communication" (Pelias & Shaffer, 2007, p. 11)—is concerned with performance as, all at once, the subject, method, and sometimes the means of presenting research. In other words, we regularly study different kinds of performance or cultural phenomena *using* performance. When the text-centric conventions of presenting research in academic journals or books fail to fully capture or convey our findings, we use performance again as the means of communicating what we have discovered. As a mode of embodied experimentation through performance, my experiences with dance and my opportunities to assess critically the dance-intensive experiences of others have become the catalyst for the observations and insights presented throughout this chapter.

This chapter addresses and is concerned, broadly, with the cathartic capacity of the dance process; more specifically, with the ways in which working, developing, learning, embodying, coordinating, and somatically socializing through dance can alleviate otherwise unrelated frustrations, anxieties, tensions, and so on. In the sections that follow, I alternate between critical analyses of the dance production process and critically reflexive references to personal experiences within said process, in part by recalling direct dialogues with other dance practitioners whose similar and particular experiences with the process more fully illustrate its capacity for catharsis and comfort. That is, because I often take the opportunity to engage my colleagues and past collaborators from the world of dance to discuss our mutual experiences with its benefits, I have had the opportunity to learn more comprehensively about the factors and moments that motivate practitioners to enter and to remain within that world.

Throughout the following observations and analyses I refer to specific dance practitioners—each of whom has graciously offered me their permission to reference our past dialogues—initially by their full names, and then exclusively by their first names in order to differentiate their contributions from the formal scholarship I reference throughout as well. Colleagues and collaborators with whom I have had the privilege to exchange rich dialogues on the topic of therapeutic dance practice include: Jamie Risch, a visual artist who has spent several years also immersing herself in staged performance practices including traditional and physical theatre, and who at one point also participated in a contemporary dance production that premiered in Santa Monica, California, in 2017; Montana Smith, a fellow Performance Studies researcher and practitioner with nearly two decades of extensive modern dance experience, both as a performer and choreographer; Edwin Siguenza, an experienced dancer and member of a renowned Los Angeles–area dance company with whom he has performed in several large-scale contemporary dance productions both in Los Angeles and on international tours; and Carson Lambing, a stage actor who has now twice embraced opportunities to perform as part of contemporary dance productions in the Los Angeles area, and who has expressed interest in pursuing such opportunities further. My references to each of these performers' dialogues aim specifically to reinforce the analysis throughout this chapter; that is, to demonstrate how lived experiences indeed reflect the insights gained through critical inquiry.

DANCE AS A VIBRANT NETWORK OF STIMULI

As Ann Cooper Albright (2010) indicates in her oft-cited *Choreographing Difference: The Body and Identity in Contemporary Dance*, experienced dancers are intimately familiar with the practice's "psychic consequences" (p. 32). The dance production process as a whole, like other artistic practices, comprises several distinct processes and elements that complement and rely on one another. A skeletal overview of everything dance production entails reveals several parts of the process, from training to rehearsal to performance, and a great deal more, as I further describe below. Performers of virtually all disciplinary creeds reveal often how performing for a public audience can produce both excitement and relief, as if the act of fully and unapologetically expressing oneself invigorates the body and mind while letting go of all of the muscular and cognitive tensions that otherwise and often remind us that we are socially limited from taking self-expression *too far*.

Yet, those practitioners who engage actively with any given role of the dance process learn quickly that the end product—the performance and the moment to which many performers point as a powerful instance of relief—is only one manifestation of catharsis the dance process affords. Though many audiences (and even some practitioners) primarily or exclusively recognize dance as the artistically-calculated, tightly-rehearsed staged performance (that is, the performance *product*) within and preceding the dance product is an exhaustive and complex series of processes. Put another way, the former (the dance product) is not independent of the latter (the network of processes that allow the dance performance to materialize). As Richard Boon and Jane Plastow (2006) note in *Theatre and Empowerment: Community Drama on the World Stage*, "Any arts process reducible to a simple and repeatable formula has to be wrong" (p. 10). Additionally, as Reba Gostand (1980) comparably observes, "Everything the audience sees or hears [in performance] is a symbol of some reality being conveyed" through the work (p. 2). The reality Gostand (1980) identifies should be understood as more than the representation of a story or some other symbolic meaning intended for the audience; it is a representation of all the work and internal processes that allow the performance ultimately to manifest.

To elaborate on only a fraction of everything comprising the dance process, we can note:

- Dancers' training involves physical conditioning alongside the development of technique and phrase work, short choreographic sequences.
- Choreography is developed, taught, and learned, and sometimes all at once, such as through a collaborative devising process.
- Choreographers, dancers, and many adept stage managers spend time developing repertoires of aesthetic staging compositions, determining how best to position bodies in relation to the audience.
- Casting for dance involves both audition and selection processes assessing performers' technical ability within a given style, as well as their readiness to work in an ensemble or with a particular choreographer.
- Dancers, choreographers, and production managers rehearse collaboratively and often for weeks or months on end through an exhaustive process of repetition and refinement of the work.
- Larger productions require both choreographic and directorial leadership, such as for dance festivals featuring work by multiple artists whose collective performances need to be carefully curated.
- Lastly, the performance products themselves succeed only as dancers, directors, production managers, technical experts, designers (lighting, music, costume, scenic, etc.), choreographers, event organizers, and audi-

ences converge cohesively to each play their role in the presentation of the work.

While I and a great many practitioners I know have immersed ourselves at different times in almost every element of dance described above, not all dance practitioners need take on every compounding demand of the process, and can instead focus primarily on ensemble performance, or on choreography, or on solo work, or on production. Further, such a rich web of practices translates understandably into a similarly vibrant network of stimuli and experiences for dance practitioners. After all, as just indicated, each individual element of the dance process still entails multiple practices, each of which provides opportunities for alleviating stress, anxiety, frustration, and so on. While some aspects of the dance process are clearly more technical than others (for example, the exhaustive repetition of rehearsal), each element or stage of the process requires the practitioner to calculate artistically how best to apply their training and unique strengths in a way that complements effectively each *other* element or stage of the process. That is, to engage actively and pointedly (focused on select elements) with the dance production process is to understand oneself as a valued force helping to provoke and to shape the identity and virtue of the work as a whole.

Karen Barbour's (2008) position that those who study and practice dance "can experience empowerment in the process of exploring their own embodied identities" (p. 8) takes on especially rich meaning when we recognize that the source of "empowerment" in dance is more than merely the practice itself (as in the actual *act* of dancing). Rather, empowerment through dance is achieved as practitioners navigate the network of demands that constitute the practice, because in doing so we become aware of the very fact that we are a necessary part of the network. Jamie, as an artist whose primary expertise leans toward creative practices *other* than dance, noted that preparing for the production in Santa Monica "was almost like learning a different language." As her choreographer for that production, I can also attest that Jamie devotedly navigated the process, not only working rigorously to rehearse her own choreography, but actively working to ensure her execution of the performance would complement and connect with the rest of the cast. Both Jamie's readiness and ability to learn that "different language" demonstrate how we can experience validation in dance as we embody the reality that our capacity to process and execute the work is inextricably tied to the work's success.

Similarly, Montana aptly expressed how she realized years ago that "dance was more about what it does for [her], rather than [just] for the consumption of other people," demonstrating how success in dance is about much more than how "flawless" or how "profound" the performance product ultimately appears. Indeed, just as dance is constituted by a vibrant network of stimuli, so too does the practice have the capacity to generate multiple outcomes. Boon and Plastow (2004), discussing the place of empowerment in theatre more broadly, note, "There is no one way, form or kind of content that is 'right'" when crafting performance that can empower (p. 10). As we understand dance as a network of stimulating practices and processes, we should assess also how each practitioner's relation to said network is distinct, not only because each performance has different demands (as to the content and intentions of the work), but because each dance practitioner understands and engages the process uniquely. Echoing Jamie while reflecting on the capacity of dance to extend beyond itself (as in beyond the act of dancing), Montana further expressed, "Whether it is building community, creating identity, catharsis, a way of understanding the world, or a way of investigating the world, dance has become the language I use to speak with others and myself."

Dance production harnesses the expressive and compositional potential of the human body, beyond its socially defined parameters, to capture or even to generate the interests of an audience, whether those interests derive from a desire to be entertained or from a need for intellectual or emotional stimulation. The performers on stage, whose sequenced and rhythmic physicalities (usually) enhance and are enhanced by other elements of performance such as lighting and musical ambience, displace for audiences their own unfulfilled expressive impulses or desires. As noted by Craig Gingrich-Philbrook and Jake Simmons (2015), "In performance, we make things to make things happen; we interact with them to produce, not merely to represent, worlds and worldviews" (p. 340). Connecting with and attending to the needs or the appetites of others (other participants in the process, audiences, etc.) thus becomes a part of the motivation to embrace our own artistically expressive impulses. Such embrace affords an opportunity to understand anew the breadth of our own bodies, and consequently an opportunity to feel more free of those restrictive social conditions we have learned simply to accept, even if we feel such freedom for only a moment.

EMOTIONAL RELEASE AND THE BREADTH OF BODY

While my own work in dance eventually evolved to account actively for the ways in which the practice might interrogate and even create new understandings of simply expressively *being* in the world, I initially embraced the practice for the foundational, built-in opportunity to better understand my own body's expressive reach. That is, I sought to learn more fully all that my body is capable of, not in terms of extreme feats of physical exertion, but in terms of *expressive* capability. For instance, many classically trained ballet artists are capable of performing intricately flexible and difficult-to-balance dance phrases. My concern, though, became less about how I might sculpt my body to perform at that same level of physical ability, and more about how I might open myself up to discovering possibilities for embodiment I had never before experienced. Jane C. Desmond (1993) asserts that "we should not ignore the ways in which dance signals and enacts social identities in all their continually changing configurations" (p. 57). As if in response to Desmond, I would learn over time, especially as I began leaning more into choreographic practice than actively dancing myself, that the body's expressive potential is constantly at odds with our own deeply conditioned and socially learned apprehensions.

Consider the creative habits of younger children at play: the possibilities for self-expression often appear endless; that is, endlessly loud, endlessly vibrant, if not wild, and endlessly *adaptable* to the whims of rapidly evolving and radically malleable imaginations. As we age and adapt instead to the rewards and punishments built into systems of social norms, we forget or even willfully suppress the impulse to just expressively be in the world. Dance, therefore, serves for many as an outlet through which we can alleviate the tension created between our expressive impulses and our learned tendencies to keep our bodies contained. Further, because dance often occurs socially—not just in terms of social dance rituals like clubbing and line dancing, but also in terms of the socializing that takes place among cast members—it offers practitioners a sense of validation that one is not alone in seeking to reacquaint themself with the body's breadth of expressive possibilities.

To elaborate, the socially conditioned body carries tensions, traumas, and stressors in many forms, and in doing so siphons its own energy and stamina. In turn, dance production provides individuals with the opportunity to collaboratively galvanize the body's willingness to embrace its self-expressive impulses. Such embrace redirects the energy and stamina, normally used to contain the body, toward creating new and powerful possibilities for self-expression while allowing for catharsis (relief of those tensions, traumas, and stressors). Laura Steckley (2017) explains, "Catharsis is associated with intense expression of emotions, which are often integral to situations requiring *physical restraint*" (p. 1648; emphasis mine). That is, processes of catharsis are necessary when the body exerts itself to withhold, rather than to allow for the natural expressive release of our feelings, especially those more abrasive sensitivities compounded by any number of social rules that target bodies for ridicule or other forms of social consequence.

For his part, Edwin noted, "At times I get all bottled up with anger, sadness, [and] frustration due to daily life issues, but dance has allowed me to embrace those feelings," going on to express, "Learning how to be self-aware through dance makes me feel at ease because I am allowed to let go of those feelings." Carson also explained, "[Dance] allows me to get outside of my head, to shift focus from whatever's been troubling me to the rest of my body." Yet, almost paradoxically, though dance can be understood as the commingling of artistic expression and physical exertion, we cannot ignore how dance is also defined as a practice that intentionally exposes bodies for judgment. As expressed in the previous section, different elements or stages of the dance process contain different opportunities for mitigating anxieties and achieving comfort or catharsis. Douglas S. Risner (1992) explains how a process of "movement investigation" precedes rehearsal, noting that while dancers are still learning and refining their choreography they are in a process that "does not generate the judgement and scrutiny that appear in the pure rehearsal stage and in the actual dance performance" (p. 62).

Those of us who have worked through devising processes for dance understand intimately the value that comes with knowing at a visceral level that our bodies' expressive possibilities are far reaching. The eventual dance product is almost always certain to deviate from the norms of expression that attempt to restrain our physicalities in everyday public life, but even the final product itself is bound to the decided-upon choreographic sequencing that makes the performance more or less repeatable for an audience. Bodies need time and room to recognize how they feel to move differently; to explore, experiment, and discover what self-expression feels like under conditions that celebrate rather than diminish the body's creative capacity. As performance "participants develop a sense of faith and trust in the [dance] process itself" (Risner, 1992, p. 62), they ultimately invigorate and strengthen the final performance product with their own new discoveries and motivations, but more importantly, in doing so they have the opportunity to release, purely through expressive experimentation, any number of "immediate or repressed" (Steckley, 2017, p. 1650) abrasive feelings that so consistently otherwise weigh us down.

As Steckley (2017) further reinforces, the emotional release made possible through catharsis is a "physiological, motor discharge" that alleviates "physiological tension" resulting from emotional suppression (p. 1650). As Julia F. Christensen and Beatriz Calvo-Merino (2013) note as well, dance "movements embody a communicative intention" marked most often by "a strong emotional component" (p. 20). To invest the body in the capital of catharsis rather than the capital of compounding traumas and everyday frustrations can free us of the circumstances from which we become stressed, frustrated, anxious, and so on. Put another way, dance fails *deliberately* to adhere to socialized rules about what a body can and cannot do, and rather than restricting the body's expressive potential, embraces it. Additionally, unlike other forms of artistically calculated performance, such as stage or film acting, dance prioritizes more ambiguous expressive utterances. For example, the meaning behind a dance phrase or choreographic sequence is consistently much more difficult to denote than the lines in a play or a movie that are designed cohesively to advance an equally cohesive narrative. By allowing for ambiguity in the way the dance product will eventually be interpreted by audiences, performers become more independent of the culturally coded systems (language, narrative structure, etc.) that too closely reflect culturally defined standards for other forms of public expression. The ambiguity of dance thus facilitates its own capacity for emotional release.

Jamie explained how working in dance involved "so much emotion and strength that had to be put into each movement that I was able to completely envelop myself in the" performance. Edwin described his approach to dance practice as "allowing [emotion] to self-manifest outward in the choreography." Carson expressed that the dance "process becomes cathartic . . . when I'm able to attach emotions to [the] movement." Montana reflected back on a number of experiences she was able to work through using the choreography process as a way to better understand hers and others' circumstances, noting specifically her parents' divorce: "I took these emotions and moments and put them into my body." She expressed further that dance "really did become like a therapy session, except dance was my doctor." The body in dance becomes the medium for internalized anxieties, frustrations, uncertainties, and any number of discomforts that need to be displaced—unapologetically physicalized—in order to be processed; so they might no longer weigh on us, or at least that they might become lighter, more manageable.

In *Teaching Dance from Contextual Perspectives in the New Zealand Curriculum*, Linda Ashley's (2010) observation that one's "own understanding is pivotal to teaching dance from a contextual perspective" (p. 139) underscores how the dance process inherently is one that necessitates a concern for (or embodiment of) empathy, an understanding beyond oneself. Cynthia F. Berrol (2006) notes of dance practice how, at a cognitive level, even "the same sets of neurons are activated in an observer"—such as a dancer who is learning the work—"as in the individual actually engaged in dance" (p. 303)—the choreographer conveying and teaching the work, for example. After all, those who teach dance as choreographers need not only determine how best to communicate the logistical demands of a dance performance—how, when, and at what pace to move—but must also determine (in the case of original work) or identify (in the case of borrowed or adapted work) the intentions that allow the movement of dance to convey both physical and emotional qualities. In turn, dancers need to work to translate as accurately as possible the logistical, physical, and emotional demands of the work while also opening themselves up to embodying newly understood emotional states.

The emotional intentions embodied in dance, translated carefully between choreographer and performer through a rich empathetic exchange, can serve one of two purposes. First, the emotional intentions inherent in the dance process may contrast with dancers' current or preexisting emotional states of being. In other words, to practice dance actively is to allow oneself the opportunity, momentary as it might be, to feel differently, not so much to distract from or to suppress one's feelings, but to spur new feelings that surface and become priority for as long as the production process is taking place. For example, depending on the particular demands of the work, dance performers might need to find ways of embodying a sense of *energetic joy*, even though they may enter the process feeling a sense of *apathy and despair*, experiences clearly at odds with one another. Certainly, that dancers can learn to embody, for the sake of the work, more uplifting emotional states of being does not mean that practicing dance allows one to attain at will any emotional state they desire. Yet, doing so reminds the body it is capable of feeling differently, more positively.

In contrast to the previous example, dance performance may at times demand dancers embody emotional states that convey intentionally to audiences a sense of anger, or frustration, or deep sadness. A second function of the embodiment of emotional intention in dance, then, is to teach dancers how to employ the body as a vehicle for navigating their feelings more fully. Dance can teach, at a visceral level, that the process of shifting between despair and optimism, sadness and joy, frustration and satisfaction is a process over which we have perhaps more agency than we would otherwise consider, should we never reintroduce ourselves to the body's expressive breadth. Just as we are often taught to intellectualize our feelings through thoughtful reflection or meditation so that we might make sense of and eventually process (or overcome) those feelings, dance reminds us of the *body's* intelligence, of our somatic intuitions that grasp what we are feeling, and why, well before we have consciously articulated as much.

DANCING DELIBERATELY: COMMUNITIES OF THERAPEUTIC PRACTICE

During the initiation stage for a new cast or new production, I always ask performers to acknowledge—for themselves, and only to whatever extent they are comfortable doing so, out loud for one another—their current frustrations, anxieties, concerns, *and* excitements, all pertaining to their lives outside the dance process. Acknowledging the latter (their excitements, joys, moments of daily reprieve, etc.) helps to ensure production processes not only mitigate adverse outlooks and experiences that might inhibit their willingness to participate fully, but also can build on their existing readiness to recognize positive qualities about themselves, or their readiness to embrace dance's therapeutic offerings. Simply put, even when practitioners begin the process with any number of personal concerns weighing on their minds, asking them to identify and reflect on positive possibilities otherwise overshadowed by their concerns brings positivity to the forefront of the process.

Momentarily acknowledging the former (their frustrations, anxieties, etc.) can help dancers connect a desire to overcome abrasive qualities of life with the dance process in which they are immersing themselves. Further, doing so can help dancers more readily embrace dance's network of stimuli and its capacity to facilitate emotional release through expressive experimentation.

Openly acknowledging the former (frustrations, anxieties, concerns, etc.) can help other cast members feel validated in actively bringing their own frustrations into the process. As such, Albright (2010) points out how "dance takes place in a *social* situation" (p. 32; emphasis mine), indicating that we seek validation from others during the production process akin to how we seek affirmations from within our everyday social circles. The dance process, in turn, often becomes a communal site of therapeutic practice wherein the shared goal of exploring expressive physicality is navigated through the socializing act of self-disclosure. The socializing act of self-disclosure, as indicated by Jean-Philippe Laurenceau, Lisa Feldman Barrett, and Paula R. Pietromonaco (1998), can produce deeply intimate bonds between participants (p. 1239). Sharing negative experiences, however, can sometimes be difficult for practitioners unaccustomed to divulging anything but positive details about their lives, even when the result of doing so proves to be empowering. Yet, Boon and Plastow (2004) connect empowerment in performance processes with "the liberation of the human mind and spirit, and with the transformation of participants who see themselves" as less than (p. 7). If empowerment is reached in part through honest reflection by practitioners on their qualities of life, then such a practice ought to be encouraged from the very beginning, and sustained throughout the process.

When Montana recounted some of her earlier experiences with "dance as a process, instead of an end product that we perform for other people," she explained how she has used dance to better understand and process her "adoption, [the concept of] death, gendered norms, space for women," and more. Montana, more so than Jamie, Carson, and Edwin, has significant experience as a choreographer. As mentioned above, she further explained how she also used the choreographic process to better understand her parents' divorce and to develop a sense of empathy for what they were going through. "Through [a] six-week process I entered studios by myself and spent hours using my body as a way to understand all angles of my parents divorce. . . . Then, I had to teach this dance to another dancer." She went on to explain, "I learned a lot about myself by watching someone else 'be my body.' The empathy of dance does that to you. I finally got to see the story in front of my eyes and empathize with myself." In other words, not only acknowledging an abrasive quality of life at any given time, but also thoughtfully embracing it through dance and with the help of another dancer, can serve practitioners quite well.

Instead of attempting to repress (or perhaps reject or somehow dissolve) their hindrances, uncertainties, frustrations, and anxieties, dancers can begin the production process with a sense of validation for their lives beyond the fleeting instances when we meet to rehearse, refine, and perform. While the technical foundation of dance work often demands a degree of shared precision, such as dancers moving in-sync with and explicitly in response to one another, achieving precision is largely still an individual task. Choreographers, production directors and managers, and fellow members of an ensemble can encourage each other's personal processes of dance development, or invite others into their own process. No other member of the production process, however, can navigate another member's hindrances on their behalf. Members of any given production's community of practitioners can, of course, help mitigate each other's frustrations as the act of bonding through performance work is largely and often a positive experience. Montana also mentioned, for instance, that her "very first reason for joining a dance studio was community," explaining how, when she was younger, she viewed the dance process explicitly as an opportunity to interact with others in a process of shared creativity. The act of bonding through performance work can redirect our focus or render our immediate concerns less significant and daunting in the face of a complex and rewarding process of collaboration.

Susan Kozel (2007) remarks in *Closer: Performance, Technologies, Phenomenology* "that bodies are the sites of difference and diversity, of pain and pleasure" (p. 306), and Jenny Roche (2019) observes, "Dancers are particular in that they carry their body of knowledge with them" (p. 85)—a body of knowledge that presumably includes experiences of difference, diversity, pain, and pleasure. Thus, when dancers form communities of therapeutic practice simply by together taking part in the production process, each bring with them their own unique experiences and perspectives. Yet, dance practitioners certainly need to account carefully for one another's differences, valuing each other for their strengths rather than diminishing them for perceived weaknesses. In turn, depending on who practitioners are working with, the dance production process can, in fact, magnify rather than alleviate anxieties and frustrations.

At times, some ensemble members and choreographers may simply be difficult to work with—such as those who are excessively critical and demanding, or those who are critical and demanding in non-constructive (for example, poorly communicated) ways. I can readily recall, for instance, performing for several years with a Los Angeles–based dance company about which I had strongly mixed feelings. In one respect, the company was essentially characterized by how emphatically they encouraged deep exploration of self, and company members were actively supported in both their professional and personal endeavors beyond dance. These were positive facets of the company about which we were constantly reminded. In another respect, notions of self-discovery and self-expression were strictly defined by the company's leadership. Any deviation from the dance group's standards of behavior was met with overt and vocal disapproval or with passive aggressive comments about company members' personal life choices, whether or not those choices had any bearing on our work as dance artists. Sometimes, failure to perform (socially and on stage) according to company leadership's expectations could even be met with abrupt dismissal from the group, no matter how slight the perceived infraction. For myself, the former qualities of the company ultimately came nowhere close to outweighing the latter. Under such or similar circumstances, dance practitioners may choose to seek out other opportunities to immerse themselves in their craft, but within more thoughtful and holistically encouraging environments.

In *An Introduction to Community Dance Practice*, Diane Amans (2017) observes that dance practice "requires cooperation and communication, a sharing of physicality and mental agility that may precipitate creative energy and communal feeling in the moment of dance" (p. 15). Amans' (2017) framing of dance practice as communal signals how any kind of ensemble work, in order to be both aesthetically productive (pleasing to an eventual audience) *and* cathartic/comforting for practitioners, needs always to account for practitioners' somatic individuality, for ways in which each body in the ensemble carries unique experiences, impulses, and conditions. As Dana Mills (2017) contends, "The body is not a one dimensional entity. It is a symbolic web of meanings which create intersections and conflicts; it enables methods of signification to become intertwined but also to struggle over power of inscription" (pp. 66–67). In other words, any choreographer or ensemble director who attempts simply and entirely to "inscribe" performers with her will dismisses the richness of experiences not her own, demanding that somatic individuality be suppressed. Ensemble dance is a unique art form in that the primary materials of production are the autonomous bodies of others, unlike paint or clay or wood that can be splattered or stretched or carved without concern for the will or desire of the materials themselves. As Mills (2017) further expresses, "The body remembers joy and pain; triumph and loss; grief and exhilaration" (p. 75), qualities that necessitate, per Amans' argument, communal collaboration.

While *Cicadas*, for example, was developed with the somewhat selfish intention of helping me to process my own struggles adapting to the unfamiliar physical and cultural environments of Louisiana, I also paid special attention to the experiences, impulses, and conditions of my cast. To the best of my ability, I opened dialogues with them to ensure they found the work accessible and stimulating in their own rights. Though the choreography was always designed to physicalize the back-and-forth between tension and relief—through those shifts from near-violent convulsions to more soft and loosely-controlled full-body gestures—I tailored said convulsions and gestures to suit the other performers' unique needs. Because I always ask members of any cast to reflect on their anxieties, frustrations, and joys outside of dance, I pose at the beginning of the rehearsal process the following: How does your *body* want to respond to the ways you feel as you reflect? *Cicadas* opens with myself and the others standing upstage, equidistant from one another, feet widely separated and knees bent, one hand hanging low and the other slowly twisting and folding in all directions as it floats around our heads, our eyes following the motion intently under faded lighting. This opening sequence is a moment of comfort, meant to preempt and punctuate the oncoming moments of violent tension. When teaching this part of the choreography, I asked the other performers to reflect again on their joys and excitements separate from the dance process, and to then allow their bodies to answer the previous question: How does your body want to respond right now? Consequently, the knee-bent, soft hand-floating opening sequence became and appeared distinct for each of us, threaded together only by our similar positioning and by a shared intention to both feel and express genuine comfort. We could maintain a togetherness that served the aesthetic of the work while allowing ourselves to *feel* as individuals. That is, we achieved synchronicity by honoring individual experience, expression, and need.

In much the same way that attuning oneself to the specific demands for synchronicity of a given performance is a task dancers can only undertake for themselves, identifying and seeking dance opportunities that facilitate comfort and catharsis by valuing (rather than admonishing) individual identity are goals only individual practitioners can pursue. Nevertheless, most communities of dance practitioners already have built in to their group cultures an active, even if not explicitly intentional or formalized, concern for the capacity of dance to facilitate therapeutic experiences. Desmond's (1993) characterization that "dance signals and enacts social identities in all their continually changing configurations" (p. 57) reflects such efforts by dance groups to view practitioners' identities and experiences as valuable to the overall process, rather than exclusively viewing the commodity of practitioners' technical skills.

Additionally, more and more often choreographers and other experienced dance practitioners are *intentionally* working to facilitate immersive dance opportunities that are more radically accessible, welcoming myriad participants and not only those with significant training or experience. By taking advantage of the expressive readiness of the *non-dancer*—one without formal training or significant experience navigating the dance production process—choreographers and directors can begin to access uniquely expressive repertoires of physicality. That is, those who have *not* been taught only to dance within the rigidly coded standards of a particular style or discipline may be even more open to performing in ways yet unseen. Such a practitioner not only has the opportunity to pursue comfort and catharsis by learning to express herself beyond culturally conditioned standards of physicality, but beyond virtually *any* predetermined standards of expression. A community of dance that is welcoming of such a practitioner might help her first to discover her own distinct expressive strengths, and then to magnify and elaborate on those strengths. An inclusive community might guide performers through systematic processes that break down those inhibitions weighing on the social body, creating institutionalized opportunities for exploring dance as a vibrant network of stimuli, and as an avenue through which to experience emotional release and a more authentic, more unreservedly expressive breadth of one's body.

In turn, we can also consider how such processes of expressive therapeutic practice facilitated by dance communities can be applied in the classroom. Certainly, expressive arts educational programs (dance, theatre, music, etc.) lend themselves explicitly to similar forms of community building. Yet, a range of educational settings or programs that are not labeled traditionally as "artistically expressive" can also benefit significantly by actively valuing students' unique lived experiences, and by prioritizing expressive accessibility and openness over absolute adherence to the rigid limitations of technique. As education journalist Katrina Schwartz (2019) notes in her reporting on a California elementary school wherein collaborative "art is at the center of learning" (par. 1), integrating artistic practices into the teaching and learning process—regardless of the subject of study—"gives students a way to think about the world differently, to make connections, and to contemplate their [own] place within it" (par. 13). Two such experiences integrating artistic expressive practices specifically derived from dance come to mind.

First, when I taught kindergartners for a year while working as the coordinator and lead instructional developer for an afterschool enrichment program, in addition to teaching a weekly youth contemporary dance class, we frequently played games that would prompt students to create new expressive gestures accompanied by expressive vocalizations (they were specifically asked to create "funny" sounds we had never heard before). Students seemed especially to enjoy how these games would follow the rigidity of their usual seven-hour school day routine, during which instructions to "sit still and be quiet" often took priority over allowances to expressively play. Yet, as students were still learning to negotiate between the demand for stillness/quiet and the motivation to play uninhibited, they often seemed to hold themselves back during these games. They had been learning, after all, that classroom time was exclusively about following directions (hence, *not* about creativity). Somewhat in line with their other classroom experiences, my weekly afterschool dance class would cover very basic principles of modern dance technique, as students would learn essential positions, phrases, and transitions designed to sharpen developing motor skills. I would also incorporate, however, simple choreography for the students to learn. Notably, as the school year progressed and the students became more and more comfortable with and excited about the expressive gesture and vocalization games we would play (meaning they were less reserved when playing), they also demonstrated a capacity to learn choreography that was more and more complex. The dance sequences they were achieving near year's end used very little formal technique, and instead relied on their own readiness to move about in stimulating, exciting new ways.

Second, almost immediately after transitioning from teaching kindergartners to teaching Communication Studies to college students, I incorporated very similar games that relied even more heavily on expressive physicalities to be played properly. The most important difference was that I was now working with students who had spent over a decade in mostly conventional educational settings that similarly and often aggressively associated the classroom experience with stillness and relative quiet. A willingness to become more powerfully expressive is paramount in many Communication Studies courses, especially introductory courses like Public Speaking that are designed to help students build effective and in-demand communication skills for the workplace. Because my college students proved generally to be much more reserved when prompted to participate in activities that require a *lack of reservation*, a series of games was transformed into a structured workshop (Langner, 2017/2018) that the older participants found more digestible/accessible. Students participating in the workshop would progress from an exercise asking them to reflect positively on their own future potential, to positioning and gesturing in ways they had never before experienced—one limb at a time—until they discovered new physically expressive sequences that activated as much of the body as they were able. I have noticed over several years that whenever I find the time to teach the workshop more than once throughout a semester, students demonstrate an observably greater willingness to apply the principles of the workshop to other tasks, to be more powerfully expressive when delivering a speech, presentation, mock interview, and so on.

CONCLUDING THOUGHTS

Dance honors our communicative capacities as they can exist beyond the rigidity of coded and easily reproducible verbal and textual language. The critical reflections offered in this chapter address dancers' experiences with the whole of the dance production process, from casting and rehearsal, to opening through final performances, and everything in between. My own personal reflections as a dancer and choreographer, as well as my critical recollections of dialogues with other practitioners, underpin both the unique and overlapping ways in which dance serves so often and so dynamically as a therapeutic practice. From personal performance experiences, and from an immersion in different dance scenes around the world, I can state with confidence the foundational claim that the dance production process is, indeed, quite often a powerful and multifaceted tool for achieving comfort and catharsis. The opportunity to critically uncover, more effectively and with greater nuance, exactly *how* the dance production process proves itself emotionally and cognitively beneficial to practitioners is an exciting avenue, one within reach and with potential implications well beyond the observations made here.

REFERENCES

Albright, A. C. (2010). *Choreographing difference: The body and identity in contemporary dance*. Middletown, CT: Wesleyan University Press.

Amans, D. (2017). *An introduction to community dance practice* (2nd ed.). London, UK: Palgrave Oxford Macmillan Education.

Ashley, L. (2010). *Teaching dance from contextual perspectives in the New Zealand curriculum: Concerns, dilemmas and opportunities in theory and practice* (Doctoral dissertation). Music University of Auckland, Auckland, New Zealand. Retrieved from https://pdfs.semanticscholar.org/2a12/e9078d1800707d2cb89373bc9a37c34b3e84.pdf

Barbour, K. (2008). Standing strong: Pedagogical approaches to affirming identity in dance. *Dance Dialogues*. Reprint. *AusDance*. Retrieved from https://ausdance.org.au/articles/details/standing-strong-pedagogical-approaches-to-affirming-identity-in-dance#toc-_acknowledgements

Berrol, C. F. (2006). Neuroscience meets dance/movement therapy: Mirror neurons, the therapeutic process and empathy. *Arts in Psychotherapy*, *33*(4), 302–315. https://doi.org/10.1016/j.aip.2006.04.001

Boon, R., & Plastow, J. (Eds.). (2004). *Theatre and empowerment: Community drama on the world stage*. Cambridge, UK: Cambridge University Press.

Christensen, J. F., & Calvo-Merino, B. (2013). Dance as a subject for empirical aesthetics. *Psychology of Aesthetics, Creativity, and the Arts*, *7*(1), 76–88. https://psycnet.apa.org/doi/10.1037/a0031827

Desmond, J. C. (1993). Embodying difference: Issues in dance and cultural studies. *Cultural Critique*, (26), 33–63. https://doi.org/10.2307/1354455

Gingrich-Philbrook, C., & Simmons, J. (2015). Reprogramming the stage: A Heuristic for posthuman performance. *Text and Performance Quarterly*, *35*(4), 323–344. http://doi.org/10.1080/10462937.2015.1075169

Gostand, R. (1980). Verbal and non-verbal communication: Drama as translation. In O. Zuber (Ed.), *The Languages of Theatre: Problems in the Translation and Transposition of Drama* (pp. 1–9). Oxford, UK: Pergamon Press.

Kozel, S. (2007). *Closer: Performance, technologies, phenomenology*. Cambridge, MA: MIT Press.

Langner, G. (2017/2018). Breaking bodies: Performing subversion in the communication classroom. *Journal of the Communication, Speech, and Theatre Association of North Dakota*, *30*, 46–51. https://drive.google.com/open?id=1SLVEtJ7119zwyaf2-KCZDK5SCSQkpb1C

Laurenceau, J. P., Barrett, L. F., & Pietromonaco, P. R. (1998). Intimacy as an interpersonal process: The importance of self-disclosure, partner disclosure, and perceived partner responsiveness in interpersonal exchanges. *Journal of Personality and Social Psychology*, *74*(5), 1238–1251. https://doi.org/10.1037//0022-3514.74.5.1238

Mills, D. (2017). 3. The Body Remembers: Dance, Discourses of Citizenship, Phenomenology and Memory. In K. Lindroos & F. Möller (Eds.), *Art as a Political Witness* (pp. 65–78). Opladen; Berlin; Torono, CN: Barbara Budrich Publisher.

Pelias, R. J., & Shaffer, T. S. (2007). *Performance studies: The interpretation of aesthetic texts*. Dubuque, IA: Kendall.

Risner, D. S. (1992). Exploring dance rehearsal—The neglected issues revealed. *Journal of Physical Education, Recreation & Dance*, *63*(6), 61–65. https://doi.org/10.1080/07303084.1992.10606621

Roche, J. (2019). Traces from elsewhere: Dancing together across distance and time. *Text and Performance Quarterly*, *39*(1), 74–88. https://doi.org/10.1080/10462937.2018.1527390

Schwartz, K. (2019, October 14). How art can help center a student's learning experience. *KQED News*. Retrieved from https://www.kqed.org/mindshift/54370/how-art-can-help-center-a-students-learning-experience?fbclid=IwAR1ypbxP6esjT3GyraTlZlO6lrTN0Fr4Dve2SiWulRA25GnPEi-WdRXKf8I

Steckley, L. (2017). Catharsis, containment and physical restraint in residential child care. *British Journal of Social Work*, *48*(6), 1645–1663. https://doi.org/10.1093/bjsw/bcx131

Chapter Ten

The Art of Love

Using Participatory Community Arts Engagement to Facilitate Relational Maintenance among Couples with Dementia

Anna K. Griggs, Meara H. Faw, and Laura H. Malinin

Memory related illnesses affect millions (Ferri et al., 2005; National Institute on Aging, 2019) and by 2050, Alzheimer's disease or related dementias (ADRD) will likely affect one in eighty-five people (Brookmeyer et al., 2007). Researchers are scrambling to determine what causes the disease and, while treatments may slow its progression, there currently is no cure (Ferri et al., 2005). Thus, it is important to focus efforts on nonpharmacological ways that people can maintain quality of life. Arts engagement programming, given its creative and tactile nature, can stimulate memory, create social networks, enhance mood, and maintain relationships, along with several other positive effects for people with ADRD (Basting, 2006; Camic & Chatterjee, 2013; Flatt et al., 2015). This chapter places relational maintenance, arts engagement, and the effects of dementia on family and spouses in conversation with one another to more fully realize the relationship-building potential of arts engagement.[1] Our research examined care partners' (CPs) experiences with participatory community arts engagement (PCAE) as one avenue for promoting connection with their loved one with ADRD. While ample research supports the mental and physical health benefits of PCAE, little research considers how it impacts communication between participants. Through our research, we highlight the unique role of therapeutic PCAE on relational maintenance among partners managing ADRD.

ALZHEIMER'S DISEASE OR RELATED DEMENTIAS' EFFECTS ON COMMUNICATION

With the rising prevalence of ADRD, researchers have sought to investigate what causes the illness and its effects on the people with ADRD and their CPs, family members, and friends. According to the Centers for Disease Control and Prevention (CDC), ADRD involves a decline in cognitive function that will eventually render a person incapable of completing the daily tasks of living, as well as remembering family and friends (CDC, 2019). Early symptoms of ADRD include difficulty remembering newly learned information, but ADRD is degenerative, meaning that as it progresses, a person may face mood and behavior changes, confusion, general disorientation, and difficulty swallowing, speaking, and walking (Alzheimer's Association, 2019). Alzheimer's disease is the sixth leading cause of death in the United States, and people with ADRD live an average of eight years after diagnosis, requiring extensive care as the disease progresses (Alzheimer's Association, 2019; National Institute on Aging, 2019).

One of the main challenges a person diagnosed with ADRD may face is communication (Stone, 2013). Changing communicative patterns of people who are experiencing ADRD negatively impacts the person, family, and caregivers (Stone & Jones, 2009), including the nature of relationships, which can be a painful process for all members involved. For spouses, an ADRD diagnosis can greatly change marital relationships. Spouses tend to care for their partner until it becomes unmanageable and the caregiver's burden is often significant, causing stress, anger, or other negative emotional states (Butcher, Holkup, & Buckwalter, 2001). In one study, husbands and wives who served as a CP reported diminished intimacy in many forms (for example, sexual, emotional, social, physical) (Hayes et al., 2009). Additionally, women are more likely than men to report that they struggled with their own identity within the marriage as their husbands' diseases progressed (Hayes et al., 2009). Many CPs described the process of caring for a loved one with ADRD who is slowly losing capabilities as "heartbreaking," highlighting the painful grief process that accompanies an ADRD diagnosis (Butcher, Holkup, & Buckwalter, 2001).

PARTICIPATORY COMMUNITY ARTS ENGAGEMENT AND RELATIONAL MAINTENANCE

PCAE typically consists of interactive and hands-on creative activities for community members (Flatt et al., 2015). For those dealing with life-altering health illnesses, art can serve as a way to express complex emotions and process difficult diagnoses (Camic & Chatterjee, 2013). PCAE can take place in hospitals and clinics, but research increasingly suggests that art museums and galleries may be better suited for effective PCAE (Camic & Chatterjee, 2013). Several studies have examined the effects of therapeutic PCAE for people with ADRD and CPs (for a review, see Beard, 2012). In a review article, Anne Davis Basting (2006) explained, "where rational language and factual memory have failed people with dementia, the arts offer an avenue for communication and connection with caregivers, loved ones, and the greater world" (p. 17). When a person may no longer be able to communicate their thoughts as they used to, PCAE programming can work to fill at least a piece of that gap. In her systematic review, Justine Schneider (2018) argued that creativity is not dependent upon memory, claiming that art can remain accessible despite memory loss due to its multi-sensory nature. Carol M. Johnson and Eileen M. Sullivan-Marx (2006) found that for people with ADRD, art is a "visual reminder that they can still accomplish and learn new things despite limited mobility or cognition" (p. 312).

Ample research documents negative effects that ADRD can have on family and spousal communication, though research also suggests that PCAE might provide one avenue for promoting positive interactions among CPs and adults with ADRD. For example, evidence points to the efficacy of PCAE in facilitating feelings of connection and of closeness between CPs and adults with ADRD, enhancing their relationship in positive ways (Clair, 2002; Corbeil, Quayhagen, & Quayhagen, 1999). Similarly, PCAE can provide new avenues for older adult pairs (dyads) to engage in communication patterns such as reminiscing and participating in activities together, which have been shown to positively influence communication among CPs and adults with ADRD (Astell et al., 2010; DiLauro et al., 2017).

Given the evidence outlining the potential for PCAE to promote positive communication, it is also possible that PCAE might enhance relationship dynamics by creating new avenues for *relational maintenance*. Daniel J. Canary and Laura Stafford (2003b) define relational maintenance as "actions and activities used to sustain desired relational definitions" (p. 5). That is, people use behaviors to ensure that their relationship continues as they want it defined, as noted in the edited volume *Communication and Relational Maintenance* (Canary & Stafford, 2003a). They argue that all relationships require maintenance. Stable relationships are not static—rather, changes in relationships are worked through and adapted to fit the needs of both participants—and individuals spend more time maintaining relationships than they do initiating or dissolving them (Duck, 1988). People use five primary communicative strategies to maintain relationships. *Positivity* involves using prosocial behaviors, such as being encouraging, polite, friendly, and kind toward another person (Canary & Stafford, 2003b). *Openness* refers to self-disclosing and communicating about the nature of a relationship (Weigel & Ballard-Reisch, 2001). *Assurances* includes using expressions of love, typically implying that the relationship has a future (Canary & Stafford, 2003b). *Shared networks* describes efforts to surround the relationship with friends and family who provide support (sustaining relationships across different networks), and participate in activities together (Weigel & Ballard-Reisch, 2001). Finally, *tasks* involves equitable sharing of relationship responsibilities, household obligations, etc. (Canary & Stafford, 2003b).

Relational maintenance strategies can be strategic or routine (Canary & Stafford, 2003b). Research suggests people use strategic behaviors intentionally to connect with another, whereas routine behaviors are mundane and occur at a lower level of consciousness (Greene, 1984). While many studies highlight relational maintenance behaviors that are predominately prosocial, more recent research has examined various anti-social relational maintenance strategies (Goodboy et al., 2017). Alan K. Goodboy (2017) and colleagues outline five anti-social relational maintenance strategies: *jealousy induction* (showing interest in someone other than partner); *avoidance* of important conversations or of each other; *spying* on one another; *infidelity*; and *destructive conflict*. Anti-social strategies can occur in conjunction with prosocial relational maintenance behaviors, highlighting the complexity of maintaining long-term relationships. This may be particularly true for partners managing ADRD, yet little research has investigated how relational maintenance might change with ADRD, which can affect how individuals communicate and experience their relationship. Additionally, very limited work has explored how relational maintenance might be encouraged and enhanced through formal programming like that experienced in PCAE.

METHODS

Given the extensive research underscoring the value of creative expression for individuals dealing with ADRD and their caregivers (Beard, 2012; Camic & Chatterjee, 2013; Chancellor, Duncan, & Chatterjee, 2014; Johnson & Sullivan-Marx, 2006), our study explored the potential of PCAE specifically within the context of enhancing relational maintenance, as researchers have yet to explore how PCAE might facilitate relational maintenance behaviors for adults with ADRD and their CPs. With this in mind, we posed the following research question:

> What relational maintenance behaviors do people with ADRD and their CPs use while engaging in PCAE?

To answer this question, we used observations from two, four-week long workshops in which couples created masks designed to promote connection and cognitive stimulation. The first series of workshops took place during spring 2017, and the second occurred in autumn 2018. All sessions took place in the same local art museum, and each workshop was led by a certified therapist. Participants included dyads, comprised of a person with ADRD and his/her informal CP (spouse or close friend).

Each workshop lasted about one and a half hours. In the first week of class, the therapist gave each dyad an undecorated clay mask. Dyads looked through magazines together for inspiration and documented ideas. Class two involved creating the first layer of the masks. For example, some participants used tissue paper, whereas others painted or drew on the masks. In the third and fourth sessions, participants continued working on their masks using a variety of techniques (for example, applying beads or tissue paper, painting, or hot gluing paper or other supplies to the mask).

Participants

To protect participants' privacy, all participants were given pseudonyms for use in data reporting. All participants in our study were recruited through a larger study. In total, six dyads participated: four in 2017 and two in 2018 (see table 10.1). However, in 2017, two dyads were unable to complete all four weeks of the workshop. All other dyads attended all workshop sessions. Five of the dyads were male-female partners (spouses), and one was a female-female dyad (life-long friends). Participants were predominantly white, only one dyad consisted of non-white individuals. Participants ranged from 69 to 79 years old. In 2017, all spousal partners lived together; the life-long friend dyad lived separately. In 2018, one dyad lived separately because the person with ADRD lived in a long-term care facility. Participants with ADRD had varying levels of functioning and different communication abilities.

Table 10.1. Study of Participant Background and Demographic Information

Names	*Ages*	*Race/Ethnicity*	*Relationship*	*Former professions*	*Basic description*	*Year*
Jan and Lewis (ADRD)	Unknown	White	Married	Art teacher and professor	Jan was vocal and talkative with the group. She helped Lewis with the mask. Lewis was quiet but comedic when he did speak. They talked about their lives together as a married couple.	2018
Carol and Bruce (ADRD)	Unknown	White	Married	Unknown, and former statistical process controller, training manager, and truck driver	Carol was quiet and did not help Bruce with the mask. Her husband, Bruce, was kind and liked to talk. Bruce was creative and had plenty of ideas for the mask. He rarely accepted help.	2018
Emily and Deb (ADRD)	Unknown, 79	White	Best Friends	Unknown, and former nurse	Emily was talkative with her partner	2017

Names	***Ages***	***Race/Ethnicity***	***Relationship***	***Former professions***	***Basic description***	***Year***
					and with the rest of the group. Emily and Deb are best friends of 40 years. Deb was quiet and spoke mostly to Emily.	
Louise and Aaron (ADRD)	Unknown, 69	Latina and Black	Married	Unknown, and former medical research illustrator	Aaron had many of his own ideas, and Louise would brainstorm with him. Aaron and Louise did not talk extensively to each other but would talk with other participants.	2017
Jessica and John (ADRD)	Unknown, 70	White	Married	Unknown, and former pilot	Jessica and John only attended one week. John was social with other participants. Jessica was quiet but engaged with her partner. John made jokes and	2017

Names	***Ages***	***Race/Ethnicity***	***Relationship***	***Former professions***	***Basic description***	***Year***
					engaged most with Charles.	
Sharon and Charles (ADRD)	Unknown, 69	White	Married	Unknown, and former ironworker	Sharon and Charles only attended one week. During that time, Sharon helped him with everything. Charles was agitated during the class and did not seem to enjoy his time.	2017

Source: This is a recap of data collected from workshop participants through video recording and field notes, taken in 2017–2018.

Data Collection and Analysis

Data was collected at each workshop through video recording and field notes.

In each workshop session, one or two video cameras were set up on opposing sides of the space. Throughout the 2018 workshop sessions, a member of the research team took approximately fourteen pages of field notes, which were included in the analysis. Researchers interacted with participants before and after the workshop but sought to be unobtrusive during creative activities. Approximately twelve hours of video recordings were obtained across both years of workshop sessions. Analysis of the videos stemmed from a grounded approach to thematic analysis (Braun & Clarke, 2006). The important concepts that emerged from the data were woven together with Canary and Stafford's (2003a, 2003b) relational maintenance typology to identify appropriate themes. Additionally, we considered three criteria when constructing themes: (1) the recurrence of ideas, (2) the repetition of terms, and (3) the forcefulness of concepts (Owen, 1984).

Specifically, for this project, data analysis included a constant comparative analysis of the video footage through six steps (Braun & Clarke, 2006). First, researchers familiarized themselves with the data. Second, they created a general observational protocol to differentiate between relational maintenance behaviors for the initial coding. After identifying initial codes, the codes were then grouped together through a round of axial coding into preliminary themes (Glaser & Strauss, 1967). These themes were then reviewed and named (Braun & Clarke, 2006). Throughout the process, reflexive coding through conversation among the research team helped develop thoughts and challenge assumptions to ensure proper analysis (Lindlof & Taylor, 2011).

RESULTS

We found that participants used *touch*, *reminiscing*, *positivity*, *networks*, *shared tasks*, *openness*, *assurances*, *avoidance*, and *other anti-social behaviors* in their interactions (table 10.2).

Table 10.2. Study of Participant Use of Relational Maintenance Behaviors

Behavior	*Group more likely to use behavior*	*Explanation*
Touch	Care Partner	Touch was used more frequently by the care partner as they asked the participant with ADRD to respond to their question or used touch to assist their partner in a task or encourage them to continue working on that task. Participants with ADRD were less likely to use touch but when they did, it was largely to affirm another person with ADRD.
Reminiscing	Care Partner	Reminiscing was introduced more frequently by care partners, but participants with ADRD engaged in the act of reminiscing when prompted. While the behavior was typically shared equally, it was commonly stimulated by the care partner in order to create conversation or stimulate their partner's memory as they worked.
Positivity	Shared Equally	While care partners did most of the positivity to affirm everyone in the workshop, participants with ADRD used jokes more frequently than the care partners. These jokes were commonly at their own expense. Therefore, of the two purposes behind each behavior, care partners used positivity to affirm, and participants with ADRD used positivity to joke.
Shared Tasks	Care Partner	Like reminiscing, care partners were more likely than the participants with ADRD to begin

Behavior	*Group more likely to use behavior*	*Explanation*
		the relational maintenance behavior of shared tasks. However, once asked to share the task, several people with ADRD readily engaged in the relational maintenance for an extended period, particularly in relation to sharing tasks to brainstorm. Sharing tasks to assist was exclusively associated with the care partner as they helped the person with ADRD complete a task that they would otherwise by unable to do alone.
Networks	Care Partner	Networks created with other workshop participants were used by people with ADRD when they would talk and ask each other questions but appeared more frequently between care partners as they shared experiences and advice with one another. Additionally, networks created by family and friends outside of the workshop were usually brought into conversation by care partners as they remarked on how friends and children would enjoy seeing the creations.
Openness	Care Partner	Throughout the interactions, care partners were much more likely to disclose information about themselves, their partner, or their relationships than people with ADRD. When people with ADRD did disclose, it was nearly always as a result of a care partner asking them a question about themselves.

Behavior	***Group more likely to use behavior***	***Explanation***
Assurances	Care Partner	Although infrequent in interactions, assurances were used almost exclusively by care partners as they commented on how the mask could be used outside of the workshop while making the mask with their partner. Only one person with ADRD commented on how he saw the mask being displayed in the home he shared with his care partner.
Avoidance	Shared Equally	Avoidance appeared for two reasons in this research: by being disengaged and by rejecting help. Care partners were more likely to be disengaged in the mask making process and subsequent conversation whereas participants with ADRD were exclusively the people who would reject help either from their care partner or the therapist.
Anti-social behaviors	Care Partner	There were few, if any, instances in which a person with ADRD used sarcastic comments with their partner. Instead, this behavior appeared in how some care partners reacted to the participant with ADRD rejecting their help or becoming agitated in the mask-making process.

Source: This is a recap of relational maintenance strategies used by care partners and participants with ADRD taken from workshop video recording and field notes, taken in 2017–2018.

Touch. *Touch*, defined as making intentional physical contact with another person (Canary & Stafford, 2003b), was an important relational maintenance behavior used throughout the workshops. Participants used touch *to affirm*, *to assist*, and *to elicit a response*.

To affirm. Affirmation was the most common form of touch used by all six CPs and usually consisted of a CP encouraging their partner with ADRD. Affirmative touch was often paired with another relational maintenance behavior, like positivity. For example, CPs would tap their partner on the back, shoulder, or hands while telling them "good job."

Touch as affirmation was prevalent during the few times in the workshop sessions where individuals with ADRD became upset or agitated. For example, without prompting, Sharon smiled at Charles and patted him on the leg as they received instructions on how to make their mask. Soon after, she wrapped her arms around Charles to talk to him after he had hesitated to answer questions asked by one of the researchers. When he did not immediately answer her questions, Sharon moved her body so that she was right in front of Charles and looked him in the eyes while keeping her hands on his shoulders. In this instance, she used touch to encourage him to talk with her about his feelings and to affirm that she was physically near him to support him.

In another instance, Emily brought a poem to the workshop session that Deb had recently written so that they could attach it to their mask. After reading it, the therapist asked if she could use Deb's poem for marketing material. Emily was excited for Deb, and she patted her on the back to affirm Deb. Deb responded positively to Emily's touch in the interaction. When partnered with positivity, touch often worked to affirm the person with ADRD.

To assist. Although less common, four dyads used touch *to assist*. Most often, CP used touch as assistance in response to a need of their partner with ADRD. For example, Jan would hold Lewis' wrist as he painted to steady his hand. Carol similarly held Bruce's wrist as he used a marker to draw a face on his mask. This touch served to help the person with ADRD complete their task. Emily would position herself beside Deb and hold her arms as she stood to make sure that Deb was stable. Due to the relationship between the care partner and their loved one with ADRD, *touch as assistance* played a unique role in this setting because not only did the behaviors act as a form of connection for partners, but also in many cases, the art workshop likely would have been less effective for several participants had their partners not been there to assist.

To elicit a response. Three of the six CPs used *touch to elicit a response* from their partners. For example, during the first workshop, Sharon was trying to get Charles to look through photographs or to attach tissue paper to their mask. When he refused, she would tap him to remind him that she was asking him to do a task. Other times, she would ask him a question and then tap his hand when he did not respond. Usually, he would respond to that touch with a brief answer. Jan also used this technique with Lewis when he had trouble answering questions. She would ask him a question, look at him, and if he did not respond, she would tap his wrist and re-ask the question. Touch to elicit a response was used by CPs to facilitate interaction, which could lead to further connection between the partners.

Reminiscing. Another common relational maintenance behavior that occurred during the workshops was *reminiscing*. Reminiscing involved participants reflecting on their shared past either with their partner or other workshop participants. Reminiscing manifested in two ways: *to encourage conversation* and *to trigger a memory.*

To encourage conversation. Across both workshop cohorts, all twelve participants used reminiscing as a conversation starter. This behavior was most common among CPs and occurred both between dyads as they worked together as well as among the group of workshop participants. For example, Jan and Lewis talked about their lives together many times during the 2018 workshops. In one interaction, they talked about where they had traveled:

Jan: Does that remind you of anything? Where were we when we saw that?

Lewis: Uh, Africa.

Jan: Remember that special place that we went then?

Lewis: (nodded his head)

Jan: What does that remind you of? See anything so far? I've got a few pictures but I want you to choose some. Try and pick out some animals. Maybe some trips that we have been on. Some fishing, football.

Therapist: I am curious about your trip to Africa. Where did you go in Africa?

Lewis: Well we flew into South Africa.

Jan: No, we flew into Kenya first. Remember we flew in and did the safari first in Kenya because remember that was the year Obama got elected that year? We had signs in our car and people cheered as we were going through their town. Then where else did we go after that? Tanzania? And then what you said. What was the place you just said, the place you really liked?

Lewis: South Africa.

Jan: What did you like about South Africa? Do you remember?

Lewis: It was everything that I did not expect.

Jan: That's a good answer. It was a really big, beautiful city right?

The two then smiled at each other and continued looking through magazines. Although the conversation was short, the act of reflecting on past experiences in the unique setting of an arts workshop allowed for a conversation that later informed how Jan and Lewis designed their mask.

Another example of reminiscing and its important role in the arts workshops took place as Emily and Deb looked at the photographs they had decided to attach to their mask. When asked about one photo, Emily said:

Emily: That was when we moved to [location] in 1981 and we had the house built. Then we build the deck around it.

Therapist: So, you built the deck yourselves?

Emily: Yeah, we have developed decks on nearly every house we have had pretty much.

Deb: That's what we do.

Emily: We made a nice floor and a walk out dining room from our kitchen onto the porch too and uh the ceiling. We have done it all.

By talking about their lives together, Emily created conversation with Aaron and Louise. This created a welcoming and collaborative environment in the workshop where participants talked with one another or the therapist as they worked instead of sitting silently.

To trigger a memory. Reminiscing *to trigger a memory* worked as a way for all participants to gather inspiration for their mask. For example, early in the first workshop session, Jan asked Lewis several times what specific photographs reminded him of, and he would respond. In one instance, Jan asked Lewis what a specific photo looked like and he responded:

Jan: (pointing at photograph in magazine) What does that remind you of?

Lewis: [City Name].

> Jan: Yes! Good for you. Boy, that's a word you haven't said in a long time. We used to go fishing in [State]. Wow, that certainly brought up a memory.

Jan continued to tell the therapist that Lewis used to love to fish and be outdoors. Seeing this photograph clearly sparked a memory for both of them.

Sharon also used reminiscing to trigger a memory with her partner, Charles. Charles also enjoyed fishing, and Sharon made sure to choose photographs related to his hobbies and to where they used to live. She told Jessica and John, "I brought some photos and green tissue paper because he loved to fish and be outdoors since we lived up in the mountains for a long time." Emily and Deb also focused on reminiscing through their mask, as they used a photo collage from their lives as its main focus. As they selected photographs and attached them to the mask, Emily would ask Deb if she remembered certain aspects of her life as depicted in the photographs. Each of these examples illustrate the ways that reminiscing allowed participants with ADRD to briefly remember and discuss aspects of their lives with their care partner.

Positivity. Another relational maintenance behavior used by all participants was positivity. Positivity included the use of prosocial behaviors such as being upbeat, friendly, polite, and encouraging (Canary & Stafford, 2003b). Throughout the workshops, positivity took two distinct forms: *jokes to add levity* and *affirmations.*

Jokes to add levity. Participants enjoyed making jokes as they worked on their masks. For example, at one point, Bruce and Carol had the following exchange:

> Bruce: [pointing at a picture in a magazine] You ever think about crocheting these things?
>
> Carol: Well you can crochet . . .
>
> Bruce: [interrupting Carol] No I cannot!

Bruce's joke about being unable to crochet made both chuckle. When looking through magazines early in the process, Jan made a comment about liking a photo. Lewis then looked at the photo, smiled, and said it reminded him of something she liked to do. When Jan inquired about his comment, he responded, "Spend money." They both laughed in response. These short interactions were important to how the participants related to one another and allowed for levity and connection.

To affirm. Another way that participants communicated positivity was through *words of affirmation* specifically about their masks. Across all workshops, every participant talked about how they liked their mask and were having a nice time. Participants also made an effort to connect with others during the workshop. As participants arrived at each session, they would say hello to one another and to the therapist. Emily was particularly good at positivity. At one point, Aaron remarked:

Aaron: I just am not that creative.

Emily: I disagree, and I don't even know you! He could have fooled us, couldn't he, Deb?

Deb: Yes, he did!

In another example, John told Sharon and Charles that he liked their work. These words of affirmation created a welcoming environment where participants asked about and encouraged one another as they all worked on their masks.

Shared Tasks. Shared tasks included the equitable sharing of responsibility during workshop activities (Canary & Stafford, 2003b). Although CPs tended to do more work than the participants with ADRD, there were several instances where pairs shared tasks. Shared tasks took two forms: sharing tasks *to ideate* and *to assist.*

To ideate. Throughout the mask-making process, four of the six CPs asked their partner to help ideate. For example, Jan and Lewis worked together to discover inspiration for their mask through looking at photographs in magazines.

Jan: This is a pretty photo. We could do something with that.

Lewis: It is pretty.

Jan: It is a toucan. We could do a bird theme for our mask. Something about travel with bright colors and feathers.

Lewis: Okay.

While some participants could have come up with ideas for the mask on their own, sharing the task of ideation allowed for all to engage with the process and have a voice in what they created.

To assist. For all dyads, shared tasks arose from a need for the CP to help their loved one with ADRD with physical tasks. While *touch to assist* focused on the pair making physical contact, *sharing tasks to assist* meant doing tasks the person with ADRD could not do but did not include physical contact. For example, near the end of the mask making, Carol held Bruce's mask up as he walked around the room and examined his work. In another example, Jessica held John's mask in place so he could continue painting it without it wiggling on the table. Jan also took an active role in the mask-making process with Lewis as he had limited physical capabilities. For example, she would pour the paint for him since he could not lift the container himself. As all of the participants with ADRD suffered from cognitive and (in some cases) physical limitations, every care partner needed to assist at some point throughout the workshops. Through sharing tasks to *ideate* and *assist*, the CPs established a process of teamwork with their partners, allowing for extensive focus on the art-making process.

Networks. Networks as a relational maintenance behavior are typically understood as surrounding the relationships with family and friends who support the relationship (Canary & Stafford, 2003a; 2003b). For the purposes of this research, networks included each dyad's discussions about the relationship that they shared with their partner or others. Although the class did not get to meet extended family or friends (except for Aaron's daughter who accompanied him to one workshop), participants frequently discussed their loved ones. Thus, networks as relational maintenance presented in two ways: *network created by workshop participants* and *network created outside of workshop.*

Network created by workshop participants. All participants worked to create community within the workshops by talking to and asking questions about each other. A common manifestation of network creation included CPs offering each other information that might help them care for their partner with ADRD. For example, Jan told Carol about a ride share program. Additionally, Emily invited Louise and Aaron to come to another program she and Deb attended. Interactions like these highlighted how CPs could use the workshops as an opportunity to glean potentially important information from one another.

Participants also used conversation throughout the workshop to create a shared network. For example, John and Charles talked frequently about their shared interest in cars. Additionally, the 2018 group had a conversation about phone number area codes at one point. This conversation revealed personal information about each participant and where they lived or had lived previously. Through getting to know one another, participants created a network among themselves.

Networks created outside of workshop. While external network members did not attend the workshops, four of the six dyads talked about important people from their broader network. In many cases, participants talked about their children and how they looked forward to telling them about the mask-making experience. For example, members of the 2018 workshop cohort talked about their anticipation for sharing their creations with others:

Jan: We need to get a photograph of you [Lewis] with your mask so that I can send it to your kids. They would love to see this.

Lewis: Okay.

Carol: Bruce, do you want me to take a photo to send to [daughter's name]?

Bruce: Yeah, she would like that.

In this instance, both participant dyads wanted to share what they had done with their children. The inclusion of these external networks is important as it signals that the work created in the art workshops connected to the dyads' larger lives.

Openness. Openness is traditionally defined as discussions people have about their relationship (Canary & Stafford, 2003a; 2003b). In this research, openness was broadened to include present-focused self-disclosure. Four dyads used this relational maintenance behavior.

To disclose personal information. Throughout the workshops, several participants disclosed personal information to either their partner or, more often, to the larger group. Their disclosure was typically related to their mask, but also manifested in organic conversations. Four dyads disclosed personal information, talking about where they lived, the activities they enjoyed, how they were feeling, etc. Across both cohorts, Emily was the most open participant. At one point, she talked about how she and Deb lived by a reservoir in a house that they had built together. In the 2018 cohort, Jan was also very open, discussing her and Lewis' life. She talked about how they were retired, how they enjoyed being outdoors, and how Lewis liked to joke.

While most of the participants with ADRD did not self-disclose without prompting, rare instances of unprompted self-disclosure occurred. One notable instance came from Bruce after the therapist stated that she liked his sketch:

Therapist: Bruce, I love the shading you have done here.

Bruce: You want to know my secret? It is a technique called "the shakes" (laughs). My Parkinson's . . .

Therapist: Oh, well it looks good!

In this instance, he was making a joke (a form of positivity) about his tremors while also self-disclosing its cause.

Assurances. Assurances were the least common form of prosocial relational maintenance behaviors. Assurances include expressions of love that explicitly or implicitly indicate that the relationship has a future (Canary & Stafford, 2003b). Only three dyads explicitly discussed the future of their relationship through conversations about *how the mask could be used outside of the workshop.*

To emphasize how the mask can be used outside of the workshop. A few participants talked about how they would display the mask in their home. These instances functioned as assurances, because they showed that their mask would not go unappreciated. Jan and Lewis were the most vocal about how they would use their mask. Since they had based the mask on their life together, they both mentioned that they would display it in their house (where only Jan lives). In another instance, Bruce had run out of ideas for the mask, showing visible agitation. In response, Carol said:

> Carol: You don't have to do that right this minute, Bruce. I have hot glue at home.
>
> Bruce: Okay.

Later in the same workshop, Jan made a similar remark, mentioning, "We are thinking we might add some beads once we get home since we forgot them." These remarks emphasized the future of the relationship outside of the workshop and its continued existence, a unique form of assurance.

Avoidance. Although negative relational maintenance behaviors were not common during the workshops, two dyads used *avoidance*. Avoidance involved intentionally failing to address a conversation or task. Typically, avoidance appeared in two forms: *by being disengaged in conversation* and *by rejecting help.*

By being disengaged in conversation. At certain points in the workshop, some participants became disinterested in conversing. At one point, Bruce showed Carol a photo that he liked. Instead of responding, she simply looked back down at a magazine, and he went back to work. In this instance, she did not engage in conversation with her partner. A similar incident occurred between Sharon and Charles when he seemed uninterested in helping Sharon decorate the mask. While this could represent a larger problem he was having on this day, he was unable or unwilling to engage with his partner.

By rejecting help. Throughout the mask-making process, all of the CPs asked their loved ones if they needed help. While participants accepted help at times, two participants (Aaron and Bruce) preferred to work alone. Both Aaron and Bruce had higher levels of functioning than other participants, and each rejected help from their partners (Louise and Carol) several times during the workshops. They were not unkind in their rejection, but simply made it clear that they did not need or desire assistance.

Anti-social behaviors. At times, participants would use anti-social behavior that created distance between partners. While uncommon, this typically took the form of *making sarcastic comments to their partner.*

Making sarcastic comments to partner. Bruce and Carol were the only dyad who made sarcastic remarks to one another, though this happened several times over the course of the four weeks. One example took place when Carol asked Bruce for help. When he responded that he did not need help, she said "Okay. I'll shut up and leave you alone," with a sarcastic tone. Bruce did not acknowledge this remark and kept working, creating an environment where the two did not interact.

DISCUSSION

Alzheimer's disease and other related dementias (ADRD) are an increasing public health concern in the United States. While ample communication research illustrates the effects of ADRD on those diagnosed with the disease as well as their relationship partners, few studies have sought to understand how the use of relational maintenance behaviors influence the experiences of people with ADRD and their CPs. Additionally, very little research has explored how PCAE interventions might provide unique opportunities for relational maintenance among people with ADRD and their CPs. This research identified nine relational maintenance behaviors (*touch*, *reminiscing*, *positivity*, *shared tasks*, *networks*, *openness*, *assurances*, *avoidance*, and *anti-social behaviors*) that were used by interactants in a PCAE setting. These strategies represent both confirmation of existing relational maintenance typologies, while also adding to the literature by identifying new behaviors and the influence of participatory community arts engagement (PCAE) as a unique context for interaction.

Prosocial Relational Maintenance Behaviors. Results from the study showed that some relational maintenance behaviors appeared in interactions within the PCAE environment more frequently than others, and that the environment itself created unique opportunities for relational maintenance. For example, the process of making a mask was inevitably a *shared task* for most participants as they worked together on the project. Since they were engaged in a shared task, participants were required to communicate with each other. The PCAE environment differs from the household setting commonly associated with Canary and Stafford's (2003a, 2003b) relational maintenance typology. In the PCAE setting, participants were required to work on their mask, and the role of the CP was to assist their partner in the process. The fact that the space was not their own and the tasks went beyond household chores highlights the unique opportunities to invest in their relationship by engaging in PCAE together. In this context, PCAE worked to take participants out of their normal routine and asked them to do tasks that required both physical and mental concentration. As a dyad, the participants had to negotiate this process while also navigating each other's personal limitations.

The act of participating in the workshop created a *network* for participants where they could form new relationships and explore the challenges of managing ADRD. In alignment with previous research, much of the caretaking process involves patience and kindness toward a loved one suffering from ADRD (Hayes, Boylstein, & Zimmerman, 2009), and participants in this research used *positivity* to affirm and support their loved one. For example, when a participant with ADRD contributed their ideas to the mask, hearing that it looked good or being asked by others what it symbolized showed that their ideas were understood and respected by others. Since ADRD is associated with isolation of the person with dementia (Burgener et al., 2015), these positive remarks and the creation of networks may serve as a piece of temporary reprieve from isolation as they deal with the effects of their illness.

Although less prevalent, participants also used *assurances*, *openness*, *avoidance*, and *anti-social behaviors* to maintain their relationship during the art workshops. The fact that these behaviors appeared less frequently is important as it better explains the role of CPs in the art-making process and the influence of ADRD on a dyad's ability to complete the mask. According to Canary and Stafford (2003a, 2003b), *assurances* aim to affirm to a loved one that the relationship has a future. Though people with ADRD can live for years past their initial diagnosis, there is no cure for the disease (Ferri et al., 2005). This creates a unique tension, as talking about the future can be difficult for loved ones of those with ADRD since they often experience uncertainty regarding the illness and the person's life expectancy (Hellström & Torres, 2016). Instead, Ingrid Hellström and Sandra Torres (2016) argue that loved ones focus on the present or the past challenges they have already overcome instead of on the future. When exploring the use and effects of assurances in this PCAE context, it is important to note that the same conditions that encouraged positivity and shared tasks might have limited the communication of assurances given the future's charged and uncertain status among CPs and adults with ADRD.

The use of *openness* in the workshops was interesting, as some participants disclosed a great deal whereas others did not. Previous research highlights social isolation as one of the main issues associated with ADRD (Burgener et al., 2015). Given that self-disclosure and openness are essential relational building blocks (Altman & Taylor, 1973), it stands to reason that people would use openness during PCAE to potentially create new relationships. However, research also notes the uncertainty and vulnerability associated with ADRD, particularly as it relates to feeling stigmatized (Stone & Jones, 2009). If a person fears being stigmatized, they might choose to withhold openness in an act of self-defense both for themselves and for their partner. Additionally, participants might refrain from openness because of the pressure to reciprocate associated with self-disclosure (Perion & Steiner, 2017). For those who may already feel isolated, both self-disclosing and reciprocating disclosures could cause undue stress (Stone, 2013). This presents a challenging dynamic for participants in that the behaviors needed to form new relationships and combat isolation (openness and self-disclosure) might feel too risky for those with ADRD and their CPs. Future research should explore how small adjustments to the PCAE experience, such as asking participants to share their approach toward mask-making, might help them overcome barriers to openness and create greater potential for relationship-building.

Anti-Social Relational Maintenance Behaviors. Given the collaborative nature of the art workshops, the lack of negative relational maintenance behaviors is consistent with social norms, which generally dictate that people act politely toward one another (Griffin, Ledbetter, & Sparks, 2014). When participants did engage in anti-social behaviors, it was only with their partner and not with other participants in the PCAE workshops. While these terse comments or moments of avoidance temporarily changed the collaborative dynamics between dyads, these behaviors did not create tension among the larger group. It was as though CPs knew that their partner needed to do some actions alone to assert some measure of independence during a time in life when that independence might feel like it is slipping away (Camic, Tischler, & Pearman, 2014). Future research should explore how anti-social relational maintenance behaviors might be associated with desires for independence as well as with the circumstances that might help these behaviors promote the relationship (as was possible during the PCAE workshops) rather than detracting from it.

New Relational Maintenance Behaviors. Previous relational maintenance typologies did not fully capture all of the behaviors present in the PCAE workshops. As such, we outlined two additional relational maintenance behaviors: *touch* and *reminiscing. Touch* highlights the importance of nonverbal communication for those with ADRD (Gleeson & Timmins, 2004). Touch was particularly salient given that ADRD is associated with loss of language and limited communication (Stone, 2013). As a result, nonverbal communication becomes essential for people with ADRD and their families (Gleeson & Timmins, 2004). The importance of touch also underscores the value of PCAE for adults with ADRD, as these workshops create space for CPs and adults with ADRD to incorporate new forms of touch to maintain their relationship and accomplish tangible tasks together. The prevalence of touch also highlights how CPs intentionally seek new ways to connect with their partners with ADRD, demonstrating their commitment to relational maintenance in the face of challenges.

Similarly, *reminiscing* was prevalent in the workshops, yet it did not fit neatly into the original relational maintenance typology. On the one hand, *assurances* look toward the future of the relationship, which can be difficult for couples dealing with the uncertain future of ADRD. Reminiscing, on the other hand, could fill the gap in relational maintenance behaviors. Reminiscing has been found to decrease caregiver burden and increase the person with ADRD's perception of being loved (Fletcher & Eckberg, 2014). Previous research also supports that reminiscing connects CPs and adults with ADRD to one another in profound ways not accomplished through future visioning (Astell et al., 2010; Fletcher & Eckberg, 2014). Including reminiscing as a form of relational maintenance is essential within the context of ADRD, and future research should continue to explore how PCAE can facilitate reminiscing in ways not experienced in normal day-to-day routines, and how this form of relational maintenance can strengthen the relationship between CPs and adults with ADRD.

Retention of Relational Maintenance Behaviors. In general, the results from this research highlight that people maintain their relationships regardless of their cognitive capacity. Even the participants with the most limited communication abilities demonstrated relational maintenance through their interactions. For example, Lewis, who suffered severe language deficits, was able to use the PCAE context to ideate and reminisce with his wife, to offer positivity to others, and to share mask-making tasks with his partner. This is particularly striking given that loved ones of people with ADRD often express concerns about communication barriers resulting from the disease (Stone, 2013). For CPs, these results offer insight into how communication with a loved one with ADRD can change but also how this communication can still be meaningful and relationship enhancing.

Arts Engagement as a Unique Context

Aside from the known benefits of PCAE, creating art as therapy is a unique experience for people with ADRD given the mix of both cognitive and physical stimulation inherent in the activities (Camic, Tischler, & Pearman, 2014). PCAE requires a person with ADRD to plan and to develop ideas for their art in addition to physically creating a final product. This is important as it engages several skill sets that ADRD may threaten or diminish. In this research, the physical creation of the mask served as a way for participants to process their feelings, engage in different movement, and connect with others (Stone, 2013). Importantly, this context also presented unique and meaningful opportunities for relational maintenance. The prevalence of relational maintenance strategies such as positivity, touch, reminiscing, and sharing tasks illustrate how PCAE can help CPs and adults with ADRD explore and maintain their relationship in ways that might not present themselves in everyday interactions.

Limitations and Future Directions

Although this research provides important considerations regarding the capacity of PCAE to facilitate relational maintenance behaviors, it is not without limitations. First, it is important to note that this study included a small number of participants. Throughout the two different cohorts, only three dyads attended every session. Two dyads only attended the first workshop session and a third dyad attended all four workshop sessions, though both participants were not present at every session. Though this methodological approach provided an in-depth look at the experience of CPs and adults with ADRD, it merely touches on the surface of the issue. Future research should look to explore the impact of PCAE among larger, more diverse cohorts.

Another important limitation of this research was the fact that all of the CPs were women, and only one of the participants with ADRD was a woman. This is particularly interesting given that two thirds of people living with ADRD are women (Alzheimer's Association, "Women and Alzheimer's," n.d.). While it is also true that more than 60% of ADRD caregivers are also women (Alzheimer's Association, "Women and Alzheimer's," n.d.), the fact that no male CPs participated in this research might limit its findings, as the way that men and women use relational maintenance might differ (Ragsdale, 1996). To address this disparity, programming changes might be necessary to better engage male CPs. Since men are less likely to access social support programs (Doward, 2016), programmers might consider creating workshops specifically targeting male CPs.

CONCLUSION

When beginning this research, we sought to better understand the utility of PCAE among CPs and adults diagnosed with ADRD. While only the first step in this process, the observations of and interactions with participants have highlighted both when PCAE is fruitful and where it can be limiting for CPs and adults with ADRD. As the prevalence of life-altering illnesses like ADRD continues to rise, research examining experiences related to enriching activities like PCAE can help us understand and manage some of the negative effects of these illnesses on relationships and communication.

NOTE

1. We would like to thank and recognize the following individuals for their contributions to this research: Beth Gherardi, Education and Outreach Coordinator for the Fort Collins Museum

of Art; Alison Cope, occupational therapist; Lisa Hatchadoorian, Executive Director of the Fort Collins Museum of Art; Sarah Harlow, Home Instead; Cyndy Luzinski, Dementia Friendly Communities; Angel Hoffman, Banner Health; and Dawn Paepke, Kaiser Permanente. This research was supported by Colorado State University's Office of the Vice President for Research Catalyst for Innovative Partnerships Program. The content is solely the responsibility of the authors and does not necessarily represent the official views of the Office of the Vice President for Research.

REFERENCES

Altman, I., & Taylor, D. A. (1973). *Social penetration: The development of interpersonal relationships.* New York, NY: Holt, Rinehart, & Winston.

Alzheimer's Association. (n.d.). Women and Alzheimer's. Retrieved May 14, 2019, from https://alz.org/alzheimers-dementia/what-is-alzheimers/women-and-alzheimer-s

Alzheimer's Association. (2019). What is Alzheimer's disease? Retrieved from https://alz.org/alzheimers-dementia/what-is-alzheimers

Astell, A. J., Ellis, M. P., Alm, N., Dye, R., & Gowans, G. (2010). Stimulating people with dementia to reminisce using personal and generic photographs. *International Journal of Computers in Healthcare*, *1*(2), 177–198. https://doi.org/10.1504/IJCIH.2010.037461

Basting, A. D. (2006). Arts in dementia care: "This is not the end . . . it's the end of this chapter." *Generations*, *30*(1), 16–20. https://www.ingentaconnect.com/content/asag/gen/2006/00000030/00000001/art00004

Beard, R. L. (2012). Art therapies and dementia care: A systematic review. *Dementia*, *11*(5), 633–656. https://doi.org/10.1177%2F1471301211421090

Braun, V., & Clarke, V. (2006). Using thematic analysis in psychology. *Qualitative Research in Psychology*, *3*(2), 77–101. http://dx.doi.org/10.1191/1478088706qp063oa

Brookmeyer, R., Johnson, E., Ziegler-Graham, K., & Arrighi, H. M. (2007). Forecasting the global burden of Alzheimer's disease. *Alzheimer's & Dementia*, *3*(3), 186–191. https://doi.org/10.1016/j.jalz.2007.04.381

Burgener, S. C., Buckwalter, K., Perkhounkova, Y., & Liu, M. F. (2015). The effects of perceived stigma on quality of life outcomes in persons with early-stage dementia: Longitudinal findings: Part 2. *Dementia*, *14*(5), 609–632. https://doi.org/10.1177/1471301213504202

Butcher, H. K., Holkup, P. A., & Buckwalter, K. C. (2001). The experience of caring for a family member with Alzheimer's disease. *Western Journal of Nursing Research*, *23*(1), 33–55. https://doi.org/10.1177/019394590102300104

Camic, P. M., & Chatterjee, H. J. (2013). Museums and art galleries as partners for public health interventions. *Perspectives in Public Health*, *133*(1), 66–71. https://doi.org/10.1177/1757913912468523

Camic, P. M., Tischler, V., & Pearman, C. H. (2014). Viewing and making art together: A multi-session art-gallery-based intervention for people with dementia and their careers. *Aging & Mental Health*, *18*(2), 161–168. https://doi.org/10.1080/13607863.2013.818101

Canary, D. J., & Stafford, L. (Eds.). (2003a). *Communication and relational maintenance* (1st ed.). Bingley, UK: Emerald Group Publishing.

Canary, D. J., & Stafford, L. (2003b). Maintaining relationships through strategic and routine interaction. In D. Canary & L. Stafford (Eds.), *Communication and relational maintenance* (1st ed., pp. 3–22). Bingley: Emerald Group Publishing Limited.

Centers for Disease Control and Prevention (CDC). (2019). Alzheimer's disease and healthy aging. Retrieved from https://www.cdc.gov/aging/aginginfo/alzheimers.htm

Chancellor, B., Duncan, A., & Chatterjee, A. (2014). Art therapy for Alzheimer's disease and other dementias. *Journal of Alzheimer's Disease*, *39*(1), 1–11. https://doi.org/10.3233/JAD-131295

Clair, A. A. (2002). The effects of music therapy on engagement in family caregiver and care receiver couples with dementia. *American Journal of Alzheimer's Disease & Other Dementias*, *17*(5), 286–290. https://doi.org/10.1177/153331750201700505

Corbeil, R. R., Quayhagen, M. P., & Quayhagen, M. (1999). Intervention effects on dementia caregiving interaction: A stress-adaptation modeling approach. *Journal of Aging and Health*, *11*(1), 79–95. https://doi.org/10.1177/089826439901100105

DiLauro, M., Pereira, A., Carr, J., Chiu, M., & Wesson, V. (2017). Spousal caregivers and persons with dementia: Increasing participation in shared leisure activities among hospital-based dementia support program participants. *Dementia*, *16*(1), 9–28. https://doi.org/10.1177/1471301215570680

Doward, J. (2016, November 5). Men much less likely to seek mental health help than women. *Observer*. Retrieved from https://www.theguardian.com/society/2016/nov/05/men-less-likely-to-get-help--mental-health

Duck, S. (1988). *Relating to others*. Chicago, IL: Dorsey Press.

Ferri, C. P., Prince, M., Brayne, C., Brodaty, H., Fratiglioni, L., Ganguli, M., . . . Alzheimer's Disease International. (2005). Global prevalence of dementia: A Delphi consensus study. *Lancet*, *366*(9503), 2112–2117. https://doi.org/10.1016/S0140–6736(05)67889–0

Flatt, J. D., Liptak, A., Oakley, M. A., Gogan, J., Varner, T., & Lingler, J. H. (2015). Subjective experiences of an art museum engagement activity for persons with early-stage Alzheimer's disease and their family caregivers. *American Journal of Alzheimer's Disease & Other Dementiasr*, *30*(4), 380–389. https://doi.org/10.1177/1533317514549953

Fletcher, T. S., & Eckberg, J. D. (2014). The effects of creative reminiscing on individuals with dementia and their caregivers: A pilot study. *Physical & Occupational Therapy In Geriatrics*, *32*(1), 68–84. https://doi.org/10.3109/02703181.2014.880863

Glaser, B. G., & Strauss, A. L. (1967). *The discovery of grounded theory : Strategies for qualitative research*. Hawthorne, NY: Aldine de Gruyter.

Gleeson, M., & Timmins, F. (2004). Touch: A fundamental aspect of communication with older people experiencing dementia. *Nursing Older People*, *16*(2), 18–21. https://doi.org/10.7748/nop2004.04.16.2.18.c2302

Goodboy, A. K., Dainton, M., Borzea, D., & Goldman, Z. W. (2017). Attachment and negative relational maintenance: Dyadic comparisons using an actor-partner interdependence model. *Western Journal of Communication*, *81*(5), 541–559. https://doi.org/10.1080/10570314.2017.1302601

Greene, J. O. (1984). A cognitive approach to human communications: An action assembly theory. *Communication Monographs*, *51*(4), 289–306. https://doi.org/10.1080/03637758409390203

Griffin, E., Ledbetter, A., & Sparks, G. (2014). *A first look at communication theory* (9th ed.). New York, NY: McGraw-Hill.

Hayes, J., Boylstein, C., & Zimmerman, M. K. (2009). Living and loving with dementia: Negotiating spousal and caregiver identity through narrative. *Journal of Aging Studies*, *23*(1), 48–59. https://doi.org/10.1016/j.jaging.2007.09.002

Hellström, I., & Torres, S. (2016). The "not yet" horizon: Understandings of the future amongst couples living with dementia. *Dementia*, *15*(6), 1562–1585. https://doi.org/10.1177/1471301214565673

Johnson, C. M., & Sullivan-Marx, E. M. (2006). Art therapy: Using the creative process for healing and hope among African American older adults. *Geriatric Nursing*, *27*(5), 309–316. https://doi.org/10.1016/j.gerinurse.2006.08.010

Lindlof, T. R., & Taylor, B. C. (2011). *Qualitative communication research methods* (3rd ed.). Thousand Oaks, CA: Sage Publications.

National Institute on Aging. (2019). Alzheimer's disease fact sheet. *NIH.gov*. Retrieved from https://www.nia.nih.gov/health/alzheimers-disease-fact-sheet

Owen, W. F. (1984). Interpretive themes in relational Communication. *Quarterly Journal of Speech*, *70*(3), 274–287. https://doi.org/10.1080/00335638409383697

Perion, J., & Steiner, V. (2017). Perceptions of reciprocity in friendship by community dwelling people with mild to moderate dementia. *Dementia*, *18*(6), 2107–2121. https://doi.org/10.1177/1471301217742503

Ragsdale, J. D. (1996). Gender, satisfaction level, and the use of relational maintenance strategies in marriage. *Communication Monographs*, *63*(4), 354–369. https://doi.org/10.1080/03637759609376399

Schneider, J. (2018). The arts as a medium for care and self-care in dementia: Arguments and evidence. *International Journal of Environmental Research and Public Health*, *15*(6), 1151–1162. https://doi.org/10.3390/ijerph15061151

Stone, A. M. (2013). Dilemmas of communicating about Alzheimer's disease: Professional caregivers, social support, and illness uncertainty. *Journal of Applied Communication Research*, *41*(1), 1–17. https://doi.org/10.1080/00909882.2012.738426

Stone, A. M., & Jones, C. L. (2009). Sources of uncertainty: Experiences of Alzheimer's disease. *Issues in Mental Health Nursing*, *30*(11), 677–686. https://doi.org/10.1080/01612840903046354

Weigel, D. J., & Ballard-Reisch, D. S. (2001). The impact of relational maintenance behaviors on marital satisfaction: A longitudinal analysis. *Journal of Family Communication*, *1*(4), 265–279. https://doi.org/10.1207/S15327698JFC0104_03

Chapter Eleven

Storying Clinical Interactions

Narrative Medicine as an Artistic Intervention in Medical Training and Education

Elizabeth Spradley

> I try to talk to them, I try to understand like the nurses do, like the psychiatrists do, but I can't. I can't understand the shattered minds, the broken spirits, the mix of fantasy and reality. I don't know what to say, how to react. I ask questions, probing for rationality and so often find none. I struggle to find the humanity here. I want so badly to connect with these patients, to know their worlds and navigate through them. Although I'm ashamed to admit it, most days I just see animals . . . restless, prowling, lurking, and sulking. I fail again and again to relate. I sympathize, but I cannot find empathy. I wonder if this rotation is bound to be a failure for me. If I memorize the side effect profiles of antipsychotics but cannot find the humanity in those taking them, what will I have accomplished? (Fyfe, 2017, p. 2)

This excerpt is taken from a piece in the medical humanities journal *Intima: A Journal of Narrative Medicine* and demonstrates retrospective sensemaking of the author's rotation as a medical student in a psychiatric hospital. To begin with this story and lingering question is to foreground the role of narrating clinical experiences in medical training and education. Storying clinical experiences is the act of narrating lived experience from clinical rotations, whether as healthcare providers or as students. Narrative medicine embodies the storying of clinical experiences, as the practice of narrative medicine requires the enactment of communication skills as both a storyteller and an audience member. At its inception, narrative medicine strove to "recognize patients' lived experiences," understanding that in doing so medical practitioners would become increasingly aware of their own roles in their patients' stories (Charon & Hermann, 2012, p. 2). Narrative medicine has a short but rich history in medical education in the United States, resulting in pockets of educators promoting storytelling through written reflection and patient-provider interaction.

With the emphasis on patient-provider interactions, a lingering question remains to be fully explored with regard to how narrative medical practices can be integrated in medical education as an interventional strategy to promote a storytelling community for the well-being of the student-practitioner in provider-provider interactions? This chapter explores narrative medicine, its practices, and its influence on medical training and education, and argues that narrative medical practices should be more fully developed to generate storytelling communities for the enhancement of both provider-provider and patient-provider relationships. To investigate how such a community can be constructed, this chapter analyzes stories submitted and published in the medical humanities journal *Intima* that engage in clinical storytelling. Analysis considers the functionality of storying clinical experiences and how such functions could be realized through oral and written storytelling in clinical practice. Now, attention turns to the literature in narrative medicine and health communication that has advanced narrative medical practices.

NARRATIVE MEDICINE

> Narrative medicine reminds us that illness unfolds in stories, that our bodies, being more than machines or vehicles, live through our lives with us, perform our lives, carry our scars, our bliss, and our memories, simultaneously both limiting and expanding our lives. Narrative medicine recognizes that the central events of health care are the giving and receiving of accounts of self. (Charon, 2009, p. 120)

Narrative medicine could be reduced to a definition that simply argues health is storied—*the giving and receiving of accounts of self.* But to do so would eschew the nuanced ways in which story is experienced, performed/communicated, elicited, and interpreted as well as the rich literature that has shaped narrative practices that have, in turn, shaped patients' and providers' lives, and even deaths. Rita Charon's (2006) work with narrative medical practices from the classroom to the hospital room have challenged the traditional epistemology of the biomedical model and the provider-patient communication patterns that support it.

Narrative Medicine's Narrative Framework

The narrative medicine model is best understood in relation to its (1) narrative framework and (2) narrative practices. In an article in the *Journal of the American Medical Association*, Charon (2001) articulated a model of narrative medicine that challenged taken-for-granted epistemologies that valued science over lived experiences of patients and their clinicians. This article integrated concepts and practices from influential scholars and medical practitioners, as well as clarified an approach to medicine with which Charon has largely been credited. Her narrative framework channels Aristotle's notion of *phronesis*, a type of lived-in or experiential wisdom (Charon & Wyer, 2008). Explaining the rationale for a narrative framework, Rita Charon and Peter Wyer (2008) write,

> Whether the issue arises from the laboratory, the clinic, or the polis, we do not serve ourselves or our patients well by underestimating their complexity. To face them fully, one needs at one's disposal a way of knowing that exceeds the technical or the theoretical, that is equipped to absorb and comprehend the situated, unruly, contradictory, meaning-saturated levels of experience. One needs charts and soundings to navigate fraught channels, but only the seasoned river pilot has the lived-in wisdom to find the way safely through. Aristotle calls this kind of wisdom *phronesis* while philosophers and clinicians call it narrative knowledge or reflective practice-it is a way of knowing that recognises the known/knowable, the unknown/unknowable, the universal, the particular, the body, and the self. (Charon & Wyer, 2008, p. 296; italics in the original)

In other words, narrative medicine values a plurality of ways of knowing—science-based evidence through diagnostic testing and the lived experience of patients and clinicians. Thus, what constitutes valuable information from a narrative framework includes the patient's story.

Narrative Medicine's Narrative Practices

At its core, narrative medical practices hinge on narrative competence, which Charon (2001) defines as "the competence that human beings use to absorb, interpret, and respond to stories" (p. 1897). Over time, Charon and colleagues have expounded on specific communicative competencies that constitute narrative competence in healthcare relationships, including: eliciting narratives, close reading, and medical charting. The first two competencies relate to attention, whereas the last competency relates to representation (Charon, 2005). First, to elicit narratives is to invite storytelling. While eliciting a medical history is a familiar set of skills taught in medical education (Kalitzkus & Matthiessen, 2009), eliciting a patient's story requires an invitation and attentiveness. Charon (2005) explains how she elicits patients' stories:

> I find that I have changed my routines on meeting with new patients. I simply say, "I'm going to be your doctor. I need to know a lot about your body and

> your health and your life. Please tell me what you think I should know about your situation." (Charon, 2005, p. 264)

This open-ended invitation permits the patient to construct a narrative of relevant stories that contextualize the patient's symptoms. Then, practitioners from a narrative medicine framework must make sense of the narratives shared with them, but to do so requires attentiveness as an audience member. Second, close reading of narratives implies a particular kind of listening that guides narrative interpretation. To know how a practitioner attentively listens to a patient's narrative, Charon (2005) recounts her own listening practices:

> I sit on my hands so as not to write or reflexively call up their medical record on the computer. I sit and pay attention to what they say and how they say it: the forms, the metaphors, the gaps and silences. Where will be the beginning? How will symptoms intercalate with life events? I listen, not with Freudian or Lacanian or gestalt frameworks of meaning-making, but with narratological ones. (Charon, 2005, p. 264)

Third, narrative competence results in a medical chart that reflects a narrative framework and represents the patient's narrative. The narrative medical chart parallels a traditional chart to include the clinician's reflection and representation of the patient's narrative, but it may also contain additional narrative components, such as mementos or pictures, that help construct—even if only a fragmented version of—the patient's narrative. Health communication scholar Lynn M. Harter's (2009) work with pediatric oncologists at MD Anderson demonstrates the interpenetrating narratives of patient, patient's family, and provider in charts that contain pictures. The narrative chapter in *The Routledge Handbook of Health Communication* also illustrates how a pediatric cancer patient and her family contributed to and, in part, curated the patient's chart through scrapbooking (Sharf et al., 2011). To better illustrate how a narrative medical chart may read, here is an excerpt from a clinician's note regarding a 52-year-old male stroke patient. Charon (2005) wrote this about her patient: "Man of tremendous courage. Last year, was in good health, worked full-time in the post office, played soccer, met his friends to play dominos, enjoyed life" (p. 264). She goes on to record details of his stroke and its long-term effects on his abilities, but she also includes his current emotional reactions to loss of ability and reactions to familial relationships, saying, "His wife and sons are still at home, but is very difficult for them all. This has been a horrible ordeal for the whole family. The patient feels all his losses. He sometimes feels pitied by his wife" (p. 265). Then, Charon (2005) explains that she reads the note to the patient and provides the patient a copy so that he not only knows how she is representing him in his chart but also so that he can be the curator of his own patient narrative. Through the attentiveness and representation narrative competencies, Charon

(2005) argues that affiliation develops and deepens between patient and provider.

Charon and colleagues have advanced the framework and practices of narrative medicine so as to influence medical education and training programs to include electives in narrative medicine, and medical humanities programs have emerged that weave narrative medicine into their curriculum. Such courses and programs can be self-selected by interested students, but they are typically not mandatory for healthcare practitioners (Arntfield et al., 2013). Given these advances, there are pockets of research that have suggested that narrative medicine has value beyond the patient-provider relationship and is also beneficial to the relationships between providers. From this rich literature expounding on the theoretical framework and practice of narrative medicine, a number of lines of inquiry remain underdeveloped in terms of the value of storying clinical encounters and the nuanced ways to implement storytelling in medical practice for varied purposes, including educational interventions for student-practitioner well-being. Consider how explorations of the following research questions would contribute to the current body of literature on narrative medicine.

> RQ1: In what ways does clinical storytelling benefit the storyteller?
>
> RQ2: How do sharing these stories construct a storytelling medical community?
>
> RQ3: How can storytelling be woven into medical training as a way to develop storytelling practices for long-term use for patient-provider and provider-provider communication?

This chapter begins to answer these questions by analyzing published stories of clinical interactions and the storytellers' motives for engaging in storytelling. If we can learn more about why people share stories from clinical experiences, we can begin to shape storytelling practices in medical education and training to capitalize on these motivations.

NARRATIVE METHODS OF DATA COLLECTION AND ANALYSIS: TOWARD AN UNDERSTANDING OF NARRATIVE FUNCTION

Narrative function is revealed as storytellers recount events, characters, and scenes in their discourse. To clarify how terms are used in subsequent sections, this section offers definitions for story and for narrative. While scholars define (when they decide to differentiate story and narrative at all) story and narrative differently, this study assumes a delineation similar to Linda C.

Garro and Cheryl Mattingly's (2000) description of story and of narrative. Story is a term delineating action or sequencing of events in situ, whereas narrative is a term delineating the discursive act of communicating a story. Thus, for stories to become narratives, a storyteller is needed to discursively recount a story to an audience. This chapter is primarily interested in the functionality of clinical stories as revealed through published narratives circulated among an audience of other health practitioners.

In a similar way as Barbara F. Sharf and Marsha L. Vanderford (2003) set out to delineate the functions of illness narration (which included sense-making, asserting control, transforming identity, warranting decisions, and building community), this study delineates the functions of clinical storytelling by analyzing published narratives about clinical interactions and experiences. The interdisciplinary medical humanities journal *Intima* is a site *par excellence* to collect stories of clinical encounters. Published semiannually since 2011, *Intima* publishes art, multi-media art, poetry, fiction, non-fiction, field notes, and academic works aimed at "promoting the theory and practice of Narrative Medicine, an interdisciplinary field that enhances healthcare through the effective communication and understanding between caregivers and patients" (*Intima*, 2019, para. 1). The journal's audience varies, but is comprised primarily of medical students, medical humanities students, and healthcare practitioners ranging from medical doctors, nurses, clinical psychologists, and physical and occupational therapists. Since its inception through Columbia's Master of Science program in Narrative Medicine, *Intima* has published a total of 270 narratives in the submission categories of Non-fiction and Field Notes that chronicle clinical encounters and present patient-provider interactions. These narratives reveal how storytelling functions from the perspective of the narrator/author, who tends to be a medical student, healthcare practitioner, or patient, with the majority of authors in the category of medical student or healthcare practitioner. For this chapter, all 165 narratives from Non-fiction and 105 narratives from Field Notes categories over an eight-year span were collected, coded, and analyzed.

While there are different approaches to narrative analysis (see Riessman, 2008), the approach applied in this study was to examine each of the narratives thematically. To begin, stories were coded designating narrative components consistent with Deanna D. Sellnow's (2018) instruction on examining the text: narrator, characters, plot/events, scene, temporal relations, causal relations, audience, motive, and moral. Like other forms of thematic coding (see Charmaz's work with constructivist grounded theory in 2000, 2005, and 2006), early stages of narrative coding resembled an open and iterative practice, in which I went back and forth between the narratives and codes, refining the codes with each iteration. This open and iterative process allowed me to see how narrative components were emphasized and placed in relation to one another, thus determining emergent thematic narrative functions. Themes were related to narrative function, specifically as the narrator was emphasized and as the motive and moral were either implicitly or explicitly narrated. Across the 270 total stories, the predominant themes of clinical storytelling were identity management, resistance, reflection, practice, therapy, and community.

FINDINGS ON NARRATIVE FUNCTION IN CLINICAL STORYTELLING

Identity Management

To begin, the identity management function of clinical storytelling was evident in each of the 270 coded stories in varying degrees with different identity management themes. In one sense, all storytelling performances construct characterizations of the actors (including the narrator) that function to manage identity, which is loosely defined as the public performance of self (Goffman, 1978). The stories in *Intima* explored identity struggles and role conflict, as well as asserted particular identities such as the "good" doctor, the "bilingual" doctor, the "faithful" nurse, and the "hardworking" medical student. In this section, the focus turns to the storied identity struggles voiced by narrators as they recall their clinical experiences. Identity struggles varied based on narrators, scenes, and other characters, but one particular thematic struggle that threaded through pieces was a *struggle of becoming but not yet there*. *Intima* authors narrated concerns that they felt as if they would be competent, prepared, and experienced medical practitioners one day, but that day was a future projection of themselves. The *becoming* identity management function theme harkens to sociologist Arthur W. Frank's notion of *becoming* with one major distinction. Frank (1995) foregrounds the role of the patient as storyteller narrating their illness stories, thus (re)shaping their identity in relation to their illness, and the medical practitioners narrating their clinical experiences in the pages of *Intima* are (re)shaping their professional identities in relation to their patients and other medical professionals.

Becoming is voiced in a plurality of ways, with linguistic indicators like *acting*, *imposter*, *charlatan*, and *evolution*. To illustrate, one *Intima* contributor writes, "I didn't feel like it or look it, but I was ready to keep acting the part of a doctor and mother until I became real at each one" (McManus, 2019, para. 32). This contributor and others voice the liminality of medical education for the practitioner as the *in between* period. In the liminal *in between period*, she does not feel that she has fully embodied the professional self that she must perform in her rounds.

> Medical school has a way of making one feel like a charlatan. Often, standing before a patient as part of a healthcare team, the medical student is the only

> one wearing a white coat, often the only one taking extensive notes, and nevertheless amusingly the least useful person in the room. . . . At least for the first two years, going to the clinic feels like some kind of a theatre production, memorizing lines and trying to look convincing to patients who may themselves be acting for the purposes of our education. (Jayanti, 2017, para. 1)

For this author, even wearing the white coat symbolizes an identity as a medical "charlatan," but for others, the length of the white coat gives them away. Wearing the white coat symbolizes medical authority, but the length of the white coat symbolizes a class of medical practitioner. Most medical students' white coats are shorter, reminding them of the liminality of their professional selves while in medical school and residency. In her own struggle with the length of her white coat and uncertainty of self in a neurology rotation, one author writes, "It was being there, within arm's reach, ready to embrace my own need to protect and comfort my patient that put me on the road from 'doctorsita' to 'Doctor'" (Bracho-Sanchez, 2015, para. 8). In another piece, the narrator uses a mixed metaphor of metamorphosis and aliens to describe the struggle of becoming a medical practitioner but not having arrived.

> As I observe, I see that Residency is a bit of a metamorphosis—violent stretching, yanking mutation of humans into aliens. It is not a pretty process. But in many ways it speaks to the resiliency of these beings. Placed in extreme conditions—they adapt and evolve. (Little, 2014, para. 2)

Becoming a medical practitioner is fraught with identity struggles, wrestling with the occupational identity that one must assume in clinical rotations yet knowing that one has not been credentialed or experienced. Storying clinicals functions as a means to explore and voice these identity struggles with others that may share them.

Resistance Function

Second, narrators used their stories to resist taken-for-granted meanings and practices embedded in the practice of medicine. While scant examples of this theme appeared explicitly in the stories of non-fiction and field notes, examples appeared nonetheless and demonstrated that a valuable function of clinical storytelling includes voicing resistance. In one case, a family medicine doctor in a hospital describes "exhaling [her] judgment in the space between" her and a patient, whom the charge nurse had just reported confiscating a crack pipe from (Scott, 2019, para. 49). Defying the charge nurse's insistence that the patient had decisional capacity to discharge herself, the narrator questions the decision capacity and the wisdom of a nurse with over twenty years of experience juxtaposed to her two years of experience as a doctor.

Similarly questioning, and ultimately defying, medical practices, a recently credentialed psychiatric nurse is faced with a dilemma. She narrates her encounter with a young, pregnant cocaine addict, writing, "I am not supposed to care so much about her. My case manager and I try to get her into an inpatient rehab, but they won't accept crack. Only alcohol. I lie" (Gabby, 2015, para. 5). Questioning authority, challenging traditions, and offering alternative practices are not typically associated with practicing medicine, especially if that practitioner is inexperienced or still a student. Storying resistance enables the narrator to explain and justify resistance, as well as to provide perspective on the outcome of the resistance.

Reflexive Function

Third, narrators embraced self-awareness, reflexively exploring their roles and the meanings of their stories. Narrative medicine has lauded self-awareness in medical practice, as storytelling unlocks the potential for practitioners not only to better understand and relate to their patients but also to understand and relate to oneself.

> Reflection can be understood to be an active interior state that uses cognitive, affective, imaginative, and creative means to perceive, represent in language, and thereby undergo one's lived experience. . . . The reflecting self is one with the attentive self, the present self, the feeling self, the self with the sense of story. (Charon & Hermann, 2012, p. 3)

Putting to pen their reflections, one particular theme stood out within the reflexive function of clinical storytelling—humanizing. Self-aware of tendencies to grow callous or treat patients as their symptoms, pieces in *Intima* demonstrated narrators' reflexive concerns with humanizing themselves and their patients. For example, a doctor recalls her interactions with a *non-compliant* patient needing an amputation for a neglected infection in the left leg: "A little peppermint oil helped me find the person underneath the pathology. It helped me remember the vulnerability that unites all of us" (Bruckner, 2019, para. 20). Peppermint oil masked the odor and facilitated a humanizing effect that the doctor described in relation to the patient's *non-compliance*, but the writing of the story also helped the doctor be more reflexive about her own humanity.

> I've felt frustrated when patients damage their health through neglect or denial, but then I remember all the times I wished I could just forget my cancer for a while. I've been annoyed when someone won't take the medication I prescribe, yet I remember when I skipped days of my own pills. I've resented patients for not being thankful or kind, but then I remember when my own fear, anger, or pain took precedence over any gratitude I felt toward my doctors. (Bruckner, 2019, para. 19)

Humanizing reflections also surfaced in writing that called into question clinical reasoning and decision making, demonstrating concern for the influence of decisions on patients' well-being. One contributor raises such reflections in his piece that draws attention to the role of a radiologist in healthcare:

> Yes, I agree. We overdiagnose, and I sometimes doubt our motives. Are we doing all these tests because we want to help our patients as much as possible? Or is it because we're uncomfortable with uncertainty? Perhaps we're doing more harm than good with some of these guidelines. Like attacking a fly with an axe. (Tahvildari, 2017. para. 22)

By posing questions to oneself either in the story or in the telling of the story, narrators of their clinical encounters used reflexivity to humanize themselves and their patients and to explore alternative meanings, decisions, or communication patterns. Health communication scholar Harter (2013) describes the reflexive function well: "Storytelling works simultaneously as an agent of self-discovery and creation, constituting knowledge of self and others" (p. 18). The reflexive function of clinical storytelling foregrounds the way learning crystalizes in characters, plots, scenes, and motives, and subsequently beckons the storyteller to circulate this retrospection with an audience who may likewise glean meaning to inform their clinical practice and roles.

Practice-Based Function

The fourth narrative function of clinical storytelling demonstrated the need to explain or justify medical practices and decision-making. Simulations and clinical experiences in medical education are valuable. These experiences immerse students in situations that require clinical reasoning, decision-making, and practice enactment. Narrating those experiences is another way for students to make sense of their reasoning and decisions as well as to argue for particular practices. Because *Intima* is a journal that advances the practice and research of narrative medicine, it is not surprising that storytellers of non-fiction and field notes wrote about their narratively-based reasoning, decisions, and practices. To illustrate, one contributor explains why and how he chose to share a personal narrative with a patient: "I weigh the pros and cons and decide that a way forward for this mother might be for me to share a bit of my life" (Deady, 2018, para. 26). While other types of reasoning, decisions, and practices emerge in the stories told, the practice-based function, similar to the resistance function, did not feature as prominently in storytelling as did other themes. Generally speaking, the practice-based function of clinical storytelling was embedded in the plot as a way to move along the storyline but did not appear to be the author's primary function in writing the story.

Therapeutic Function

> Exposure to suffering is a formative piece of students' clinical experience. Through every rotation, we encounter it in various incarnations: on OB/GYN, the would-be-mother struggling with the aftermath of stillbirth; on primary care, the carpenter crippled by chronic pain; on neurology, the CEO robbed of speech by stroke; on pediatrics, James [an 8 month old with multiple fractures from abuse]. (Nanda, 2015, para. 8)

Fifth, the therapeutic function of storytelling emerged as writers narrated stories of challenge, difficulty, and trauma in three distinctive ways: (1) recalled traumatic clinical experiences, (2) penned stories of personal trial and loss, or (3) wrote about how a clinical experience caused traumatic/difficult memories to surface. To begin, clinicians narrated stories of trauma that they experienced through their work with patients in healthcare scenes.

While what constituted trauma from one narrator to the next differed, death consistently emerged as a traumatic clinical experience. Writing about her transition from labor and delivery to emergency room nursing, a nurse recalls questioning where to tag an adult body: "I still can't remember on which ankle and which wrist the death tags go on. But I know how to tie them now" (Belc, 2018, para. 4). As in this nurse's narrative, death came "again and again" and one by one, but in a different author's narrative, death came in wave by wave.

> Like our daily walks and routine rides home with Suli, witnessing death became another pattern—rapidly, our new normal. For the first few days during my time there, I tried to write down the names of every person who'd died in our unit. As fast as empathetic fatigue set in and exhaustion became ever present, the numbers added up too quickly. The dead became a blur to me. I lost count, I lost track, I lost my bearings. (Cunningham, 2019, para. 18)

Second, clinicians wrote about personal illness, trial, and loss that contextualized their own approaches to medicine. Those that embody medical practitioner roles do so as bodies that have experienced illness, trauma, and loss. In his recollections of postponing medical school to be a caregiver to his father diagnosed with cancer, this author describes the overwhelming desire for "it to be over."

> No one tells you that you'll have thoughts about how much easier life would be if your dad would die and let you and your family move on. No one tells you that you'll furtively feel relief for your mom, for your entire family, when the funeral home shows up to your front door to take his body and you watch as the men in suits wheel out a husband, father, brother, and friend. No one tells you death smells. No one tells you these things because it hurts just to think them. (Minor, 2017, para. 8)

In writing about the loss of his father, the author ends his piece by making the moral of the story explicit: "I learned what kind of doctor I want to be, that I need to be, because I know what it means to lose, I know what it means to feel hope, to have it crushed, to look for comfort in family" (Minor, 2017, para. 9). As he thinks on the role of doctor, that role is impacted by his own story of personal loss.

Third, clinical experiences often prompt the resurfacing of traumatic or difficult personal memories, whether it be a personal illness or that of a loved one. For example, a code blue in the ER cued the memory of one author's father's death and failed attempts to resuscitate. Confronted with the memory of her father's death, she writes, "My hands shook as I filled the death and cremation certificate. A suffocating feeling of despair and deep sorrow took me by surprise. I felt caged in the ER" (Joomun, 2017, para. 9). Such stories of cued personal trauma were often accompanied by an explicit moral of what lessened the trauma, and in this case, the author goes on to explain her reaction to the code blue patient's daughter:

> I flung myself out the door where I found the girl cradled onto the staircase. She stared blankly at me. I knew what I had to do, what nobody did for me back then, what I had to helplessly figure out for myself in time. I climbed onto the step next to her. Taking her hand softly in mine, I told her that her father was already dead when he was brought in, probably for a while, judging by the flaccid limbs and the coolness of his skin. I reassured her that there was nothing she could have done. His death was never her fault. Even calling an ambulance would not have made a difference. (Joomun, 2017, para. 9)

Her father's code blue, as emotionally painful and overwhelming as the memory was, became the impetus for her compassionate and comforting communication. In the case of a different author, a medical resident, trauma was lessened by touch, so touch is what she offered another in his trauma.

> My instinct to reach out to the patient came from my own experience. At age fourteen I was the one on the gurney, shivering by myself in a pre-op area. Wearing only a thin cotton gown, I felt very small and vulnerable waiting to be wheeled into the OR. A nurse came to my bedside. I have no memory of what she looked like, or what words were exchanged. All I remember is her taking my hand in hers; the sensation of heat from her palm was immediately comforting. Her touch alone somehow conveyed the caring and support I needed in the moments before my operation. (Swain, 2019, para. 5)

Recollections of authors varied from seeing a patient pre-op being wheeled into the ER, to vomiting from chemo, to failing to respond from resuscitation attempts. Seeing these vivid cues play out in clinicals stimulates an array of emotions of varying intensity. Of interest in this set of stories analyzed is the desire for the narrator to lessen the trauma for others. These storytellers have harnessed narrative as a means to transform their own trauma, their response to others' trauma, and their storytelling community's capacity for compassion as they listen to and are shaped by the stories shared through *Intima.*

Overall, the therapeutic function of clinical storytelling is shored up in these authors' desire to put to paper and disseminate that which was difficult and, at times, tragic to endure. A nursing student in the 1950s reflects on writing a case study of insulin therapy for a schizophrenic patient: "I felt my heart contracting into a knot of sadness. Soon such a paralyzing gloom came over me that I could hardly get up from chair" (Valinoti, 2019, para. 40). Being able to write, and thus, voice such emotionally, and sometimes physically, trying situations is presumably therapeutic.

Identification or Communal Function

Finally, a sixth function of storytelling thematically emerged in field note and non-fiction writing of *Intima*—provider-provider identification or communality. Scholars suggest that the narrative form implies relationality between the narrator and the audience (Harter, 2013), and the stories of *Intima* are no exception. As the majority of non-fiction and field note stories in *Intima* are written by medical practitioners and students for a readership of mostly medical practitioners and students, the relationality between narrator and audience is primarily provider-provider communication. Subsequently, the provider-provider communication constitutes a community of students and practitioners shaping and being shaped by one another's stories. Within the identification or communal theme, mutual learning is emphasized. Whether it was the willingness to learn modeled by the narrator or the wisdom offered from the narrator to the audience, *Intima*'s storytelling community is a learning community. Modeling a humble willingness to learn, one author writes about her time in the largest slum in India:

> I shifted away from the proposal I had entered Kandivali with to: listen, learn, and then work to develop solutions together. This understanding, their stories, led me to narrative medicine—to recognizing the *power* that narratives have in the offering and receiving of effective, and more importantly, dignified care. (Khedagi, 2016, para. 16)

Other narrators elected to be more prescriptive to the learning community by explicitly providing morals to their stories intended to redress medical practice. For example, another author advises his readers to rethink their role as providers in the stories of their patients: "We are just minor parts of the innumerable chapters in the book of a patient's life. We aren't the main characters, though we hope to play protagonists in our own small ways" (Wellman, 2017, para. 5).

The thematic analysis of *Intima* clinical narratives revealed six narrative functions: identity management, resistance, reflection, practice, therapy, and communal functions. Analysis addresses both RQ1 and RQ2. The first research question asked how medical storytelling benefitted the storyteller, and narrative analysis identified six unique functions that may benefit the storyteller. Expounding upon the finding to RQ1, narrators often fulfilled multiple functions in the same narrative, demonstrating a plurality of reasons for narrating clinical experiences. The second research question asked how sharing clinical narratives constructs a storytelling community. Much like sociologist Frank's (1995) notion of witnessing in illness narration, *Intima* contributors share their stories to witness to their audience lessons learned from their clinical interactions. Narratives shared between providers are means of developing a community of providers who can learn from one another's identity struggles, acts of resistance, reflections, practice preferences, and ways of coping with trauma. At this juncture, attention turns to RQ3 to develop ways of weaving storytelling practices into clinical training and education.

RECOMMENDATIONS FOR INTERVENTIONAL ARTS

Story is not a stranger within medical education. As Charon (2009) has eloquently surmised, narrative medicine expands the interpretive range of medicine. This range of possibilities has been explored, primarily, through reflective writing.

> Can we not imagine the splendor of a medicine that does not shirk from beauty, that embraces interpretive range beyond the physical realm, that creates the known from the unknown and the speakable from the unspeakable, accepting generative mystery at the core of truth? (Charon, 2009, p. 130)

As Sayantani DasGupta and Rita Charon (2004) explain, reflective writing has long been used through exercises like critical incident reports, clinical journaling, and clinical reflections. In these types of exercises (typically written), medical students story their experiences in clinical education to enhance their empathy with illness and ill patients. Similar exercises can be co-opted in different types of health and medical education not only to enhance empathy, but also to benefit from storytelling communities and the functionality of clinical storytelling. This chapter argues that medical education in its various forms should intentionally foster storytelling communities and accomplish the aforementioned storytelling functions. Using a story-based design for clinical debriefings and discussions, medical educators are positioned to demonstrate storytelling in a communal context, elicit stories from trainees, empower storytellers, and reduce risk of storytelling (Lawrence & Thomas, 1999). From an instructional standpoint, Rita Charon and Nellie Hermann (2012) argue that teachers' and trainers' roles are to model rather than to judge or rate storytelling by: engaging in close readings of their students' stories, learning to paraphrase what is seen, helping students in their writing and telling, and facilitating multiple readership to "form strong, trusting, collaborative teams" (p. 4). Aiming to realize this vision of storytelling in a story-based design for clinical debriefings and discussions, six recommendations for storytelling praxis are unpacked: (1) encourage fragmented, open-ended stories, (2) integrate oral storytelling, (3) integrate written storytelling, (4) collaborate for group storytelling, (5) share stories, and (6) acknowledge risks of storytelling.

Encouraging Fragmented, Open-Ended Storytelling in Clinicals

To encourage fragmented, open-ended storytelling in clinicals is to recognize and value the indeterminate and disjointed nature of story and narrative. As David M. Boje (1995) argues, narratives are open-ended, fragmented plots with a plurality of interpretations, and to conceptualize this post-modern rendering of narrative, Boje (1995) offers the term "ante-narrative." Medical educators should embrace the ante-narrative, subsequently enabling students' openness to multiple interpretations of their lived stories as they tell those stories and encourage students to reframe their lived stories as ongoing.

Integrating Oral Storytelling into Clinicals

Just as Charon (2001) argued for a model of narrative medicine to develop narrative competence for doctors to reconstitute their patient-provider relationships, oral storytelling in clinical debriefings has the power to reconstitute provider-provider relationships and learning. To integrate oral storytelling into clinicals is to exercise storytelling power (Lawrence & Thomas, 1999) as a speech act. Speaking to the power of storytelling, Kristin M. Langellier (2009) writes, "The performative power in storytelling—embodied and precarious—materializes a horizon of possibility and hope" (p. 157). Such powerful communication is not necessarily embedded in clinical components of health and medical education, but structured clinical debriefings can use storied design to invite and value oral storytelling praxis in a similar way that Charon (2005) elicits patients' narratives in patient-provider interaction. A clinical debriefing facilitator training in a narrative framework and practice can ask the open-ended question of students, "What happened today in your clinical rotations?" Further promptings could include questions like, "In what ways were you constrained in your medical reasoning or decision-making with patients?" Or, "describe a situation that you would like insight on from your peers." Prompts can vary, but oral storytelling directly following clinical experiences enables students to perform the fresh events in a narrative.

Integrating Written Storytelling into Clinicals

To integrate written storytelling into clinicals is to cultivate language skills through writing-as-reflection and materialize the story for distribution to the storytelling community. Writing can be a solo activity or a collaborative activity (Charon & Hermann, 2012) generated by predetermined prompts or debriefing questions. Written stories can in turn be shared with other students to read or listen to so that their written reflections can also be used to develop listening competencies. Integrating storytelling implies integrating listening into story-based design for clinicals because story is directed to a particular audience. As David B. Morris (1998) argues, "A narrative bioethics would insist that effective listening—as an indispensable part of the doctor-patient dialogue—is a necessary skill for physicians" (p. 264). Story-based design by necessity infers the value of listening that will enable community with other providers in the immediate clinical context and enable relationship-building with patients in the long term.

Collaborating for Group Storytelling in Clinicals

To integrate collaboration for group storytelling in clinicals is to capitalize on the communal function of storytelling and practice collaborative storytelling. While we often conceive of storytelling as a monologue, storytelling can be a collective construction with additions, subtractions, edits, comments, questions, and objections (Lawrence & Thomas, 1999). Charon and Hermann (2012) explain that collaborative writing workshops benefit writers as multiple readers engage in close reading. Collaboration offers the unique interpretations of the story from different readers' perspectives. In turn, collaborative narrative production expands individual capacity to include group resources to construct narrative features such as metaphor, plot, and genre. Collaborative storytelling can be implemented with student groups on the same clinical rotation by having them reflectively write about experiences, share their writings, and edit their writings in conjunction with one another.

Sharing Stories in Clinicals

To share stories in clinicals, whether oral or written stories, is to value narrative knowledge and fabricate a culture of storytelling composed of a tightly knit group of students with shared experiences. Sharing stories enhances narrative function in a number of ways, but possibly most notably, sharing stories enables community and identification, which can reduce negative outcomes associated with stress and trauma. By facilitating storytelling groups in clinical debriefings and reflections, medical educators tap into what other practitioners in social and mental health services have known, experienced, and institutionalized—strong social support networks help people manage stress and trauma associated with care professions in order to reduce negative outcomes, including burnout (Babin, Palazzolo, & Rivera, 2012).

In terms of how to facilitate clinical storytelling communities for students, there is no one size fits all strategy. One method could include weekly meetings in small groups of students in clinicals with a facilitator trained to elicit stories from the students. In an American Medical Association online article, Dhruv Khullar explains a similar method. He met with a group of four other medical students every Sunday for an hour,

> put our smart phones away and . . . we'd talk about what went well that week, what didn't go well, difficult patient experiences, good patient experiences and that hour, to me, was tremendously enriching. . . . It's important for everyone to know they're not alone. . . . When you start opening up to your colleagues, other residents, other medical students, you'll find that most people are going through similar feelings and sensations to a lesser or greater extent. (quoted in Parks, 2016, July 13, para. 17, 18)

While Khullar's example is informal, self-selected, and voluntary, his experience sharing stories with other medical students in clinical rotations demonstrates one way to implement a storytelling community. Drawing on this example, clinical instructors could organize debriefing groups like simulation debriefing groups to function in a similar way to Khullar's group but more formal and involuntary.

Acknowledging Risks of Storytelling in Clinicals

Storytelling is an act of vulnerability (Garro & Mattingly, 2000) as narrative choices are made about what to reveal about plot, sequence, characters, scene, and motives and about what to remain silent about. Inclusions and exclusions shape the story and the way the narrator and story are perceived by the audience. Changing names of patients or other identifying characteristics of the narrative may protect the privacy of those within the story; however, narrators choose to make themselves vulnerable to the judgments of others as soon as they voice their stories and attach themselves, either in face-to-face or mediated channels, to their stories. Narrative choices are made, in part, based on the degree of vulnerability the narrator is willing to risk in relation to the audience. To acknowledge risks of storytelling in clinicals is to understand that the story and/or storyteller may experience negative consequence as a result of storying clinical experiences. Such risks may include competition, stigma, marginalization, threats to public image, or privacy violations. For example, in a study with medical students, students reported that sharing stories worked best in a safe and non-competitive environment (Arntfield et al., 2013). Ideally, clinical storytelling should include non-judgmental listening, unfixed expectations, and active participation to recognize how storytellers are using words and the different meanings they may convey (Charon & Hermann, 2012). Medical educators can design debriefing sessions and group discussions to reduce storytelling risks and maximize storytelling gains (Lawrence & Thomas, 1999).

CONCLUSIONS

The body and discourse collide in storytelling. This collision may reflect an aesthetic beauty as embodied experience melds with language to shape meaning, declare understandings, apply lessons learned, reveal identity, persuade for particular practices, and provide therapy for the storyteller. Conversely, this collision may be a chaotic, violent crashing of embodied experience and language as the storyteller is in the midst of role conflict, identity struggles, and other challenges. Narrative medicine has foregrounded the role of listening to and telling stories as means of *human communion* between patient and provider, but its capacity for *human communion* is also between provider and other providers as these medical practitioners navigate their clinical experiences and range of patient stories.

More research and pedagogical development are needed to understand how the narrative medicine practices outlined above may function toward their ends. As Megan M. Milota, Ghislaine van Thiel, and Johannes J. M. van Delden (2019) point out in their systematic review of narrative medicine articles using the Best Evidence in Medical Education Global Scale and Kirkpatrick Scale, narrative medicine has progressed, resulting in patterns that are both reproducible in pedagogy and methodology. However, little is known as to how narrative medicine influences students' communication patterns with other practitioners or patients long-term. In other words, has the storytelling ethic fundamentally altered how medical practitioners approach human relationships? Have medical practitioners begun to think and to act in stories? Another question must be added when considering the recommendations for narrative praxis in clinicals outlined in this chapter: in what ways does a storytelling ethic extending beyond education to professional relationships to transform and enable the storyteller to cope with the traumatic experiences in medicine? Story-based designs for clinical debriefings may have a positive influence on student well-being through a social support network in a storytelling community, enhanced peer learning within that community, and lessened negative outcomes from the stressors of their education. Student and practitioner stress and burnout are widely noted in medical and nursing education literature. Curriculum-based interventions have demonstrated potential in alleviating stress and burnout (see examples from van Vliet, Jong, & Jong, 2017 on mind-body curriculum and Michael J. Ireland et al., 2017) on mindfulness interventional training). Even narrative medicine interventions with students and with interprofessional medical teams have indicated that narrative medicine through reflective writing and oral storytelling was pleasureful and professionally satisfying (Arntfield et al., 2013; Miller et al., 2014; Sands, Stanley, & Charon, 2008). Clearly, there are multiple pathways moving forward to advance the scholarship and practice of story-based design in clinical medical education and training.

Additional research is needed, but in the meantime, medical educators in medical schools, nursing, pharmacy, physician assistant, dentistry, physical and occupational therapy (not an exhaustive list) should capitalize on the functionality of storying clinical experiences expressed by practitioners published in *Intima*. By examining published stories of clinical interactions, this chapter has demonstrated the varied functions that storytelling accomplishes for medical practitioners, and then uses those functions to suggest how medical educators could engage in best practices of narrative medicine during clinical training. Clinical rotations and clerkships are fundamental training experiences in medical education. Yet, these educational experiences may not sufficiently guide students to the reflective practices of storytelling. Storytelling is a means of reflecting, coping, and learning from traumatic, emotion-laden experiences of people's lives laid bare before them on an operating table, gurney, patient bed, or other apparatus. By facilitating oral and written storytelling communities, medical educators reinforce the storytelling ethic that can benefit healthcare practitioners as they cope with the stresses and trauma of clinical experiences and may reshape how medical practitioners approach human relationships long term.

REFERENCES

Arntfield, S. L., Slesar, K., Dickson, J., & Charon, R. (2013). Narrative medicine as a means of training medical students toward residency competencies. *Patient Education and Counseling*, *91*(3), 280–286. https://doi.org/10.1016/j.pec.2013.01.014

Babin, E. A., Palazzolo, K. E., & Rivera, K. D. (2012). Communication skills, social support, and burnout among advocates in a domestic violence agency. *Journal of Applied Communication Research*, *40*(2), 147–166. https://doi.org/10.1080/00909882.2012.670257

Belc, A. (2018). Getting to know dying. *Intima: A Journal of Narrative Medicine.* Retrieved from https://static1.squarespace.com/static/54bc1287e4b09cb81d8d8439/t/5aff4dab88251b629fead85f/1526681003590/Getting+to+Know+Dying+by+Anna+Belc+SPRING+2018+INTIMA.pdf

Boje, D. M. (1995). Stories of the storytelling organization: A postmodern analysis of Disney as "Tamara-Land." *Academy of Management Journal*, *38*(4), 997–1035. https://doi.org/10.5465/256618

Bracho-Sanchez, E. (2015). A familiar accent. *Intima: A Journal of Narrative Medicine.* Retrieved from https://static1.squarespace.com/static/54bc1287e4b09cb81d8d8439/t/54e54e94e4b0973657d06d74/1424314004323/A+Familiar+Accent.pdf

Bruckner, J. M. (2019). Peppermint oil. *Intima: A Journal of Narrative Medicine.* Retrieved from https://static1.squarespace.com/static/54bc1287e4b09cb81d8d8439/t/5ce30fc4b638bf0001161dd9/1558384581514/Peppermint+Oil+by+Julia+Michie+Bruckner+%281%29.pdf

Charmaz, K. (2000). Grounded theory: Objectivist and constructivist methods. In N. K. Denzin & Y. S. Lincoln (Eds.), *The SAGE Handbook of qualitative research* (2nd ed., pp. 509–535). Thousand Oaks, CA: Sage.

Charmaz, K. (2005). Grounded theory in the 21st century: Applications for advancing social justice studies. In N. K. Denzin & Y. S. Lincoln (Eds.), *The SAGE Handbook of qualitative research* (3rd ed., pp. 507–535). Thousand Oaks, CA: Sage.

Charmaz, K. (2006). *Constructing grounded theory: A practical guide through qualitative analysis*. London: Sage.

Charon, R. (2001). Narrative medicine: A model for empathy, reflection, profession, and trust. *Journal of the American Medical Association, 286*(15), 1897–1902. http://dx.doi.org/10.1001/jama.286.15.1897

Charon, R. (2005). Narrative medicine: Attention, representation, and affiliation. *Narrative, 13*(3), 261–270. http://doi.org/10.1353/nar.2005.0017

Charon, R. (2006). *Narrative medicine: Honoring the stories of illness.* Oxford: Oxford University Press.

Charon, R. (2009). Narrative medicine as witness for the self-telling body. *Journal of Applied Communication Research, 37*(2), 118–131. http://doi.org/10.1080/00909880902792248

Charon, R., & Hermann, N. (2012). Commentary: A sense of story, or why teach reflective writing? *Academy of Medicine, 87*(1), 5–7. http://doi.org/10.1097/ACM.0b013e31823a59c7

Charon, R., & Wyer, P. (2008, January 26). The art of medicine: Narrative evidence based medicine. *Lancet, 371*(9609), 296–297. https://doi.org/10.1016/S0140–6736(08)60156–7

Cunningham, T. (2019). Sulieman. *Intima: A Journal of Narrative Medicine.* Retrieved from http://www.theintima.org/sulieman

DasGupta, S., & Charon, R. (2004). Personal Illness Narratives: Using Reflective Writing to Teach Empathy. *Academic Medicine, 79*(4), 351–356. http://doi.org/10.1097/00001888–200404000–00013

Deady, B. (2018). The magic wand. *Intima: A Journal of Narrative Medicine*. Retrieved from https://static1.squarespace.com/static/54bc1287e4b09cb81d8d8439/t/5bbf9a59b208fc01e805b21d/1539283546085/THEMAGIC+WAND_BRIANDEADY.pdf

Frank, A. W. (1995). *The wounded storyteller: Body, illness, and ethics.* Chicago, IL: University of Chicago Press.

Fyfe, B. (2017). Disequilibrium. *Intima: A Journal of Narrative Medicine*. 1–2. Retrieved from https://static1.squarespace.com/static/54bc1287e4b09cb81d8d8439/t/59d527fba9db09e37f143b7f/1507141628014/Disequilibrium+Fyfe.pdf

Gabby, N. (2015). The baby on the bus. *Intima: A Journal of Narrative Medicine*. Retrieved from https://static1.squarespace.com/static/54bc1287e4b09cb81d8d8439/t/55103407e4b07f1da67cd4e6/1427125255034/The+Baby+on+the+Bus.pdf

Garro, L. C., & Mattingly, C. (2000). Narrative as construct and construction. In C. Mattingly & L. C. Garro (Eds.), *Narrative and the cultural construction of illness and healing* (pp. 1–49). Berkley, CA: University of California Press.

Goffman, E. (1978). *The presentation of self in everyday life.* London; Harmondsworth: Penguin Books.

Harter, L. M. (2009). Narratives as dialogic, contested, and aesthetic performances. *Journal of Applied Communication Research, 37*(2), 140–150. http://doi.org/10.1080/00909880902792255

Harter, L. M. (2013). The poetics and politics of storytelling in health contexts. In L. Harter (Ed.), *Imaging new normals: A narrative framework for health communication* (pp. 3–27). Dubuque, IA: Kendall Hunt.

Intima: A Journal of Narrative Medicine. (2019). Our mission & vision. *Intima*. Retrieved from http://www.theintima.org/missionandvison

Ireland, M. J., Cough, B., Gill, K., Langan, F., O'Connor, A., & Spencer, L. (2017). A randomized controlled trial of mindfulness to reduce stress and burnout among intern medical practitioners. *Medical Teacher*, *39*(4), 409–414. http://doi.org/10.1080/0142159X.2017.1294749

Jayanti, A. (2017). Taking a history. *Intima: A Journal of Narrative Medicine*. Retrieved from https://static1.squarespace.com/static/54bc1287e4b09cb81d8d8439/t/590245551b631b595f84e785/1493321081392/Taking+A+History+-+Anand+Jayanti.pdf

Joomun, R. A. (2017). My first code blue. *Intima: A Journal of Narrative Medicine*. Retrieved from https://static1.squarespace.com/static/54bc1287e4b09cb81d8d8439/t/590d12498419c2fe3de9c32d/1494028874044/Initma+My+First+Code+Blue+by+Rayda+Aaishah+Joomun.pdf

Kalitzkus, V., & Matthiessen, P. F. (2009). Narrative-based medicine: Potential, pitfalls, and practice. *Permanente Journal*, *13*(1), 80–86. http://doi.org/ 10.7812/tpp/08–043

Khedagi, A. (2016). Pedagogy by the oppressed: My journey to narrative medicine. *Intima: A Journal of Narrative Medicine*. Retrieved from https://static1.squarespace.com/static/54bc1287e4b09cb81d8d8439/t/57e22fb4b8a79b2526a49734/1474441144371/Pedagogy_Khedagi_field%2Bnotes.pdf

Langellier, K. M. (2009). Performing narrative medicine. *Journal of Applied Communication Research*, *37*(2), 151–158. https://doi.org/10.1080/00909880902792263

Lawrence, D., & Thomas, J. C. (1999). Social dynamics of storytelling: Implications for storybase design. *AAAI Technical Report* (FS-99–01). Retrieved from https://www.aaai.org/Papers/Symposia/Fall/1999/FS-99–01/FS99–01–005.pdf

Little, J. (2014). Medical metamorphosis. *Intima: A Journal of Narrative Medicine.* Retrieved from https://static1.squarespace.com/static/54bc1287e4b09cb81d8d8439/t/558349a4e4b07d6bd20672ca/1434667428068/Medical+Metamorphisis%2C+Jessica+Little.pdf

McManus, S. (2019). Learning to be real. *Intima: A Journal of Narrative Medicine.* Retrieved from http://www.theintima.org/learning-to-be-real

Milota, M. M, van Thiel, G. J. M. W., & van Delden, J. J. M. (2019). Narrative medicine as a medical education tool: A systematic review. *Medical Teacher*, *41*(7), 802–810. DOI: http://doi.org/10.1080/0142159X.2019.1584274

Miller, E., Balmer, D., Hermann, N., Graham, G., & Charon, R. (2014). Sounding narrative medicine: Studying students' professional identity development at Columbia University College of Physicians and Surgeons. *Academic Medicine*, *89*(2), 335–342. http://doi.org/10.1097/ACM.0000000000000098

Minor, J. (2017). The Crash. *Intima: A Journal of Narrative Medicine*. Retrieved from https://static1.squarespace.com/static/54bc1287e4b09cb81d8d8439/t/590b600217bffc466157899f/1493917698890/Minor_Jake_The+Crash.pdf

Morris, D. B. (1998). *Illness and culture in the postmodern age.* Berkley, CA: University of California Press.

Nanda, P. (2015). Suffer little children. *Intima: A Journal of Narrative Medicine.* Retrieved from https://static1.squarespace.com/static/54bc1287e4b09cb81d8d8439/t/55f0dee5e4b021b43f87d8db/1441849061566/INTIMA+F15+SUFFER+LITTLE+CHILDREN.pdf

Parks, T. (2016, July 13). The physician's essential art of balancing emotion and logic. *AMA*. Retrieved from https://www.ama-assn.org/residents-students/resident-student-health/physicians-essential-art-balancing-emotion-and-logic

Riessman, C. K. (2008). *Narrative methods for the human sciences.* Thousand Oaks, CA: Sage.

Sands, S., Stanley, P., & Charon, R. (2008). Pediatric narrative oncology: Interprofessional training to promote empathy, build teams, and prevent burnout. *Journal of Supportive Oncology*, *6*(7), 307–312.

Sellnow, D. D. (2018). *The rhetorical power of popular culture: Considering mediated texts* (3rd ed.). Los Angeles, CA: Sage.

Scott, A. (2019). Carlie's crack pipe. *Intima: A Journal of Narrative Medicine*. Retrieved from http://www.theintima.org/carlies-crack-pipe

Sharf, B. F., Harter, L. M., Yamasaki, J., & Haidet, P. (2011). Narrative turns epic: Continuing developments in health narrative scholarship. In T. L. Thompson, R. Parrott, & J. F. Nussbaum (Eds.), *The Routledge handbook of health communication* (2nd ed., pp. 66–81). New York: Routledge.

Sharf, B. F., & Vanderford, M. L. (2003). Illness narratives and the social construction of health. In T. L. Thompson, A. M. Dorsey, K. I. Miller, & R. Parrott (Eds.), *Handbook of health communication* (1st ed., pp. 9–34). Mahwah, NJ: Lawrence Erlbaum.

Tahvildari, A. (2017). The long ride. *Intima: A Journal of Narrative Medicine.* Retrieved from https://static1.squarespace.com/static/54bc1287e4b09cb81d8d8439/t/59daf133f7e0ab21edd2cbe1/1507520821699/The+Long+Ride+Ali+T.pdf

Valinoti, E. (2019). Th insulin unit 1954: A memoir. *Intima: A Journal of Narrative Medicine*. Retrieved from http://www.theintima.org/the-insulin-unit-1954–a-memoir

van Vliet, M., Jong, M., & Jong, M. C. (2017). Long-term benefits by a mind-body medicine skills course on perceived stress and empathy among medical and nursing students. *Medical Teacher*, *39*(7), 710–719. http://doi.org/10.1080/0142159X.2017.1309374

Wellman, H. (2017). Robes the color of saffron. *Intima: A Journal of Narrative Medicine.* Retrieved from https://static1.squarespace.com/static/54bc1287e4b09cb81d8d8439/t/59db7210a8b2b06fbe1844c2/1507553809669/Robes+the+Color+of+Saffron+by+Hannah+Wellman.pdf

Index

About the Editors and Contributors

Kamran Afary is Assistant Professor of Communication Studies at California State University Los Angeles, and holds a PhD in Performance Studies and is a Registered Drama Therapist (RDT). He is the author of *Performance and Activism: Grassroots Discourse After the Los Angeles Rebellion of 1992* (2009) and a coauthor in the following works: *Iranian Diaspora Identities: Stories and Songs* (2020); *Mollā Nasreddin and the Creative Cauldron of Transcaucasia* (2019); and "Dwight Conquergood: An Appreciation of His Intellectual Life and Contribution to Critical Gang Studies" in the forthcoming *Routledge Critical Handbook of Gangs.*

Alice Marianne Fritz received her MA in Communication Studies from California State University, Los Angeles. As a lecturer, she teaches various courses, including Social Science Research Methods. Fritz regularly presents her research at industry conventions, including the National Communication Association (NCA), International Communication Association (ICA), and the Association for Education in Journalism and Mass Communication (AEJMC) annual conferences. Her work has been published in the *Journal of Children and Media*, as well as in *Colloquy*, the journal of the Department of Communication Studies at CSULA. Her experience teaching Research Methods has allowed her to understand the importance of placing complex theoretical concepts in real-world examples and practices to enhance student learning.

Andrea Baldwin is a Lecturer of Communication at the University of Houston-Clear Lake, and holds a PhD in Communication Studies, Southern Illinois University, Carbondale. Her research explores pedagogical experiences in spaces outside of the classroom and genealogical embodied mentoring in the academy. She has a background in Performance Studies with an interest in storytelling, adaptation, and rhetoric.

Jessica Bleuer teaches in the Master of Arts Drama Therapy Program at Concordia University in Montreal, Quebec. She holds an MA and M.Ed, and is a Registered Drama Therapist (RDT) and holds a Psychotherapist Permit (OPQ). She also maintains a private practice. Her teaching and research focus on the intersections between individual wellness and larger systemic change. Her work has appeared in various journals including *Qualitative Research in Psychology* and *The Drama Therapy Review*. She has co-authored an upcoming chapter in the third edition of *Current Approaches in Drama Therapy*.

Meara H. Faw is Assistant Professor in the Communication Studies Department at Colorado State University, and holds a PhD in Communication, University of Washington. Her work explores how interpersonal communication can promote mental, physical, and social health, and her current research projects focus on the challenges and joys associated with caregiving relationships. Her work has been published in journals such as *Health Communication*, *Qualitative Health Research*, *Journal of Social and Personal Relationships*, and *Communication Studies*.

Anna K. Griggs holds an MA in Communication Studies, Colorado State University. She studied interpersonal communication and explored how engaging in creative arts can facilitate relationships. Her chapter represents work from her master of arts thesis project. She currently works as a communications specialist and intends on furthering her education in interpersonal communication in the coming years.

Travis Heath is Associate Professor of Psychology at Metropolitan State University of Denver, holds a PhD in Psychology from the University of Northern Colorado, and is a cofounder of Rocky Mountain Narrative Therapy Center (RMNTC). Health's areas of teaching and research interest are addiction, relationships, therapeutic change, sports psychology, communication, and sex and gender. He is a coauthor of *Interactive Psychology: An Introductory Workbook* (2012).

Melanie Frontz Kramer is an online College Instructor in Communication and English, and is a Workforce Initiatives Manager assisting individuals with disabilities and military veterans and spouses. She holds an MA in Communication Studies, San Diego State University, and a BA in Spanish, University of California, Los Angeles. She lives in San Diego with her husband who is active duty U.S. Navy and has twin toddlers. She is a true believer in the power of music, writing, and writing music.

Gregory J. Langner teaches in the Department of Communication Studies at Antelope Valley College and holds a PhD in Communication and Performance Studies, Louisiana State University. Langner teaches courses that include Critical-Qualitative Research Methods, Humanities Theories of Communication, Intercultural Communication in Civic Contexts, Performance of Literature, Critical Media Studies, and Queer Studies. Taking a practice-centered approach to both teaching and research, Langner's scholarship appears in several peer-reviewed book chapters and journal articles, including in *Text and Performance Quarterly* and *Liminalities: A Journal of Performance Studies*. Beyond academia, Greg is an active performance practitioner and stage director whose devised productions and solo performances have toured across the United States at venues including the New Orleans Contemporary Arts Center and Highways Performance Space in Santa Monica, California

Kurt Lindemann is Professor in the School of Communication at San Diego State University, and holds a PhD, Arizona State University. He is also Director of the Center for the Study of Media and Performance at SDSU. His teaching interests include performance studies, ethnography, critical theory, and organizational communication. He has performed his writing in numerous performance venues. His work has appeared in a variety of outlets, including *Qualitative Inquiry*, *Text and Performance Quarterly*, and *Rebel Magazine*.

Laura H. Malinin is Director of the Nancy Richardson Design Center and Associate Professor of Interior Architecture at Colorado State University, and as a licensed architect, she holds a joint PhD in Design & Planning and Cognitive Science, as well as certifications and licenses of AIA, EDAC, WELL AP, LEED AP BD+C. Malinin examines effects of designed environments on creativity, health, and well-being, including how cognition emerges through physical and social interactions in environments. She has published in psychology, business, and design research journals on topics including individual and group creativity and how spatial designs might improve cognitive processes.

Bonny McDonald is an Instructor and Director of Basic Courses in the Communications Studies Department at Louisiana State University, and holds a PhD in Performance Studies, LSU. She is a poet, performer, and teaching artist who frequently offers workshops on incorporating kinesthetic performance methods into traditional educational settings, from creative writing groups to biology classrooms. McDonald's work as a director and scholar focuses on engaging aesthetic performance as social justice practice.

Jacobo Mesa Ramirez is a student in Psychology and Human Services, as well as a rap songwriter who lives in Denver, Colorado. He believes in the power of the spoken word and that music has helped to shape generations.

Mady Schutzman is Faculty Emerita at California Institute of the Arts, and a writer, scholar, theatre artist, and filmmaker. Schutzman is author of *Radical Doubt: The Joker System, after Boal* (2019), and coeditor with Jan Cohen-Cruz of two anthologies on the intersection of theatre and cultural politics.

Elizabeth Spradley is Assistant Professor of Communication Studies at Stephen F. Austin State University, and holds a PhD in Health Communication, Texas A&M University. She teaches courses in health communication, communication theory, communication research, professional communication, and interpersonal communication. Spradley's research focuses on narrative, healthcare, occupational training, professional identity, and tensions. Her research and professional goals are to wed her scholarly and teaching work to develop narrative-based communication interventions. Serving on the editorial board for *The Intima: A Journal of Narrative Medicine* is one of the ways she seeks to advance narrative research and praxis in healthcare. Previous narrative research has been published in *The Journal of Community Informatics*. She could not do what she does without the support of her colleague and spouse, R. Tyler Spradley, and her four sons, a chocolate lab, and a flock of chickens.

www.ingramcontent.com/pod-product-compliance
Ingram Content Group UK Ltd.
Pitfield, Milton Keynes, MK11 3LW, UK
UKHW041841031026
15587UKWH00002B/930

9 781793 602688